Progress in Epileptic Disorders
Volume 1

**Cognitive Dysfunction
in Children
with Temporal Lobe
Epilepsy**

# Progress in Epileptic Disorders
## International Advisory Board

Aicardi Jean, *France*
Arzimanoglou Alexis, *France*
Baumgartner Christoph, *Austria*
Brodie Martin, *UK*
Cross Helen, *UK*
Duchowny Michael, *USA*
Elger Christian, *Germany*
French Jacqueline, *USA*
Glauser Tracy, *USA*
Gobbi Giuseppe, *Italy*
Guerrini Renzo, *Italy*
Hirsch Edouard, *France*
Kahane Philippe, *France*
Luders Hans, *USA*
Meador Kimford, *USA*
Moshé Solomon L., *USA*
Noachtar Soheyl, *Germany*
Noebels Jeffrey, *USA*
Palmini André, *Brazil*
Perucca Emilio, *Italy*
Pitkanen Asla, *Finland*
Ryvlin Philippe, *France*
Scheffer Ingrid, *Australia*
Schmitz Bettina, *Germany*
Schmidt Dieter, *Germany*
Serratosa José, *Spain*
Shorvon Simon, *UK*
Tinuper Paolo, *Italy*
Thomas Pierre, *France*
Tuxhorn Ingrid, *Germany*
Wolf Peter, *Denmark*

# Progress in Epileptic Disorders
## Volume 1

# Cognitive Dysfunction in Children with Temporal Lobe Epilepsy

*Alexis Arzimanoglou*
*Albert Aldenkamp*
*Helen Cross*
*Maryse Lassonde*
*Solomon L. Moshé*
*Bettina Schmitz*

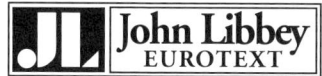

ISBN: 2-7420-0562-5
ISSN: en cours
Vol. 1.

Published by
**Éditions John Libbey Eurotext**
127, avenue de la République, 92120 Montrouge, France
Tél. : 01 46 73 06 60
Site internet : http://www.jle.com

John Libbey Eurotext
42-46 High Street
Esher, Surrey
KT10 9KY
United Kingdom

© 2005, John Libbey Eurotext. All rights reserved.

Unauthorized duplication contravenes applicable laws.
Il est interdit de reproduire intégralement ou partiellement le présent ouvrage sans autorisation de l'éditeur ou du Centre Français d'Exploitation du Droit de Copie, 20, rue des Grands-Augustins, 75006 Paris.

# Contents

Foreword ............................................................................................... VII

Workshop participants ............................................................................ IX

Neuropsychological deficits in children with temporal lobe epilepsy
    H. C. Sauerwein, A. Gallagher, M. Lassonde ........................................... 1

Effects of chronic temporal lobe epilepsy on memory functions
    C. Helmstaedter ................................................................................... 13

Attention deficit hyperactivity disorder and attentional problems in children with temporal lobe epilepsy
    D.W. Dunn, W. Kronenberger ............................................................. 31

Brain maturation and development of socio-cognitive perception and neural damaging process
    A. Laurent, A. Arzimanoglou, S. de Schonen ........................................ 47

Autism spectrum disorder in children with temporal lobe epilepsy
    J.H. Cross, A. McLellan, S. Davies, I. Heyman ..................................... 67

Temporal lobe and social abilities
    M. Zilbovicius, I. Meresse .................................................................... 75

Input of structural and metabolic MRI techniques in understanding neuronal dysfunction in temporal lobe epilepsy
    F. Cendes .............................................................................................. 95

Temporal lobe epilepsy and cognition in children: will fMRI be of some help for a better understanding of the mechanisms involved?
    D.A. Weber, M.M. Berl, E.N. Moore, G.A. Gioia, E.K. Ritzl, N.B. Ratner, C. Vaidya, W.D. Gaillard ...................................................................... 105

Temporal lobe epilepsy and cognitive dysfunction: what do we learn from PET studies in children?
    E. Asano, H.T. Chugani .................................................................................. 127

What future for neuroimaging techniques in evaluating cognition in children?
    P. Ryvlin, A. Montavont, A. Arzimanoglou ...................................................... 141

Age-dependent consequences of seizures and the development of TLE in the rat
    A. Nehlig ........................................................................................................ 153

Maturation of synchronised activities and epileptogenesis: when is as important as what!
    Y. Ben-Ari ...................................................................................................... 171

Temporal lobe epileptogenesis and epilepsy in the developing brain: bridging the gap between the laboratory and the clinic
    H.J. Hasson, J. Veliskova, S.R. Haut, S. Shinnar, S.L. Moshé ........................ 183

Does epileptic activity influence speech organization in temporal lobe epilepsy?
    J. Janszky, A. Ebner, M. Mertens, C. Gyimesi, H. Jokeit, F.G. Woermann ....... 203

Cognitive side-effects of antiepileptic drugs
    A.P. Aldenkamp, H.P. Bootsma ...................................................................... 217

Mood effects of antiepileptic drugs
    B. Schmitz ..................................................................................................... 233

Can we expect a specific correlation between the type of partial epilepsy, etiology and neuropsychological deficits?
    H. Jokeit, M. Schacher .................................................................................. 251

Restored cognitive functions: what can we expect following resective surgery?
    I. Tuxhorn, H. Freitag, H. Holthausen ........................................................... 265

Temporal lobe epilepsy in children and cognitive dysfunction: comprehensive methodologies for a comprehensive research and care
    A. Arzimanoglou ............................................................................................ 277

# Foreword

"Cognitive dysfunction in children with temporal lobe epilepsy", inaugurates *"Progress in Epileptic Disorders"*, a series of books edited by the journal *Epileptic Disorders* and the John Libbey Eurotext publications.

Much has been written about cognitive function in children with epilepsy, particularly children suffering from epileptic encephalopathies. Even more has been devoted to the neuropsychological status of patients, mainly adults, with intractable temporal lobe epilepsy. The latter is certainly due to the fact that temporal lobe epilepsy is very common, accounting for about 70% of all non idiopathic focal epilepsies, and often amenable to surgical treatment. However, temporal lobe epilepsy is not a homogeneous entity (early or late implication of various neuronal networks, several types of associated lesions, characteristics of ictal and interictal activity). Longitudinal studies are lacking and data available mostly derives from adult patients evaluated rather late in the course of their disease, usually as part of the pre- and post-surgical evaluation. Furthermore, although neuropsychological development in children is influenced by a number of similar factors as in adults (age at seizure onset, duration of the epilepsy, interictal EEG activity, medications, underlying pathology), other important factors, such as the role of early damage and modification of cerebral organization and the interruption of the learning process, most probably influence outcome.

The present book is the fruit of a workshop, designed as a multidisciplinary discussion forum with the participation of experts from all over the world. All participants had an active role, as speakers or discussants, and extensively reviewed available data from both clinical and fundamental research studies. The manuscripts were available for the workshop and were reviewed by the authors before publication, to include pertinent remarks and conclusions of the meeting. As clearly reflected in the chapters that follow, the workshop highlighted those domains that need further research and those for which immediate established techniques for a better care can be undertaken.

During the last decade, early epilepsy surgery has become a valid option for epilepsy care in children. Issues related to the natural history of temporal lobe epilepsy and those related to cognitive development are already in the frontline. The quality of the debates and the valid contributions of all authors ensure that the book encompasses current knowledge and provides the basis for the elaboration of collaborative comprehensive research projects.

On behalf of *Epileptic Disorders*, I would like to sincerely thank my co editors, the scientific committee of the workshop all the participants for their valuable contributions, the ILAE Commission on Psychobiology, as well as UCB for having supported the workshop with an unrestricted educational grant.

Alexis Arzimanoglou
*Epileptic Disorders* Editor-in-Chief

# Workshop on cognitive dysfunction in children with temporal lobe epilepsy
# Rome, March 2005

*Scientific Committee:*
Albert Aldenkamp (The Netherlands), Alexis Arzimanoglou (France),
Helen Cross (United Kingdom), Edouard Hirsch (France),
Philippe Kahane (France), Maryse Lassonde (Canada), Solomon L. Moshé (USA),
Philippe Ryvlin (France), Bettina Schmitz (Germany)

# List of Participants

**Aldenkamp Albert P**, Professor Dr, Ph.D. Neuropsychologist, Epilepsy Centre Kempenhaeghe and Department of Neurology, University Hospital of Maastricht, PO Box 61, NL-5590 A.B. Heeze, The Netherlands
aldenkampB@kempenhaeghe.nl

**Arzimanoglou Alexis**, MD, Head of the Epilepsy Program, Child Neurology & Metabolic Diseases Department, University Hospital Robert-Debré, 48 Boulevard Sérurier, 75935 Paris Cedex 19, France
alexis.arzimanoglou@rdb.aphp.fr

**Asano Eishi**, MD, PhD, Assistant Professor of Pediatrics and Neurology, Director of Electroneurodiagnostics, Division of Pediatric Neurology, Children's Hospital of Michigan, 3901 Beaubien Street, Detroit, MI 48201, USA
eishi@pet.wayne.edu

**Ben-Ari Yehezkel**, Director of INMED, Director of Research Classe Exceptionnelle at CNRS, INMED/INSERM, Parc scientifique de Luminy, 163 route de Luminy, 13273 Marseille Cedex 9, France
ben-ari@inmed.univ-mrs.fr

**Besag Franck**, Consultant Neuropsychiatrist, FRCP FRCPsych FRCPCH, Bedfordshire and Luton Community NHS Trust, Twinwoods Health Resource Centre, Milton Road, Bedford, Beds MK41 6AT, UK
FBesag@aol.com

**Boddaert Nathalie**, MD, PhD, Neuroradiologist, Department of Pediatric Radiology, University Hospital Necker-Enfants Malades, 149 rue de Sèvres, 75015 Paris, France
nathalie.boddaert@nck.aphp.fr

**Brovedani Paola**, Doctor in Psychology, Child Psychologist, Department of Developmental Neuroscience, Stella Maris Scientific Institute University of Pisa - Medical School, Pisa, Italy
paola.brovedani@inpe.unipi.it

**Caplan Rochelle** MD, Professor, Director, Pediatric Neuropsychiatry Program, Neuropsychaitric Institute, UCLA, 760 Westwood Plaza, Los Angeles, CA, 90024, USA
rcaplan@ucla.edu

**Cendes Fernando**, MD, PhD, Associate Professor, Neurologist/Epileptologist, Department of Neurology, University of Campinas - UNICAMP, CEP 13083-970, Campinas, Brazil
fcendes@unicamp.br

**Chilosi Anna**, MD, PhD, Child Neurologist, Department of Developmental Neuroscience-IRCCS Stella Maris Foundation, Via dei Giacinti 2, 56018 Calambrone (Pisa), Italy
a.chilosi@inpe.unipi.it

**Cross Helen** Dr, MB ChB PhD FRCP FRCPCH, Child Neurologist, Institute of Child Health, University College London, London WC1N 2AP, United Kingdom
hcross@ich.ucl.ac.uk

**Danielsson Susanna**, MD, Child Neuropsychiatry (BNK), Queen Silvia Children's Hospital, Otterhällegatan 12A, Göteborg, Sweden
susanna.danielsson@vgregion.se

**de Saint-Martin Anne**, MD, Child Neurologist, Pediatrics Department, University Hospitals, 1 place de l'hôpital, 67091 Strasbourg Cedex, France
anne.desaintmartin@chru-strasbourg.fr

**de Schonen Scania**, Professor, Director of Research, National Center for Scientific Research, CNRS, University Hospital Robert-Debré, 48 Boulevard Sérurier, 75935 Paris Cedex 19, France
schonen@psycho.univ-paris5.fr

**Dunn David W.** MD, Associate Professor of Psychiatry and Neurology, Child and Adolescent Psychiatry, Riley Hospital for Children, ROC 4300, 702 Barnhill Drive, Indianapolis Indiana, 46202, USA
ddunn@iupui.edu

**Filippini Melissa**, Psychologist, Ospedale Maggiore, Largo Nigrisoli 2, 40133 Bologna, Italy
melissa.filippini@libero.it

**Fohlen Martine**, Child Neurologist, Pediatric Neurosurgery Department, Fondation Opthalmologique Adolphe-de-Rothschild, 29 rue Manin, 75940 Paris Cedex, France
mfohlen@fo-rothschild.fr

**Gaillard William Davis**, Professor, Pediatrics and Neurology, George Washington University School of medicine, Child neurologist, Epileptologist Director, Comprehensive Pediatric Epilepsy Program, Department of Neurosciences, Children's National Medical Center, 111 Michigan Ave NW, Washington DC 20010, USA
wgaillar@cnmc.org; gaillardw@ninds.nih.gov

**Gross-Tsur Varda**, Professor, Shaare Zedek Medical Center, PO Box 3235, 91031 Jerusalem, Israel
gros@szmc.org.il; gros_fam@netvision.net.il

**Helmstaedter Christoph**, Professor, Neuropsychologist PhD, University Clinic of Epileptology, Sigmund Freud Str. 25, Bonn, Germany
C.Helmstaedter@uni-bonn.de

**Hermann Bruce**, Professor, PhD, University of Wisconsin, Madison, WI 53792, USA
Hermann@neurology.wisc.edu

**Heyman Isobel** MBBS PhD MRCPsych, Consultant Child and Adolescent Psychiatrist, Children's Department, PO Box 085, Institute of Psychiatry, DeCrespigny Park, London SE5 8AF, United Kingdom
i.heyman@iop.kcl.ac.uk

**Hirsch Edouard**, Professor, Neurologist-Neurophysiologist, Epileptology Service, Neurology Department, University Hospitals, 1 Place de l'Hôpital, 67091 Strasbourg Cedex, France
Edouard.Hirsch@chru-strasbourg.fr

**Janszky Jozsef**, Dr, Neurologist, Associate Professor, Department of Neurology, University of Pecs, Rét U.2., 7623 Pecs, Hungary
janszky@index.hu

**Jokeit Hennric**, PhD, Lecturer for Neuropsychology at University of Zurich, Head of the Neuropsychology Department at the Swiss Epilepsy Centre, Bleulerstrasse 60, 8008 Zurich, Switzerland
h.jokeit@swissepi.ch

**Kahane Philippe**, MD, PhD, Neurologist, Neuro-physiopathology of the Epilepsies Unit, Neurology Department, University Hospital, BP 217X, 38043 Grenoble Cedex, France
philippe.kahane@ujf-grenoble.fr

**Kasteleijn-Nolst Trenité Dorothée**, Neurologist, Department of Medical Genetics, University Medical Centre Utrecht (UMCU), Locatie Wilhelmina Kinderziekenhuis, Lundlaan 6, de Uithof, 3584 EA Utrecht, The Netherlands
d.kasteleijn@azu.nl

**Krishnamoorthy Ennapadam**, T.S. Srinivasan Institute of Neurological Sciences and Research, Chennai 600113, India
krish@neurokrish.com

**Lassonde Maryse**, Professor, Neuropsychology, Department of Psychology, Montreal University, CP 6128, Succ Centre-Ville, Montréal Qc, Canada H3C 3J7
maryse.lassonde@umontreal.ca

**Laurent Agathe**, Neuropsychologist, Developmental Neurocognition Group CNRS, UMR 8605 - Paris 5, University Hospital Robert-Debré, 48 Boulevard Sérurier, 75935 Paris Cedex 19, France
Agathe.Laurent@univ-paris5.fr

**Loring David**, Professor, Neuropsychologist PhD, University of Florida, Gainesville, FL 32610, USA
david.loring@neurology.ufl.edu

**Mathern Gary**, Associate Professor, Neurosurgical Director, Pediatric Epilepsy Surgery Program, David Geffen School of Medicine, University of California, Los Angeles, California, USA
gmathern@ucla.edu

**Mikati Mohamad**, MD, Director, Adult and Pediatric Epilepsy Program, Professor and Chairman Department of Pediatrics, American University of Beirut, Lebanon
mamikati@aub.edu.lb

**Moshé Solomon L.**, MD, Scientist, Clinician, Departments of Neurology, Neuroscience and Pediatrics, Albert Einstein College of Medicine, 1410 Pelham Parkway South, Kennedy Center Room 316, Bronx, New York 10461, USA
moshe@aecom.yu.edu

**Nehlig Astrid**, INSERM U666, Faculty of Medicine, 11 rue Humann, 67085 Strasbourg, France
nehlig@neurochem.u-strasbg.fr

**Pereira de Vasconcelos Anne**, PhD, Laboratoire de Neurosciences Comportementales et Cognitives, CNRS, UMR 7521, Centre Hospitalier Universitaire, 1 Place de l'Hôpital, 67091 Strasbourg, France
pereira@neurochem.u-strasbg.fr

**Plouin Perrine**, Head of the EEG Department, University Hospital Necker-Enfants Malades, 149 rue de Sèvres, 75743 Paris Cedex 15, France
perrine.plouin@nck.ap-hop-paris.fr

**Ryvlin Philippe**, Professor, Department of Functional Neurology and Epileptology, Neurology University Hospital, 59 Boulevard Pinel, 69003 Lyon, France
ryvlin@cermep.fr

**Sauerwein Hannelore**, Ph.D., Centre de recherche en neuropsychologie expérimentale et cognition, Département de psychologie, Université de Montréal, Montréal, Québec
h.sauerwein@umontreal.ca

**Seegmuller Caroline**, Neuropsychologist, Neurology Department, University Hospitals of Strasbourg, 1 Place de l'Hôpital, 67091 Strasbourg Cedex, France
seegmuller@neurochem.u-strasbg.fr

**Schmitz Bettina**, Dr, Neurologist and Psychiatrist, Charité, Humboldt University, 13353 Berlin, Germany
bettina.schmitz@charite.de

**Siebelink Bart**, Dr, Academic Center Child and Adolescent Psychiatry Curium, Oegstgeest, The Netherlands
b.m.siebelink@umail.leidenuniv.nl

**Smith Mary Lou**, Professor, Ph.D. (Neuropsychology), University of Toronto and Hospital for Sick Children, Toronto, Canada
smithml@psych.utoronto.ca

**Stephani Ulrich**, Prof. Dr, Director, University - Clinic for Neuropediatrics and Epilepsy center for children and adolescents, Schwanenweg, 20, 24105 Kiel, Germany
stephani@pedneuro.uni-kiel.de

**Taylor David**, Professor Emeritus, Institue of Child Health, London, England
davidctaylor@btinternet.co.uk

**Tuxhorn Ingrid**, Dr, MD, Neurologist, Epilepsy Center Bethel, Clinic Mara, Maraweg 21, 33617 Bielefeld, Germany
Ingrid.Tuxhorn@evkb.de

**Vargha-Khadem Faraneh**, Professor, Developmental Cognitive Neuroscientist - Non medical doctorate, Institute of Child Health, University College London, United Kingdom
f.khadem@ich.ucl.ac.uk

**Zilbovicius Monica**, CR1, MD, PhD, INSERM - Service hospitalier Frédéric-Joliot, CEA, 4 place du Général-Leclerc, 91400 Orsay, France
zilbo@shfj.cea.fr

*Workshop supported by an unrestricted educational grant from UCB*

# Neuropsychological deficits in children with temporal lobe epilepsy

H.C. Sauerwein, A. Gallagher, M. Lassonde

*Centre de Recherche, Hôpital Sainte-Justine, Montréal, Canada, and Département de Psychologie, Université de Montréal, Canada*

## ■ Definition of temporal lobe epilepsy (TLE)

Temporal lobe epilepsy is the most prevalent type of focal epilepsy in both children and adults. The seizures may originate in lateral, inferior or medial regions of the temporal lobes. The disorder varies greatly with regard to etiology, age of onset, seizure type, severity and duration (for a move detailed description of TLE characteristics see Arzimanoglou in this volume). The main underlying causes are medial sclerosis, neoplasms, vascular disease and neuro-developmental disorders (*e.g.*, Brockhaus and Elger, 1995). Mesial temporal epilepsy is the most frequently encountered form of TLE. The syndrome is characterized by early onset, a history of recurrent febrile seizures and unilateral hippocampal sclerosis, which can be visualized by magnetic resonance imaging (Engel, 1992). Other types include lesional epilepsy, mainly caused by tumors or stroke, and idiopathic or cryptogenic epilepsy in which no lesion can be detected in the MRI (Engel, 1993).

### Clinical and behavioral manifestations

The clinical and behavioral manifestations of TLE are as heterogeneous as the functions subserved by the various anatomical structures of the temporal lobes and their limbic components. Ictal events such as autonomic phenomena, automatisms, visceral sensations, emotional responses, auditory or visual hallucinations, transient disturbances in memory, as well as psychotic episodes, have been found to be primarily associated with discharges originating in medial structures, notably, the hippocampus the hippocampal gyrus and the amygdala. These areas are known to be involved in learning, memory, long-term storage of experiences and regulation of emotions. In contrast, the inferior and lateral regions of the temporal lobes contain the anatomical substrate for auditory and visual processing.

Interictal or long-term manifestations of TLE are complex and depend on a number of factors, such as the location of the epileptogenic anomaly, the seizure type and the duration of the epilepsy. Seizures originating in temporal lobe structures can be simple or complex depending on the etiology and severity of the underlying pathology. Complex partial seizures of temporal lobe origin are often pharmacoresistant and present an indication for resective surgery. The majority of neuropsychological studies carried out in adults with TLE have focused on these patients. These studies have shown that memory and language functions are most frequently disturbed in TLE. Furthermore, they have pointed to material-specific deficits related to hemispheric specialization: left hemispheric foci are more frequently associated with impairment in verbal processing whereas right hemispheric foci tend to result in visuo-spatial dysfunction.

## Studies in children

Although epilepsy is primarily a childhood disorder, neuropsychological studies in children have only recently started to emerge. The findings indicate that children with TLE present deficits that are similar in many aspects to those observed in adults (Jambaqué, 2001; Jambaqué et al., 1993; Schoenfeld et al., 1999). Furthermore, the children are at risk of developing learning disabilities and behavior problems that can be related to temporal lobe dysfunction. In the following overview, we intend to address the most frequent cognitive dysfunctions observed in children suffering from TLE.

## ■ Intellectual functioning

The mental status of children with TLE depends on age at onset, etiology, seizure type and duration of the epilepsy. Simple focal seizures, starting at school age, are generally not associated with a decline in intellectual functioning. In contrast, seizures starting in infancy risk interfering with mental development at a time of maximal vulnerability. In these cases, the causal factors usually are structural lesions or other comorbid neurological conditions. For instance, Pacual-Castroviejo et al. (1996) reported severe mental retardation in a 24-year follow-up study of a patient suffering since age 5 from uncontrollable seizures associated with a temporal astrocytoma.

Like in adults, most of the investigations of the long term cognitive consequences of TLE have been carried out in children with poorly controlled complex partial seizures. Comparing the full scale IQ of children suffering from different epilepsy syndromes, Nolan et al. (2003) found that children with TLE, generalized idiopathic epilepsy and central epilepsy performed better than those with frontal lobe epilepsy and generalized symptomatic epilepsy. TLE children with right sided-foci obtained a significantly higher full scale IQ than those with left-sided foci. Furthermore, younger age at onset was associated with longer duration of epilepsy and correlated significantly with lower IQ.

Similarly, Schoenfield et al. (1999) found that early onset and longer exposure to uncontrollable seizures was associated with poorer cognitive status in children with complex partial seizures of temporal lobe origin. These authors examined 57 children, aged 7 to 16 years, with hippocampal sclerosis. The patients had no additional abnormalities in the MRI. Although their IQ was above borderline on the Peabody

Picture Vocabulary Test, they scored significantly lower than their neurologically-intact siblings on a variety of cognitive and educational measures including memory, language, problem solving ability, mental flexibility and dexterity. These results are comparable to those of Roeschl-Heil et al. (2002) who observed that half of the adult patients with chronic TLE performed more poorly than their healthy siblings in all cognitive domains. Furthermore, a third of the patients had an IQ in the low average range (85) compared to 7 per cent of their siblings. Since TLE frequently starts in childhood, these findings suggest, that in patients suffering from chronic TLE, intellecutal abilities may not develop optimally. This notion is supported by longitudinal findings reported by Bjoernas et al. (2001), which clearly show that childhood-onset TLE bears a greater risk of a decline in intellectual functions than adult-onset TLE.

Evidently, the impact of anticonvulsant therapy also enters into the equation. Although numerous studies have pointed out the detrimental effect of polytherapy on cognitive functioning (e.g., Aldenkamp and Bootsma in this volume; Aldenkamp, 2001; Aldenkamp et al., 2003; Bourgeois, 1998), the differential effect of seizure frequency and combinations of anticonvulsant drugs taken by the patient, is difficult to determine. Smith et al. (2002), in a neuropsychological study of nonsurgical children with intractable seizures, observed that children with higher seizure frequency were significantly more impaired on cognitive and academic measures such as full scale FSI, reading comprehension and arithmetic, than those with clusters of seizures interspersed with long seizure-free intervals. However, using seizure frequency as covariate, no significant effect of the number of drugs on cognitive functioning was found. The authors reasoned that the underlying brain pathology giving rise to poorly controlled seizures may outweigh the additional effect of polytherapy. They further observed that, while intellectual abilities in their sample ranged from the superior to the deficient range, the average impairment of the patients across diverse cognitive tasks was more than twice the rate of what would be expected in the general population.

Although diffuse impairments are more often documented in children (Camfield et al., 1986; Smith et al., 2002), material-specific laterality effects such as seen in adults, have also occasionally been reported. Gadian et al. (1996) combined neuroimaging with IQ measures in 22 children with intractable TLE and found a decline in verbal functions with left-sided pathology and impairments in nonverbal functions with right-sided pathology. However, this dichotomy is less obvious in children with uncomplicated, idiopathic TLE. Thus, Camfield et al. (1986) failed to observe significant left-right differences in full scale, verbal, or performance IQ scores on the WISC, or on a neuropsychological test battery in children with non-lesional TLE. Most of these children had no measurable cognitive impairment. It is, however, noteworthy that 11 of the 27 children had learning problems, irrespective of the side of the epileptic focus. These findings suggest that even idiopathic TLE risks interfering with learning and higher mental activity.

## ■ Memory and learning

Memory impairment is the most prominent symptom of TLE in adults (Helmstaedter in this volume; Helmstaedter, 2004; Helmstaedter and Elger, 2000; Milner, 1972) and children (Elger et al., 1997; Jambaqué, 2001; Jambaqué et al., 1993) Studies in children have revealed deficits in working memory, verbal memory and visuo-spatial memory (Beardsworth and Zaidel, 1994; Cohen, 1992; Jambaqué, 2001; Jambaqué et al., 1993; Hernandez et al., 2003). These problems can be exacerbated by certain anticonvulsant drugs, notably, phenobarbital and phenytoin (Thompson and Trimble, 1982).

While memory impairment is most characteristic of TLE, it does not appear to be limited to this epilepsy type. Studies in mixed samples have repeatedly documented memory deficits in a variety of seizure disorders (McCarthy, 1995; Jambaqué et al., 2001). Comparing children with various types of epilepsy on a memory battery (the BEM-144) Jambaqué et al. (1993) found that all children, except those with idiopathic generalized epilepsy, had difficulties with both learning and retrieval. Delayed verbal memory was most impaired. Delayed recall of a story was also impaired in the epileptic children studied by Smith et al. (2002). However, there is evidence that subgroups may differ with regard to the kind of memory that is most affected. For instance, McCarthy (1995) observed that children with absences tended to have more difficulties on both visual and verbal memory tasks than those with complex partial or tonic-clonic seizures.

In a more recent study, we compared the performance of children with TLE, frontal lobe epilepsy (FLE) and generalized absence seizures (GEA) on a variety of attention and memory tests (Hernandez et al., 2003), including the auditory continuous performance test, the CVLT and the Rey-Osterrieth Complex Figure. All of the children had a full scale IQ above 90 and none of them were candidates for resective surgery. In keeping with earlier studies, the results revealed that all epileptic children were impaired on the memory tasks relative to healthy controls. Overall, FLE children did more poorly than TLE children, and the latter were inferior to GEA children. However, there were qualitative differences between the groups: while FLE children were more prone to interference and had difficulties organizing the material to be learned, TLE children had greater problems recalling the information. This was particularly evident during the copy and recall of Rey's Complex Figure (see *Figure 1*). Children of all three groups also had sustained attention and working memory problems on the auditory continuous performance tasks which led us to suspect that at least part of the memory problems seen in epileptic children may be attributable to attention problems which would interfere with adequate encoding *(Figure 1)*.

Following this line of reasoning, we conducted a preliminary study in eight patients with mild left or right hippocampal atrophy (Gallagher et al., in preparation). As predicted, selective impairments on material-specific (verbal/non-verbal) memory tasks of the Children's Memory Scale were accompanied by deficits in auditory and visual attention. This observation is consistent with a previous study, which has shown that attention problems, identified on standardized tests, were the only variables that accounted for the everyday memory problems reported by the parents of children with intractable epilepsy (Kadis et al., 2004).

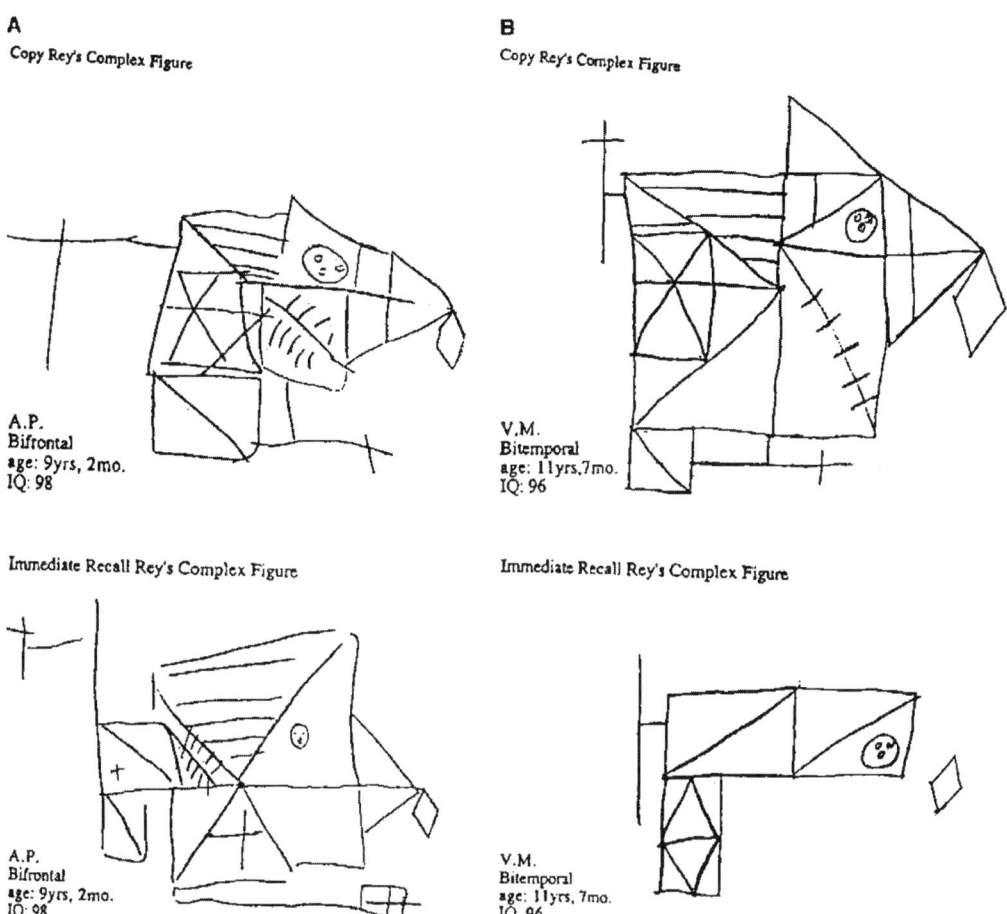

**Figure 1.** A typical example of the copy and immediate recall of the Rey-Osterrieth Complex Figure by a FLE child (A) and a TLE child (B). Reproduced from Hernandez *et al.* (2003) with permission of Elsevier.

It appears that lateralized memory problems are more readily demonstrable in patients having undergone surgery for intractable seizures (*e.g.* Hemstaedter, 2004; Lassonde *et al.*, 2000) than in nonsurgical patients (Delaney *et al.*, 1980; Elger *et al.*, 1997, Smith *et al.*, 2002). These problems can be linked to the underlying pathology, most frequently hippocampal sclerosis, and the added effect of the cortical resection (*e.g.*, Helmstaedter, 2004). Comparisons between surgical and nonsurgical candidates have shed some light on the contribution of the pathology to lateralized memory dysfunction in children with intractable seizures (Smith *et al.*, 2002). The results have revealed a high degree of shared cognitive deficits between the two groups, with delayed verbal memory (story recall) being the only measure on which group differences were obtained. Impairments were more marked in the surgical than the nonsurgical group, irrespective of the side of the epileptogenic abnormality. Most of the children had intractable seizures of temporal lobe origin. Consistent with these findings, volumetric MRI studies have shown a direct relationship between verbal memory and bilateral hippocampal volume (Reminger et al., 2004). Both left and right hippocampal volumes correlated with verbal memory, while no relationship was found between hippocampal volume and nonverbal memory functions.

Recent work suggests that the functional left/right asymmetry can be subtle and may be more qualitative than quantitative, at least as far as visual memory is concerned. For instance, applying the qualitative error analysis of the Rey-Osterrieth Complex Figure developed by Loring et al. (1988), Piquet et al. (1994), observed that while patients with both left- and right-lateralized foci obtained similar global scores in the recall condition, those with right foci made many more errors. In the same vein, significantly longer execution times in the right TLE group were the only manifestation of the typical left/right asymmetry in the patients tested by Baxendale et al. (1998) on a spatial memory battery. Finally, as pointed out by Helmstaedter et al. (1995) factors such as atypical lateralization, gender differences and task complexity can confound laterality effects.

## ▪ Language

Language dysfunction is another characteristic feature of temporal lobe epilepsy (see also Jansky et al. in this volume). Children tend to be more impaired than adults. This may be attributable to the development of atypical language representation due to partial or complete transfer of language functions to the nondominant hemisphere in case of early left hemisphere insult (Duchowny et al., 1996; Saltzman-Benaiah et al., 2003). Saltzman-Banai et al. (2003) studied a pediatric epilepsy sample and found that abnormal speech lateralization varied according to age at onset and locus of the epileptic focus. Interestingly, atypical language lateralization was more frequent in extratemporal epilepsy. With regard to age at onset, the study reaffirmed the 5-year age level as the cut-off point after which the likelihood of atypical language development decreases. However, Janszky et al. (2003) found that a relatively large proportion (close to 25%) of patients with late childhood-onset of mesial TLE presented atypical (bi-hemispheric or right hemispheric) language lateralization. These findings would provide further evidence for the notion that mesial sclerosis precedes the clinical manifestations of TLE. It may also suggest that interference of the pathological process with normal maturation may extend the window during which reorganization of language can occur.

Although interictal arrest of speech can occasionally be observed (Jambaqué, 2001), aphasic disorders are rare. One exception is the Landau Kleffner syndrome (e.g., Van Houte, 2001), a type of acquired auditory aphasia that occurs in conjunction with multifocal spike-wave activity which predominates over left temporal areas. The age of onset lies between 3 and 8 years, an age that coincides with a period of accelerated cerebral maturation. Although the seizures are infrequent, the cognitive consequences are severe and can be permanent (Beaumanoir, 1992). Receptive speech is affected first. The child may appear deaf. Expressive speech deteriorates secondarily.

More common language impairments in TLE are poor lexical knowledge, word-finding difficulties and anomia (Jambaqué, 2001; Silvia et al., 2003) There are indications that these language problems may to some extent account for the verbal memory deficits and learning disabilities associated with seizures originating in the left temporal lobe (Hermann et al., 1988). In fact, although learning problems are overrepresented in children with epilepsy compared to children with non-neurological chronic conditions, there is evidence that reading and spelling are more affected in children with TLE (e.g. Seidenberg, 1989; Stores and Hart, 1991). Children with epilepsy have been found to be approximately one year behind in their reading ability. Furthermore, children with left-sided foci tend to perform more poorly on reading tests than those with right-sided foci (Kasteleijn-Nolst Trenite et al., 1990; Stores and Hart, 1991). This is not surprising considering that the left temporal lobe is specialized in the auditory analysis of speech sounds. Functional MRI studies in normal readers have revealed activation in superior temporal gyrus and inferior frontal gyrus (Pugh et al., 1996). In contrast, dyslexic individuals show decreased activity in left temporal cortex accompanied by significant over-activity in left inferior frontal cortex during phonological processing (Shaywitz et al., 2002). Furthermore, neuroimaging and post-mortem studies in dyslexic subjects have consistently shown structural abnormalities in the language areas of the left temporal lobe (Galaburda, 1993; Geschwind and Levitsky, 1968).

Numerous studies have demonstrated the critical role of phonological skills in reading acquisition and, conversely, the common lack of phonological awareness in dyslexia (e.g., Fletcher et al., 1994; Rack et al., 1992). Individuals lacking phonological awareness are unable to break words into their phonemic components and have to rely on the visual route of word recognition. We recently had the opportunity to investigate the impact of TLE on phonological processing and reading in a pair of identical, right-handed, francophone twins, one of whom presents complex partial seizures originating from a well-localizable left temporal focus (Vanasse et al., 2003). The epilepsy was diagnosed at the age of 8 without any known precipitating factors. At the time of testing the girls were 13 years old and both attended the same grade in a regular school. While none of them was considered to be learning disabled, the affected twin reportedly had to work much harder than her healthy twin to make the grade. In particular, her French marks were much inferior to her mathematical marks. In addition, reading tests at various age levels indicated a persistent lag of approximately one year in her reading age relative to age expectations. Although her full scale IQ of 117 was well within normal range, it was much inferior to that of her twin sister, who scored in the superior range (FS: 145). This result is itself interesting in that it indicates that the impact of epilepsy on intelligence is difficult to estimate in high functioning children. In spite of her left sided focus, a difference of more than 1 standard deviation was observed between her verbal IQ and performance IQ in favor of the former.

Both twins were submitted to a phonological battery using non-words to limit lexical and semantic access. Tests included auditory discrimination, word repetition, syllable reversal, production and judgment of rhyme as well as a variety reading tasks involving oral reading of regular and irregular words and non-words. Compared to her twin sister and IQ-matched controls, the patient was found to be impaired in all functions. Furthermore, her reading age was more than two years behind expectations whereas that of her healthy twin was above age expectations. These findings underline the important role of the temporal lobes in phonological processing.

## ■ Executive functions

Although deficits in executive functions are the hallmark of frontal lobe dysfunction, several studies, including our own, have shown that children and adults suffering from TLE may present impairments that are similar to, albeit less severe than those seen in FLE patients on a number of "frontal" measures. Studying the same sample of FLE, TLE and epilepsy with generalized absence seizures (GEA) patients described above (see Hernandez et al., 2003), we found that a relatively high proportion (38-50%) of TLE children performed below age norms on tasks measuring motor coordination, verbal fluency and mental flexibility (Hernandez et al., 2002). This finding is consistent with other studies. For instance, Igarashi et al. (2002), in a cohort of TLE children with hippocampal atrophy, reported below-normal performance on the Wisconsin Card Sorting Test (WCST), a test that purports to assess concept formation and mental flexibility. Similarly, Herrmann and Seidenberg (1995) demonstrated reduced performance on the WCST in an adult sample. However, in contrast to Igarashi et al. (2002), the deficit was independent of the presence or absence of hippocampal pathology. The authors attribute these deficits to the propagation of "neural noise" associated with epileptogenic discharges in medial temporal structures to neighboring extratemporal regions, notably the frontal cortex (Hermann and Seidenberg, 1995).

## ■ Conclusion

Taken together, the reviewed studies indicate that TLE in children affects the same structures and functions as in adults, although the manifestations may not always follow the typical pattern seen in adults. Since many adult patients with chronic TLE have a seizure history that can be traced back to their childhood, these patients can be regarded as a model for the long term outcome of childhood-onset TLE.

Age at seizure onset appears to be the most reliable predictor of long term cognitive outcome. Converging evidence suggests that early onset is associated with greater and more widespread cognitive impairment. However, although children with later onset and uncomplicated TLE may have normal intelligence, many tend to have learning disabilities. These may be attributable to more subtle cognitive impairments related to an unrecognized underlying pathology. Indeed, recently, renewed interest has been directed towards the study of the so-called "benign" idiopathic epilepsies (Metz-Lutz et al., 1999). These studies have identified a number of subtle cognitive and behavior deficits which may persist long after the seizures have ceased or become rare. It seems that the term "benign" is not synonymous with absence of cognitive impairment. In the same vein, TLE children and adults with normal intelligence have consistently been found to perform more poorly than their siblings on a wide variety of neuropsychological tests. Furthermore, there is evidence of decline in intelligence with prolonged exposure to seizures. The long term manifestation of this decline is a lower IQ in adult patients with chronic TLE.

Among the typical temporal lobe functions, verbal memory and language-related functions appear to be most affected in children. There is some indication that attention and language problems may be, at least in part, responsible for the memory deficits. In turn, atypical lateralization, which is common in epilepsy, may explain some of the impairments observed in the language domain. In fact, the material specific left/right dissociation for verbal and visual processing is less obvious in children than in adults, at least in those that have not undergone focal resection. Phonological processing, which is important for reading development, is often impaired. The structural and physiological anomalies seen in the left temporal lobe of dyslexic children have been well documented and highlight the important role of this area in reading acquisition. Although children with TLE are not usually dyslexic, they may show a discrepancy between their actual and expected reading age which may interfere with academic success.

On the other hand, the diffuse cognitive deficits seen in both children and adults with intractable seizures of temporal lobe origin indicate that the impact of prolonged exposure to potentially damaging epileptic activity extends beyond the functions mediated by the temporal lobes. Findings of impaired executive functions in TLE patients tend to support the "nociferous cortex" hypothesis referring to the deleterious influence of temporal lobe seizures on extratemporal cortex (Hermann and Seidenberg, 1995). Invasive EEG procedures have shown the frontal lobes to be the preferred target of ictal and interictal spreading of epileptogenic activity originating in mesial temporal lobe regions (e.g., Emerson et al., 1995; Lieb et al., 1991; Shulman, 2000). Furthermore, consistent with the notion of extratemporal dysfunction, Hermann and Seidenberg (2002) found a reduction in total cortical volume which correlated with a wide range of cognitive deficits in patients with early-onset TLE. The volumetric decrease was most evident in white matter. Such decrease would limit intra- and interhemispheric integration of sensory information which is so important for higher mental activity.

Finally, a few temporal lobe functions still remain unexplored in epileptic children. We refer to the "what" and "where" distinction in visual object recognition and localization which are mediated by two separate visual systems. Studies in this area could provide information about which of the systems, if any, may selectively be impaired in TLE. In addition, neuropsychological studies using voice detection and face discrimination may prove useful in exploring higher-order auditory and visual processing in individuals with TLE (see Laurent et al. in this volume).

# References

Aldenkamp AP. Cognitive side effects of antiepileptic drugs. In: Jambaqué I, Lassonde M, Dulac O, eds. *Neuropsychology of childhood epilepsy*. New York: KluverAcademic/Plenum Publishers, 2001: 257-67.

Aldenkamp AP, De Krom M, Reijs R. Newer antiepileptic drugs and cognitive issues. *Epilepsia* 2003; 44 (suppl 4): 21-29.

Baxendale SA, Thompson PJ, Van Paesschen W. A test of spatial memory and its clinical utility in the pre-surgical investigation of temporal lobe epilepsy patients. *Neuropsychologia* 1998; 36 (7): 591-602.

Beardsworth ED, Zaidel DW. Memory for face in epileptic children before and after brain surgery. *J Clin Exp. Neuropsychol* 1994; 16: 589-96.

Beaumanoir A. Landau-Kleffner syndrome. In: Roger J, Bureau M, Dravet C et al., eds. *Epileptic syndromes in infancy, childhood and adolescence*, 2nd ed. London: JohnLibbey, 1992: 231-244.

Bjoernas H, Stabell K, Henriksen O, Loyning Y. The effects of refractory epilepsy on intellectual function in children and adults. A longitudinal study. *Seizure* 2001; 10: 250-9.

Black KC, Hynd GW. Epilepsy in the school-aged child: Cognitive-behavioral characteristics and effects on academic performance. *School Psych Quart* 1995; 10 (4): 345-58.

Bourgeois BFD. Antiepileptic drugs, learning, and behaviour in childhood epilepsy. *Epilepsia* 1998; 38: 913-21.

Brockhaus A, Elger CE. Complex seizures of temporal lobe origin in children of different age groups. *Epilepsia* 1995; 36: 1173-81.

Camfield PR, Gates R, Ronen G, Camfield C, Ferguson A, MacDonald GW. Comparison of cognitive ability, personality profile, and school success in epileptic children with pure right *versus* left temporal lobe EEG foci. *Ann Neurol* 1984; 15 (2): 122-6.

Cohen M. Auditory/verbal and visual/spatial memory in children with complex partial epilepsy on temporal lobe origin. *Brain Cogn* 1992; 20: 315-26.

Delaney RC, Rosen AJ, Mattson RH, Novelly RA. Memory function in focal epilepsy: a comparison of non-surgical, unilateral temporal lobe and frontal lobe samples. *Cortex* 1980; 16 (1): 103-17.

Duchowny M, Jayakar P, Harvey AS, Resnick T, Alvarez L, Dean P, Levin B. Language cortex representation: effects of developmental *versus* acquired pathology. *Ann Neurol* 1996; 40 (1): 31-8.

Elger CE, Brockhaus A, Lendt M, Kowalik A, Steidel S. Behavior and cognition in children with temporal lobe epilepsy. In: Tuxhorn I, Holthausen H, Boenigk H, eds. *Paediatric epilepsy syndromes and their surgical treatment*. London: John Libbey, 1997: 311-25.

Emerson RG, Turner CA, Pedley TA, Walczak TS, Forgione M. Propagation patterns of temporal spikes. *Electroencephalogr Clin Neurophysiol* 1995; 94 (5): 338-48.

Engel J. Surgery for seizures. *New Engl J Med* 1996; 334: 647-52.

Engel J. Surgical treatment of the epilepsies. 2$^{nd}$ edition. New York: Raven Press, 1993.

Farwell JR, Dodrill CB, Batzel LW. Neuropsychological abilities of children with epilepsy. *Epilepsia* 1985; 26: 395-400.

Fletcher JM, Shaywitz SE, Shankweiler DP, Katz L, Lieverman IY, Steubing KK, *et al*. Cognitive profiles of reading disabilities. *J Ed Psychol* 1994; 86: 6-23.

Gadian DG, Isaacs EB, Cross JH, Connelly A, Jackson GD, King MD, Neville BG, Vargha-Khadem F. Lateralization of brain function in childhood revealed by magnetic resonance spectroscopy. *Neurology* 1996; 46 (4): 974-7.

Galaburda AM. Neuroanatomic basis of developmental dyslexia. *Neurol Clin* 1993; 11 (1): 161-73.

Gallagher A, Carmant L, Sauerwein HC, Lassonde M. Material-specific short-term memory deficits in children with unilateral hippocampal atrophy. In preparation.

Geshwind N, Levitsky W. Human brain: left-right asymmetries in temporal speech region. *Science* 1968; 161 (837): 186-7.

Igarashi K, Oguni H, Osawa M, Awaya Y, Kato M, Mimura M. Wisconsin card sorting test in children with temporal lobe epilepsy. *Brain Dev* 2002; 24 (3): 174-8.

Helmstaedter C. Neuropsychological aspects of epilepsy surgery. *Epilepsy Behav* 2004; 5 (suppl 1): S45-55.

Helmstaedter C, Elger CE. Behavioral markers for self- and other-attribution of memory: a study in patients with temporal lobe epilepsy and healthy volunteers. *Epilepsy Res* 2000; 41 (3): 235-43.

Helmstaedter C, Pohl C, Elger CE. Relations between verbal and nonverbal memory performance: evidence of confounding effects particularly in patients with right temporal lobe epilepsy. *Cortex* 1995; 31 (2): 345-55.

Hermann B, Seidenberg M. Neuropsychology and temporal lobe epilepsy. *CNS Spectr* 2002; 7 (5): 343-8.

Hermann B, Seidenberg M. Executive system dysfunction in temporal lobe epilepsy: effects of nociferous cortex *versus* hippocampal pathology. *J Clin Exp Neuropsychol* 1995; 6: 809-19.

Hermann BP, Wyler AR, Steenman H, Richey ET. The interrelationship between language function and verbal learning/memory performance in patients with complex partial seizures. *Cortex* 1988; 24 (2): 245-53.

Hernandez MT Sauerwein HC, Jambaqué I, de Guise E, Lussier F, Lortie A, Dulac O, Lassonde M. Attention, memory, and behavioral adjustment in children with frontal lobe epilepsy. *Epilepsy Behav* 2003; 4: 524-35.

Hernandez MT Sauerwein HC, Jambaqué I, de Guise E, Lussier F, Lortie A, Dulac O, Lassonde M. Deficits in executive functions and motor coordination in children with frontal lobe epilepsy. *Neuropsychologia* 2002; 40: 384-400.

Jambaqué I. Neuropsychology of temporal lobe epilepsy in children. In: Jambaqué I, Lassonde M, Dulac O, eds. *Neuropsychology of childhood epilepsy*. New York: Kluver Academic/Plenum Publishers, 2001: 97-102.

Jambaqué I, Dellatolas G, Dulac O, Ponsot G, Signoret JL. Verbal and visual memory impairment in children with epilepsy. *Neurpsychologia* 1993; 31: 1321-37.

Janszky J, Rasonyi G, Clemens Z, Schulz R, Hoppe M, Barsi P, Fogarasi A, Halasz P, Ebner A. Clinical differences in patients with unilateral hippocampal sclerosis and unitemporal or bitemporal epileptiform discharges. *Seizure* 2003; 12 (8): 550-4.

Kadis DS, Stollstorff M, Elliott I, Lach L, Smith ML. Cognitive and psychological predictors of everyday memory in children with intractable epilepsy. *Epilepsy Behav* 2004; 5 (1): 37-43.

Kasteleijn-Nolst Trenite DG, Smit AM, Velis DN, Willemse J, van Emde Boas W. On-line detection of transient neuropsychological disturbances during EEG discharges in children with epilepsy. *Dev Med Child Neurol* 1990; 32 (1): 46-50.

Lassonde, M, Sauerwein HC. Jambaqué I, Smith ML, Helmstaedter C. Neuropsychology of childhood epilepsy: pre- and postsurgical assessment. *Epileptic Disord* 2000; 2 (1): 3-13.

Lieb JP, Dasheiff RM, Engel J Jr. Role of the frontal lobes in the propagation of mesial temporal lobe seizures. *Epilepsia* 1991; 32 (6): 822-37.

Loring DW, Lee GP, Meador KJ. Revising the Rey-Osterrieth: rating right hemisphere recall. *Arch Clin Neuropsychol* 1988; 3 (3): 239-47

McCarthy AM. Memory, attention, and school problems in children with seizure disorders. *Dev Neuropsychol* 1995; 1/1: 71-86.

Metz-Lutz MN, Kleizt C, De Saint Martin A, Massa F, Hirsch E. Marescaux C. Cognitive development in benign focal epilepsies of childhood. *Dev Neurosci* 1999; 21: 182-90.

Milner B. Disorders of learning and memory after temporal lobe lesions in man. *Clin Neurosurg* 1972; 19: 421-46.

Nolan, MA, Redoblado MA, Lah S, Sabaz M, Lawson JA, Cunningham AM, *et al*. Intellingec in childhood epilepsy syndromes. *Epilepsy Res* 2003; 53: 139-50.

Pacual-Castroviejo I, Garcia Blazquez M, Guitierre Molina M, Carcelle F, Lopez Martin V. 24-year preoperative evolution of a temporal astrocytoma. *Childs Nerv Syst* 1996; 12: 417-20.

Piguet O, Saling MM, O'Shea MF, Berkovic SF, Bladin PF. Rey figure distortions reflect nonverbal recall differences between right and left foci in unilateral temporal lobe epilepsy. *Arch Clin Neuropsychol* 1994; 9 (5): 451-60.

Pugh KR, Shaywitz BA, Shaywitz SE, Constable RT, Skudlarski P, Fulbright RK. Bronen RA, Shankweiler DP, Katz L, Fletcher JM, Gore JC. Cerebral organization of component processes in reading. *Brain* 1996; 119 (4): 1221-38.

Rack JP, Snowling MI, Olson RK. The non-work reading deficit in developmental dyslexia. A review. *Read Res Quart* 1992; 27 (1): 29-53.

Reminger SL, Kaszniak AW, Labiner DM, Litrell LD, David, BT, Ryan I, Herring AM, Kaemingk KL. Bilateral hippocampal volume predicts verbal memory function in temporal lobe epilepsy. *Epilepsy Behav* 2004; 5 (5): 687-95.

Roeshl-Heil A Bledowski C, Elger CE, Heils A, Helmstaedter C. Neuropsychological functioning among 32 patients with temporal lobe epilepsy and their discordant siblings. *Epilepsia* 2003; 43 (suppl 7): 185-6.

Saltzman-Benaiah J, Scott K, Smith ML. Factors associated with atypical speech representation in children with intractable epilepsy. *Neuropsychologia* 2003; 41 (14): 1967-74.

Schoenfield J. Seidenberg M, Woodard A, Hecox K, Ingle C, Mack K, Hermann B. Neuropsychological and behavior status of children with complex partial seizures *Dev Med Child Neurol* 1999; 41: 724-31.

Seidenberg M. Academic achievement and school performance of children with epilepsy. In: Hermann BP, Seidenberg M, eds. *Childhood epilepsies: Neuropschological, psychosocial and intervention aspects*. New York: John Wiley & Sons, 1989: 105-18.

Shaywitz BA, Shaywitz SE, Pugh KR, Mencl WE, Fulbright RK, Skudlarski P, Constable RT, Marchione KE, Fletcher JM, Lyon GR, Gore JC. Disruption of posterior brain systems for reading in children with developmental dyslexia. *Biol Psychiatry* 2002; 52 (2): 101-10.

Shulman MB. The frontal lobes, epilepsy, and behavior. *Epilepsy Behav* 2000; 1 (6): 384-95.

Silvia O, Silvia O, Patricia S, Damian C, Brenda G, Walter S, Luciana D, Estela C, Patricia S, Silvia K. Mesial temporal lobe epilepsy and hippocampal sclerosis: cognitive function assessment in Hispanic patients. *Epilepsy Behav* 2003; 4 (6): 717-22.

Smith ML, Elliott IM, Lach L. Cognitive skills in children with intractable epilepsy: Comparison of surgical and nonsurgical candidates. *Epilepsia* 2002; 43/6: 631-7.

Stores G, Hart JA. Reading skills in children with generalized or focal epilepsy attending ordinary school. *Dev Med Child Neurol* 1976; 18: 705-16.

Thompson PJ, Trimble MR. Anticonvulsant drugs and cognitive functions. *Epilepsia* 1982; 23 (5): 531-44.

Vanasse CM, Beland R, Jambaqué I, Lavoie K, Lassonde M. Impact of temporal lobe epilepsy on phonological processing and reading: A case study of identical twins. *Neurocase* 2003; 9: 515-22.

Van Houte A. Aphasia and auditory agnosia in children with Landau-Kleffner Syndrome. In: Jambaqué I, Lassonde M, Dulac O, eds. *Neuropsychology of childhood epilepsy*. New York: KluverAcademic/Plenum Publishers, 2001: 191-8.

# Effects of chronic temporal lobe epilepsy on memory functions

C. Helmstaedter

*University Clinic of Epileptology, Bonn, Germany*

Declarative memory processing, that is the acquisition of and the later access to newly acquired information, is one of the most essential human cognitive functions. Declarative memory establishes continuity in a steadily changing world and thus provides the basis of one's biography, identity, as well as cognitive and behavioral development. In temporal lobe epilepsy, this type of memory is characteristically impaired when mesiotemporal and associated neocortical structures are affected by lesions, ongoing epileptic activity, or undesired treatment effects (*e.g.* operative treatment). Hence, major issues are the etiology, onset and course of memory impairment in addition to the prevention of further memory decline during the course of epilepsy. The relationship between memory performance and questions regarding the course of temporal lobe epilepsy is an important one, particularly when having to determine whether epilepsy is a progressive and dementing disease, whether seizures functionally damage the brain, or which impact the treatment of temporal lobe epilepsy can have on the course of the disease.

## ■ Temporal lobe epilepsy and memory

Temporal lobe epilepsy (TLE) is very common, accounting for about 70% of all focal symptomatic or cryptogenic epilepsies. TLE is most of all characterized by the repeated and unprovoked occurrence of epileptic seizures which take their origin in temporal lobe structures. Yet, temporal lobe epilepsy is not a homogeneous cerebral disorder (see Arzimanoglou in this volume). This fact is probably best reflected by the lasting discussion as to whether TLE with hippocampal sclerosis can be considered to be a disease or a syndrome (Wieser, 2004). From a neuropsychological point of view, impaired declarative memory performance is a characteristic feature of TLE. The temporal lobes and their temporo-limbic aspects are known to be involved in the formation of new memories. Accordingly, 70-80% of the more than 1000 patients with pharmacoresistant TLE, who were evaluated in Bonn since 1988, were found to show impairment of either verbal or figural memory (performance < m –1SD). Broken down according to verbal or figural memory, 50-60% of patients showed a deficit in a specific type of memory. More precisely, it is episodic memory (*i.e.*, the acquisition of time and context dependent information) which is particularly affected in TLE. Semantic memory may also be affected but this is a much less consistent finding (Helmstaedter, 2002).

A general framework for understanding how the mesial structures are involved in declarative memory has been provided by Eichenbaum's proposal that neocortical perceptually and conceptually processed information is extendedly held by parahippocampal structures. These are bidirectionally connected to the neocortical association areas whereas the hippocampus contains properties which ensure encoding, retrieval and the linkage of experiences to stored representations (Eichenbaum, 2000).

The key-role of temporo-mesial and neocortical structures for memory in TLE has been demonstrated by a variety of functional and volumetric imaging studies, invasive electroencephalographic studies, and correlations of human hippocampal cell counts or LTP (long term potentiation) to memory performance. Memory impairment in lateralized TLE tends to be material-specific, that is, left TLE is associated with verbal memory impairment, right TLE with visual memory impairment. Moreover, neocortical temporal and mesial hippocampal structures may be differentially involved in episodic memory, indeed, the mesial structures seem to be nonspecifically involved in consolidation and retrieval, whereas neocortical structures seem to be more involved in material-specific processing of memory contents (Helmstaedter, 2001; Elger *et al.*, 2004). False lateralizing memory impairments in TLE (*i.e.* deviations from the left *versus* right or verbal *versus* nonverbal dissociations) are frequent. False lateralization in left TLE has been attributed to factors such as hemispheric dominance and gender differences. For its part, false lateralization in right TLE has been attributed to a more bilateral organization of nonverbal memory networks, covert verbalization, or the type of test and test materials (abstractness, complexity) used (Helmstaedter, 1999; Helmstaedter *et al.*, 1995) (*Figure 1*).

## ■ Cognitive impairment beyond memory

The number of TLE patients displaying memory deficits is considerable but this must not distract one from noticing that cognitive impairment in TLE exceeds the memory domain. Hermann, in his 1997 article about the neuropsychological characteristics of the syndrome of mesial temporal lobe epilepsy, noted that TLE is not only characterized by memory deficits but also by generalized cognitive impairment in terms of poor academic achievement and lower IQ scores (Hermann *et al.*, 1997). In our center about 30% of TLE patients show IQ scores below 85 and this still appears to be an underestimation. According to a recent comparison between 31 patients with mesial TLE and their healthy siblings, the degree of global impairment was much greater than was expected from previous evaluations of patients on the sole basis of test norms (Roeschl-Heils *et al.*, 2002). Thirty-six percent of the patients *versus* 7% of their siblings had an IQ below 85, but 55% of the patients negatively differed by more than one standard deviation (> 15 IQ points) from their healthy sibling. With the exception of nonverbal memory span there was no cognitive domain in which patients' performances were not significantly worse than that of their siblings' (*Figure 2*).

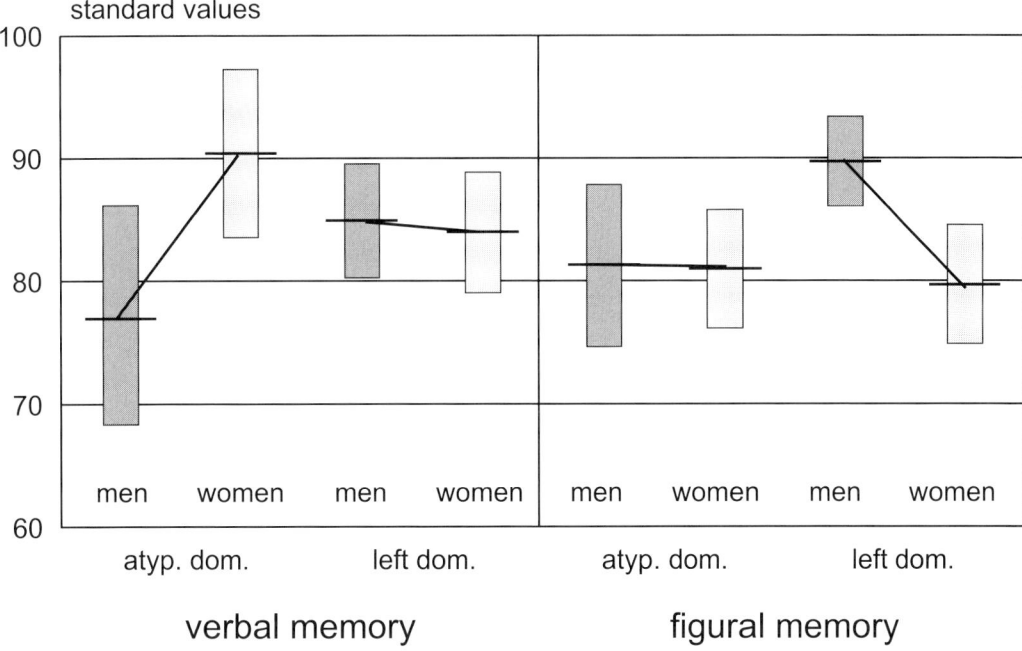

**Figure 1.** Deviations from left/right verbal/nonverbal dichotomy in patients with left TLE as a function of sex and language dominance. Only left dominant men show the expected pattern of impaired verbal and unimpaired figural memory. False lateralization by unimpaired verbal memory is observed in one group (women with atypical dominance), false lateralization by impaired figural memory is observed in three groups (atypical dominant men and women, and typically dominant women).

The number of patients who significantly differed from their sibling with respect to IQ was not different from that observed for memory. The emerging picture is similar to that reported by Oyegbile et al. in 2004 who compared TLE patients with a larger group of controls having all run through the same test battery. The observation of impairments exceeded those which would be expected from circumscribed temporal lobe lesions. This observation is at the heart of the question surrounding the effects of chronic TLE on cognition and particularly memory. Is it possible, as some argue, that not only poor memory but also general intellectual impairment are consequences of chronic TLE?

## ■ Chronic epilepsy and memory in TLE

Evaluation of the effect of chronic TLE on cognition is difficult when considering the multi-factorial nature of cognitive impairment in this disease. Apart from seizures and epileptic dysfunction, underpinning developmental disorders, acquired lesions, and negative treatment effects must be considered as factors potentially influencing cognition. In what follows, an approach to the question of the impact of chronic

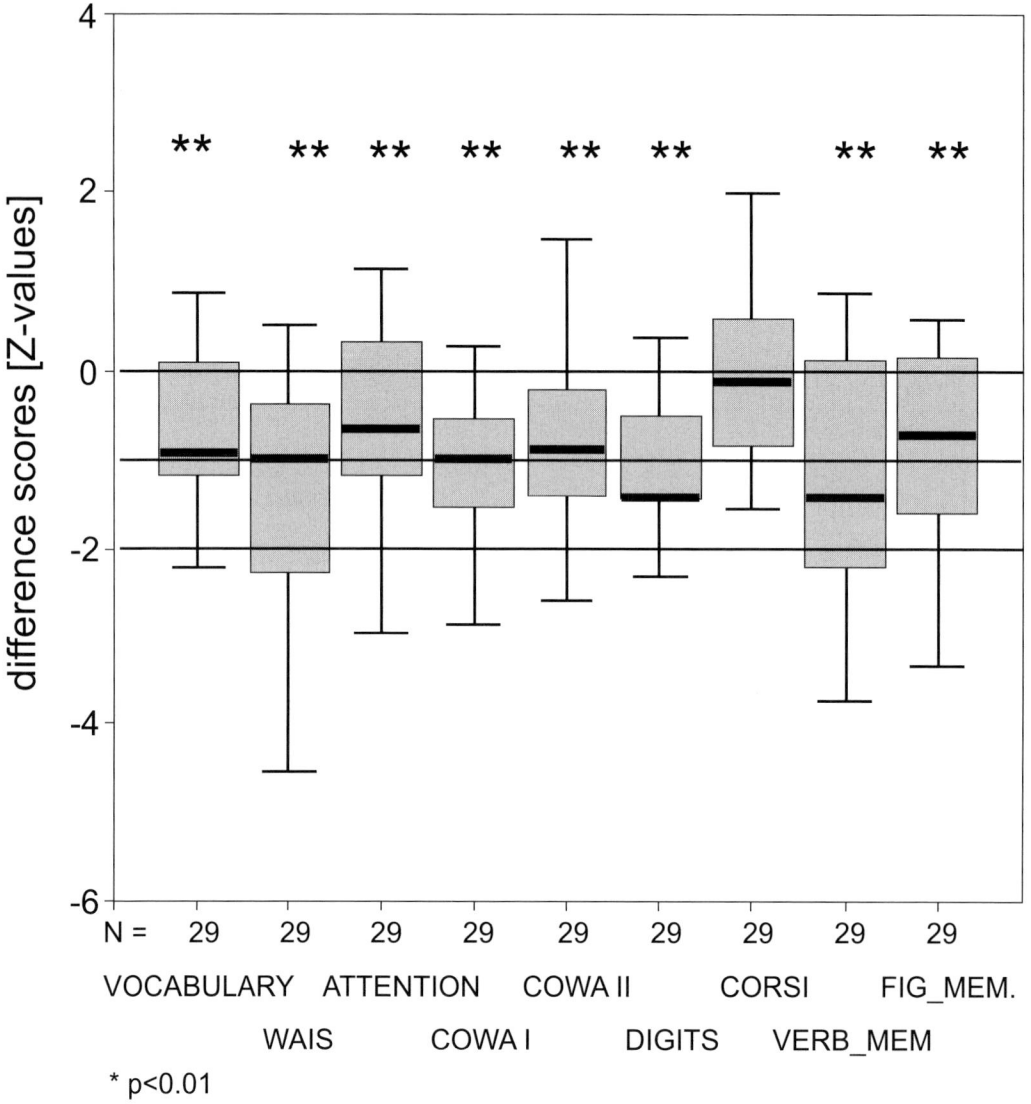

**Figure 2.** Cognitive performance in patients with mesial TLE, z-transformed with respect to the corresponding performance of their healthy siblings.
(COWA I = phonematic fluency, COWA II = semantic fluency).

epilepsy on memory is discussed. In this approach the etiological factors are explicitly placed within a developmental neuropsychological framework, which will consider the interaction and interference of epilepsy with the maturing and aging brain.

Up to now, there have been no longitudinal studies conducted on etiologically homogeneous patients with TLE starting from the very beginning of this disease and tracking those who will become seizure free *versus* those who will not. Instead we have to infer answers to our questions from reviewing a mixture of cross-sectional and longitudinal studies, most of them performed in adult and inpatients with heterogeneous pathologies.

*Initial damage* versus *chronic epilepsy*

We know cognitive impairments in epilepsy result from the complex interaction of more static and irreversible *versus* more dynamic and reversible factors. On the one hand there are impairments due to structural lesions, on the other hand there are impairments due to epileptic activity, seizures, or drug treatment. The crucial point here is that dynamic factors, despite their principal reversibility, can have a lasting negative impact on cerebral structures by causing damage, or on development by causing irreversible retardation.

It is tempting to evaluate the effects of chronic TLE on cognition by focusing on the duration of epilepsy. Duration of epilepsy is then taken as representative of the accumulation of seizures and other epilepsy related ailments during the course of the disease. However, since TLE mostly starts early in life, a longer duration of epilepsy is almost synonymous with an earlier onset of epilepsy and/or an older age, both being factors, which themselves affect the type and degree of cognitive impairment. Furthermore the age at the onset of epilepsy is heavily confounded with the etiology of epilepsy (*i.e.* early onset TLE is mostly due to developmental malformations whereas later onset TLE is more likely associated with tumors, trauma, etc.). Whether an early or late onset TLE with hippocampal sclerosis form one entity or belong to the same nosological category remains to be demonstrated (Wieser, 2004). From a developmental neuropsychological point of view, the age at the onset alone makes a significant difference (see next paragraph).

Indeed, patients with symptomatic or cryptogenic TLE either have or must be assumed to have cerebral lesions or malformations underpinning their epilepsy. These can already be assumed to be associated with dysfunctions. In addition one must assume an epileptic process that is already active before the first seizure. Thus, for patients with chronic epilepsy, the questions are, which part of the actual impairment may be due to the initial pathology and epileptic process (before or at epilepsy onset), and how much chronically occurring seizures and accumulating other noxious events add to this impairment. Evaluation of patients with new onset *versus* chronic TLE and the study of the effects of seizures and seizure control on cognition may provide some clues to answer this question.

*Cognition in newly diagnosed epilepsy*

Studies addressing the cognitive status at the onset of the epilepsy comprise either idiopathic or a mixture of symptomatic and cryptogenic epilepsies. However, these studies on children or adults with newly diagnosed epilepsy provide ample evidence that cognitive impairment and behavior problems are already present at baseline (before treatment) (Oostrom *et al.*, 2003; Austin *et al.*, 2002; Pulliainen *et al.*, 2000; Ogunrin *et al.*, 2000). In TLE patients, the comparison between newly diagnosed and chronically ill patients with left TLE shows that both groups suffer from verbal memory impairment (Aikia *et al.*, 2001). Pre-treatment impairment appears to be less specific than generalized impairment and pertains to visual motor performance, mental flexibility, memory, reaction times, and attention. This is confirmed by our own data on 29 newly diagnosed adult patients with symptomatic/cryptogenic epilepsies who, with the exception of IQ, displayed significant impairment in one or more cognitive domains in > 70% of the cases (*Figure 3*). The individual domains were affected in 36-55%, which parallels the numbers seen in patients with treated chronic epilepsies. As a trend, the subgroup of 7 patients with TLE showed the poorest performance in verbal memory. Interestingly, the duration of epilepsy before diagnosis and treatment (range 0-11 yrs, median 2.3 yrs) did not explain the degree of pre-treatment impairment. In contrast, greater impairment was associated with older age and a later onset of epilepsy (Helmstaedter et al., 2005). In later onset TLE, the mean IQ of the newly diagnosed patients observed was within a normal range (m = 102 SD = 20), and the incidence of 17% patients with an IQ below 85 was not increased.

Coming back to the already mentioned study on mesial TLE patients and their siblings, a greater difference in performances between the siblings in IQ and memory was not related to a longer duration of epilepsy but rather to an earlier age at the onset of epilepsy. This has been taken as another indicator that impairments in patients must already be present at the time of epilepsy onset (Roeschl-Heils et al., 2002). Furthermore, these results are in line with the fact that in early onset epilepsies, earlier cerebral damage has more negative consequences for cognitive development than later damage.

*Cognition and seizures*

Seizures in TLE can damage the brain, and therefore can negatively affect memory. This is most impressively demonstrated by TLE patients who became globally amnesic after a convulsive or non-convulsive status epilepticus (Dietl et al., 2004). But will each seizure do cause damage? Are all brain regions similarly susceptible to damage by temporal lobe seizures? Is there a systematic accumulation of damage with chronicity, or is there an initial homeostatic change in the beginning epilepsy followed by a more stable period? The above example of status epilepticus, not surprisingly, demonstrates that more severe seizures bear a greater risk of damage than less severe seizures. However, Dodrill, in a comprehensive review on this topic, comes to the conclusion that the literature in the field supports *definite but only mild* relationships between seizures and mental decline (Dodrill, 2004). Moreover, experimental models of TLE in animal research reveal inconsistent findings on this issue. Epilepsy inducing status epilepticus clearly damages the mesial structures but this is less clear for spontaneous seizures in the further course of epilepsy (Pitkanen et al., 2002). In another model, clear relationships between the number of induced seizures, hippocampal damage and memory loss have been demonstrated (Kotloski et al., 2002). In this respect, recent longitudinal quantitative MRI studies in new onset epilepsies are also of major importance. These studies address the question of hippocampal damage in the first years after the onset of epilepsy. Although they do not find a significant relationship between seizures and hippocampal volume changes, individual pre-treatment differences as well as individual patients, who newly developed hippocampal pathology are documented (Liu et al., 2002; Salmenpera et al., 2005). A recent report of a study conducted on 28 TLE patients with chronic epilepsies whose MRI volume

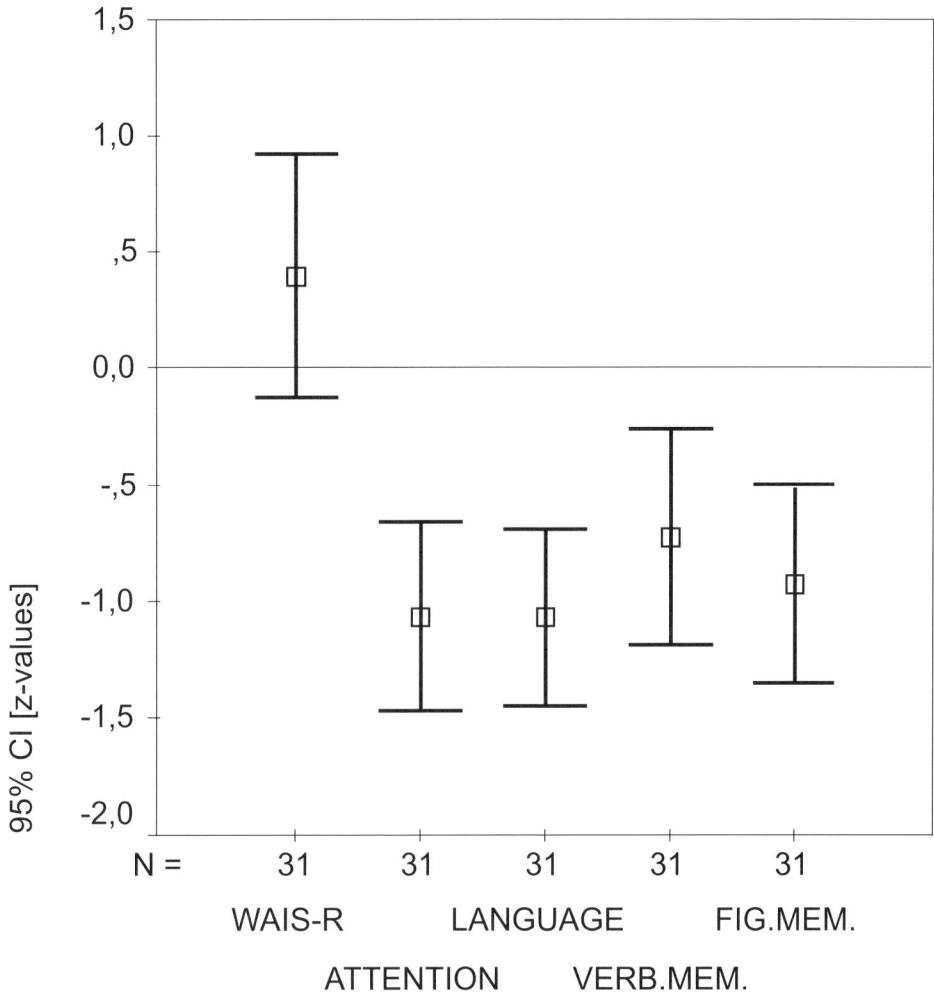

**Figure 3.** Cognitive performance in adult patients with newly diagnosed and not yet treated symptomatic/cryptogenic epilepsies indicates considerable pre-treatment impairment in partial functions. IQ in contrast appears better preserved. (data were z-transformed with regards to normative test data).

changes and performance changes were longitudinally followed (4 yrs) comes to a very similar conclusion when these changes are compared to those obtained in 21 healthy subjects (Hermann et al., 2004). Although these studies span maximally 5 years they raise evidence that there is less progress of structural damage due to chronic epilepsy than expected.

## Cognition and interictual activity

The afore-mentioned studies deal with the question of irreversible damage by lesions and seizures. More obvious, at least in the context of a seizure, is the impact of ictual epileptic dysfunction on cognition. After a temporal lobe seizure, memory impairment may last for hours despite otherwise complete recovery. This is easily demonstrated by formal postictal testing (Helmstaedter *et al.*, 1994a). The question as to whether interictual activity transiently or permanently affects cognition is less easily determined. The concept of transient cognitive impairment (TCI), which assumes a direct relationship between interictal epileptic activity and cognitive impairment has been overstressed in symptomatic focal epilepsies, where it appears to fit nonconvulsive seizures rather than single intermittent epileptic discharges (Aldenkamp *et al.*, 2004). However, interictal epileptic activity is not without an effect on cognition and memory. Cognitive improvement in seizure free patients after surgery indicates that an epileptic process was active before surgery, and caused a persistent or tonic change in cognition. Epileptic activity in TLE exerts a negative effect on distant extratemporal functions and particularly on frontal lobe functions due to their strong connectivity. Accordingly, significant recovery of mostly frontal or contralateral functions is observed within the first year after successful epilepsy surgery. Years later, recovery can also be observed with respect to the primary affected temporal lobe memory functions (Helmstaedter *et al.*, 2003). Comparable post-operative recovery has been reported with regards to behavioral disturbances in children who became seizure free (Lendt *et al.*, 2000). To assume an effect of AED withdrawal on functional recovery in seizure free patients is reasonable but remains to be demonstrated.

In summary, cognitive as well as behavioral changes after successful surgery indicate that the brain becomes functionally reorganized on different levels when seizures and epileptic activity are under control. The fact that epilepsy, beyond overt seizures, interferes with brain function leads to the assumption, that this negative influence, even if reversible, can have irreversible consequences on cognitive development in children when falling into particular sensitive periods. This also applies to negative side effects of AED. In fact, recent reports on developmental problems in children born to mothers taking valproic acid may be taken as an example (Adab *et al.*, 2004). The issue of retarded brain development leads us to the next topic.

## Mental retardation *versus* loss of acquired cognitive functions

Impairments observed at a given age may reflect loss and decline of already acquired functions and/or developmental delay or retardation. We know that the same lesions acquired at different developmental stages may present themselves as different impairments depending on the age of the patient. Children, for example, may grow into impairment, when the affected brain structures mature late. Furthermore, depending on the age of lesion onset, different functional plasticity and capacities for compensation may be observed. For example, a late onset left temporal lobe epilepsy may result in a characteristic deficit in verbal episodic memory. By contrast, an early onset left TLE can induce a shift of functions to the right hemisphere leading to largely preserved verbal memory while sacrificing originally right hemisphere nonverbal functions (Helmstaedter *et al.*, 1994b). As demonstrated in *figure 1*, a figural memory deficit instead of a verbal memory is often the consequence in this case. Finally, an early onset TLE and associated dysfunctions can be assumed to interfere negatively with the development of other cognitive functions.

According to these observations, developmental questions may be answered by focusing on the effect of the age at the onset of epilepsy on cognition or by comparing performance in children and adults with comparable pathologies. For example, memory loss after surgery in young and older patients can reveal some insight into the question of the loss of already acquired functions at different ages and the capability to compensate newly acquired damage.

## Age at the onset of epilepsy

In 1995, the Bozeman Epilepsy Consortium, which represents 8 major epilepsy centers in the USA, examined the contribution of age, age at seizure onset, duration of epilepsy, focus laterality and other variables not only on IQ but also on memory performance in 1141 patients with pharmacoresistant epilepsy. The main finding of this study was that for IQ and memory, an earlier onset of epilepsy was the only variable that predicted poorer performances (Strauss et al., 1995). However, the following data may serve as a good example for the difficulty to statistically disentangle the effects of onset and duration of epilepsy and age in such cross sectional research. *Figure 4* demonstrates IQ and memory data from a group of 74 adult TLE patients, which was broken down into patients with an onset of epilepsy = and > age 14. The onset of epilepsy made a big difference with regard to the WAIS-R IQ ($F = 16.6$, $p < 0.000$) but not with regard to a measure of delayed free recall as assessed with a verbal word list learning paradigm ($F = 0.012$, $p = 0.914$). The mean age was 38 yrs in both groups and, as can be expected from the different ages at the onset of epilepsy, there was a considerable difference in the duration of epilepsy (18 yrs; $F = 45.4$, $p < 0.000$). The results did not change when the analyses were restricted to the subgroup of 25 patients with TLE and hippocampal sclerosis.

In this example matching the patients with respect to the duration of epilepsy would have resulted in different ages at the onset of epilepsy or different chronological ages. Thus, without longitudinal data, a decision can be taken only on the basis of theoretical and practical plausibility. It makes little sense to assume that chronic TLE (*i.e.* a longer lasting TLE, more seizures, etc.) causes diffuse and generalized brain damage but no change in the primarily affected temporal lobe structures. The assumption that early onset epilepsy and its underlying etiology negatively interfere with brain development appears more adequate to explain this dissociation.

For its part, the age at the onset of TLE has a different impact on episodic and semantic memory. While no relation between performance in episodic memory and the age at the onset of epilepsy can be discerned, early acquired neocortical lesions, in particular, interfere with knowledge acquisition and the development of the semantic networks (Helmstaedter, 2002; Lutz et al., 2004). This finding nicely complements that on developmental amnesia where semantic memory acquisition is preserved despite early temporo-mesial damage (Vargha-Khadem et al., 2001).

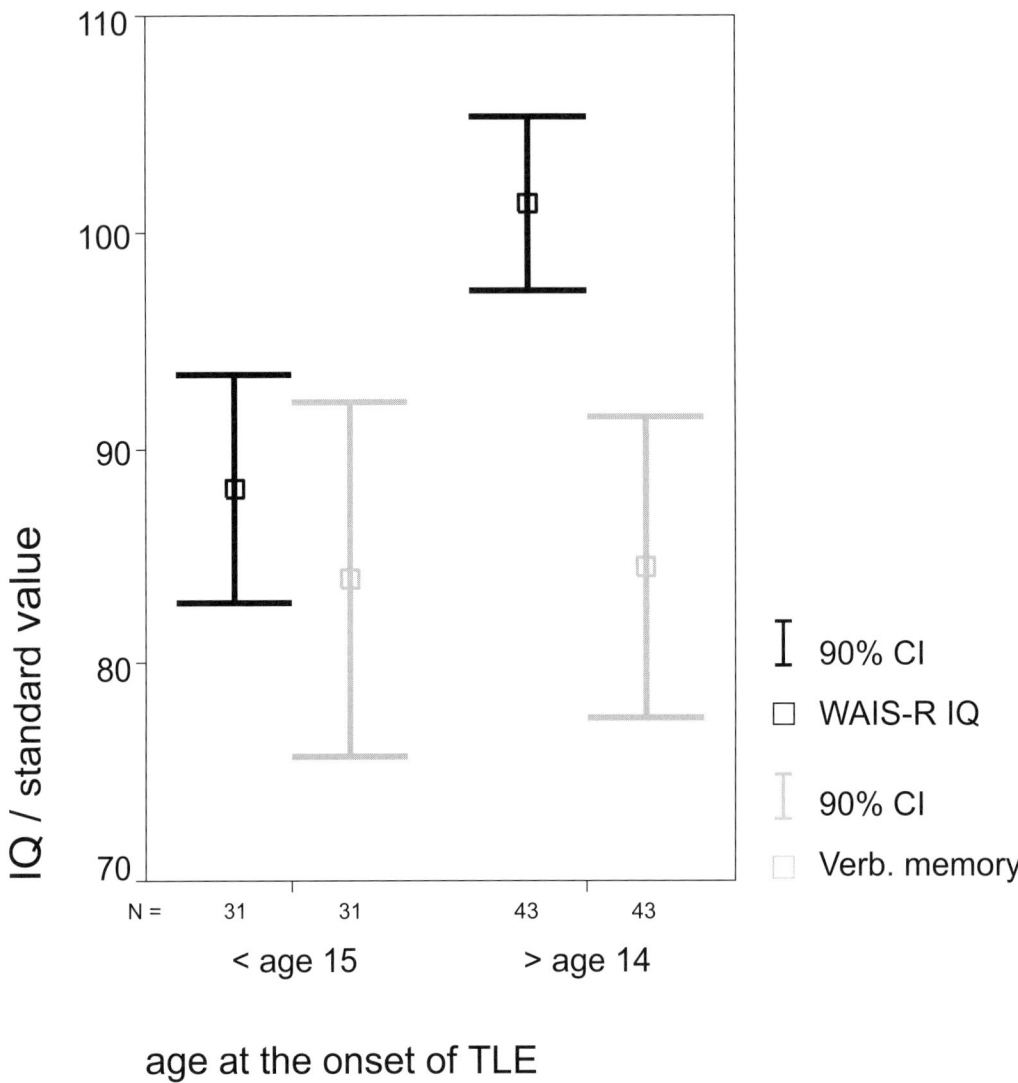

**Figure 4.** IQ and verbal memory performance in TLE as a function of the age at the onset of epilepsy within and beyond critical phases of brain development. The difference in IQ but not memory indicates developmental hindrance and retardation in the early onset group.

### Mental retardation and functional cerebral plasticity

Children with a longer duration of active epilepsy are reported to have lower IQs than children with a shorter seizure history (Farwell et al., 1985; Robinson et al., 2000). However, when children responded well to drug treatment, no intellectual decline was indicated (Bourgeois et al., 1983; Ellenberg et al., 1986). Another point of view postulates that persistent seizures in childhood probably slow the rate of cognitive and psychological development (Hirsch et al., 2000; Oguni et al., 2000). This latter view is also supported by longitudinal data on intellectual development in children and adults (Bjornaes et al., 2001).

When children and adolescents with TLE are compared, there is evidence that children are more diffusely impaired than adults. Memory problems do not represent the major impairment in children as language problems, for example, may be as common (Helmstaedter & Lendt, 2001). This result can be replicated even when children and adults with TLE are matched with regards to the underlying pathology (Gleissner et al., 2005). But why do children display greater impairments when at the same time the brain is still plastic and displays greater capacities for functional restitution and compensation than in adults? The answer to this question is that functional restitution is often achieved only at the cost of other cognitive functions which are sacrificed (Helmstaedter et al., 1994, 1997). Right hemisphere language restitution after an early left hemisphere onset epilepsy does not mean that language functions will achieve the performance level which could have been achieved without brain damage. And, developmental delays and retardation will nevertheless be the consequence of the early damage.

Positive effects of a greater functional plasticity can be observed with respect to memory outcome after temporal lobe surgery. Temporal lobe surgery, and surgery within the language dominant hemisphere in particular, bears an increased risk of causing additional memory impairment (Lee et al., 2002). The degree of postoperative loss depends on the degree of damage of functional tissues on the one hand, and the brain's reserve capacities for compensation of newly acquired damage on the other hand. Reserve capacities for the more neocortical aspects of memory (learning or short term memory) are strongly related to age (*i.e.* the outcome tends to be better at a younger age and gets worse with increasing age). The capacity to compensate unilateral damage of mesial functions (long term consolidation) in contrast, appears less age dependent (Helmstaedter, 1999 / *Figure 5*).

This finding has been explained by the more bilateral disposition of the above-mentioned processes and the lesser degree of specialization of the mesial structures for verbal or nonverbal information. The fact that only bilateral but not unilateral mesial temporal lobe resections in adults lead to global amnesia provides striking evidence for this assumption.

In summary, early onset TLE interferes with mental development although childhood is also the time of greater cerebral functional plasticity The consequence is a more generalized pattern of impairment, as compared to the more partial impairments in later onset TLE. Generalized abnormalities in cerebral grey and white matter in early onset TLE could be the structural equivalent of such generalized impairment (Hermann, et al., 2002; Arfanakis et al., 2002; Hermann et al., 2003). As for the consequences of epilepsy surgery memory impairment and losses due to temporal lobe surgery are less severe in childhood and adolescence than in adulthood. Depending on the more unilateral or bilateral disposition of mesial and neocortical memory functions, different reserve capacities must be assumed for the respective functions as dependent on the age at the time of damage. Early damage of mesial and neocortical structures furthermore has different effects on episodic and semantic memory.

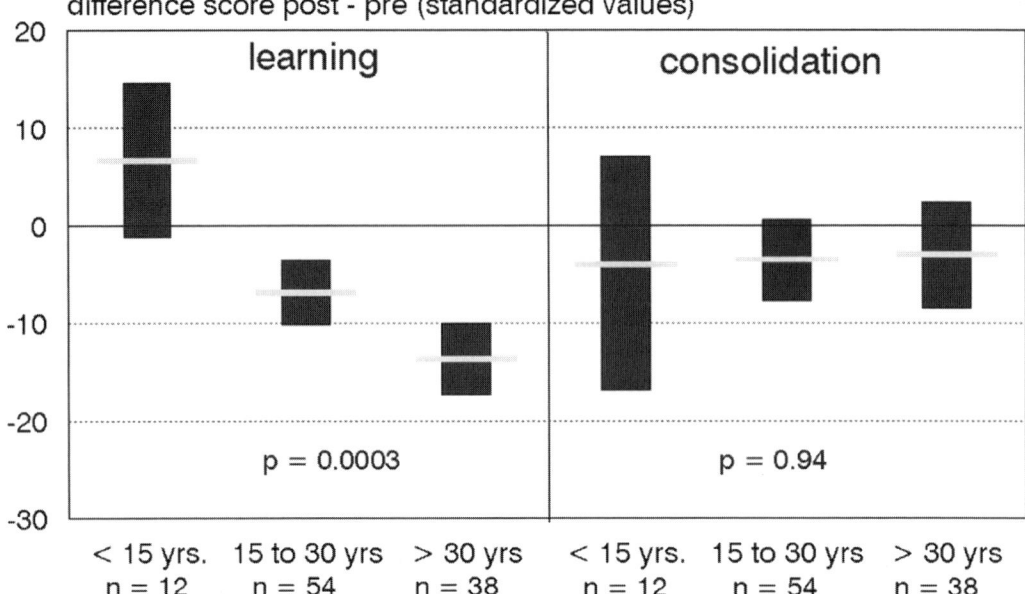

**Figure 5.** Postoperative loss of verbal learning and memory in left TLE patients as a function of age at the time of surgery. The data indicate a generally different plasticity for learning and memory. For learning, greater plasticity is indicated in patients with surgery before puberty.

## Aging *versus* chronic epilepsy

Recent cross sectional studies in TLE patients raised concerns about intellectual decline with a longer duration of epilepsy (Jokeit & Ebner, 2002). According to these findings, refractory TLE seems to induce a very slow but sustained cognitive deterioration. A high cognitive reserve capacity may postpone this deterioration, and the estimated time interval required for a significant change is greater than thirty years. This is quite a long time and raises the question of what happens with cognitive performance in healthy subjects over such an interval as well as the question of how cognitive change with a longer duration of epilepsy can be separated from that associated with normal aging.

Indeed, mental aging concerns most cognitive functions and in particular those rated as fluid intelligence (*e.g.*, functions relying on speed, flexibility, capacity, etc.). The rates of decline are similar for perceptive functions and memory (Baltes & Lindenberger, 1997; Balota *et al.*, 2000). Based on this knowledge, the comparison of age regressions of cognitive performance between patients and healthy subjects appears a reasonable approach to overcome the methodological problem to disentangle aging and duration of epilepsy in early onset TLE. If epilepsy adds to the normal mental decline, the age regression of memory in TLE patients should indicate accelerated decline as compared to the age regression observed in healthy subjects. In a study testing just this hypothesis in adult patients with left sided left mesial TLE, no accelerated decline of verbal memory performance could be discerned. Although this group of patients was considered as having high risk of memory decline with chronic epilepsy, healthy subjects and patients showed a parallel and steady decline over time (Helmstaedter & Elger, 1999). The fact that patients and controls differed to about the same degree at each age clearly favored the hypothesis of an initial difference between the groups. This initial difference can also be taken from *figure 6*, where the regression of preoperative verbal memory (learning over fife trials) in left TLE patients was related to that of healthy subjects. The significant change of the age regression after temporal lobe surgery demonstrated in this plot can well be taken as an example of how additional acquired damage in the course of epilepsy (here damage due to surgery) can accelerate mental aging (Helmstaedter et al., 2002).

While the cross sectional approach hardly supports the idea of an increasing impairment of memory with an increasing duration of epilepsy, there is nevertheless evidence of significant memory decline over time from longitudinal studies in TLE (Helmstaedter *et al.*, 2003; Rausch *et al.*, 2003). While the study of Rausch *et al.* considered operated patients only our own study with varying retest-intervals between 2 and 10 years, demonstrated a significant loss in memory also in medically treated patients. Losses due to surgery in patients one year after left temporal lobectomy were greater than those observed in medically treated patients over the long period, but some long term recovry became evident in surgical patients when seizures were successfully controlled *(Figure 7)*.

Evaluating the course of memory in medically treated and in operated patients after surgery, the correlation between memory decline and the retest interval was moderate. More decisive for the course of memory were seizure control, age, and mental reserve capacity (baseline performance and IQ). When performing analyses on an individual instead of on a group level, a large proportion of operated and non-operated patients with TLE showed individual losses in either verbal and/or verbal memory over time.

The longitudinal data support a view, also currently raised by longitudinal MRI volumetric studies, by which significant changes over time are almost individual and not the rule (Liu *et al.*, 2002; Salmenpera *et al.*, 2005). Thus no *linear* relation between time and functional decline, and thus no continuously dementing process, can be discerned in chronic TLE.

## ■ Conclusion

Considering that an epileptogenic process, lesions, uncontrolled seizures, and treatment are decisive determinants of the course of memory in chronic TLE, there is strong evidence that most impairments already exist at the onset of epilepsy or even before. Seizures, and particularly more severe seizures, can irreversibly damage the brain and cause further impairment. Additionally, there is evidence that epileptic activity in TLE can cause generalized persistent cognitive change. This change exceeds the domain of memory and is principally reversible when seizures are controlled. If TLE hits the maturing brain, epileptic dysfunctions and negative treatment

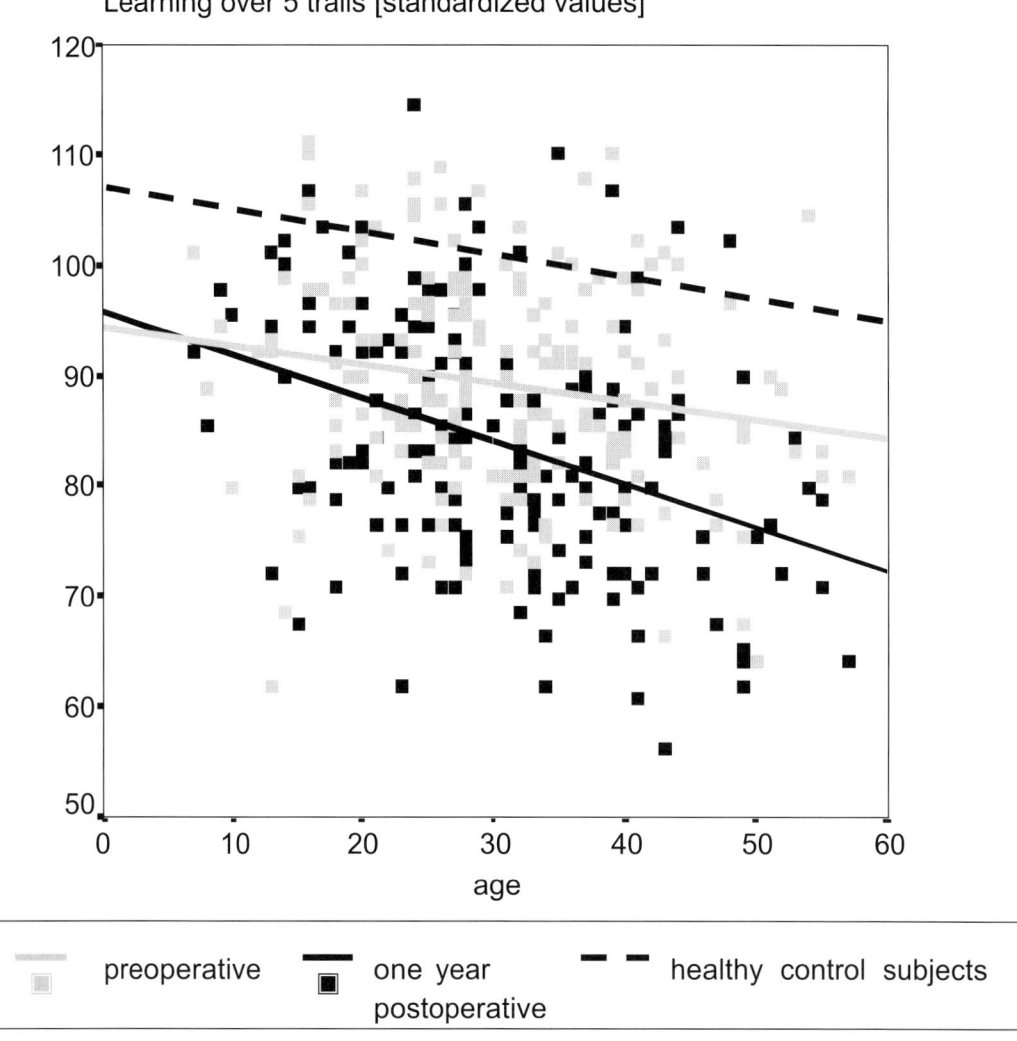

**Figure 6.** Acceleration of the age regression of verbal memory in left temporal lobe resected patients from before to after surgery. Before surgery memory decline does not differ from that observed in healthy subjects. Different performance levels at any age indicate that patients and healthy subjects differ because of the initial damage rather than because of chronic uncontrolled epilepsy.

effects, even if reversible, may cause developmental delay or retardation, thus inducing global intellectual retardation. If TLE hits the mature brain, partial impairment particularly in memory may be observed. Early and late onset epilepsies have in common that chronic uncontrolled epilepsy can add to the initial impairment. However, additional impairment in TLE appears to be an individual condition rather than the consequence of a continuously dementing process. Cognitive decline is slow and

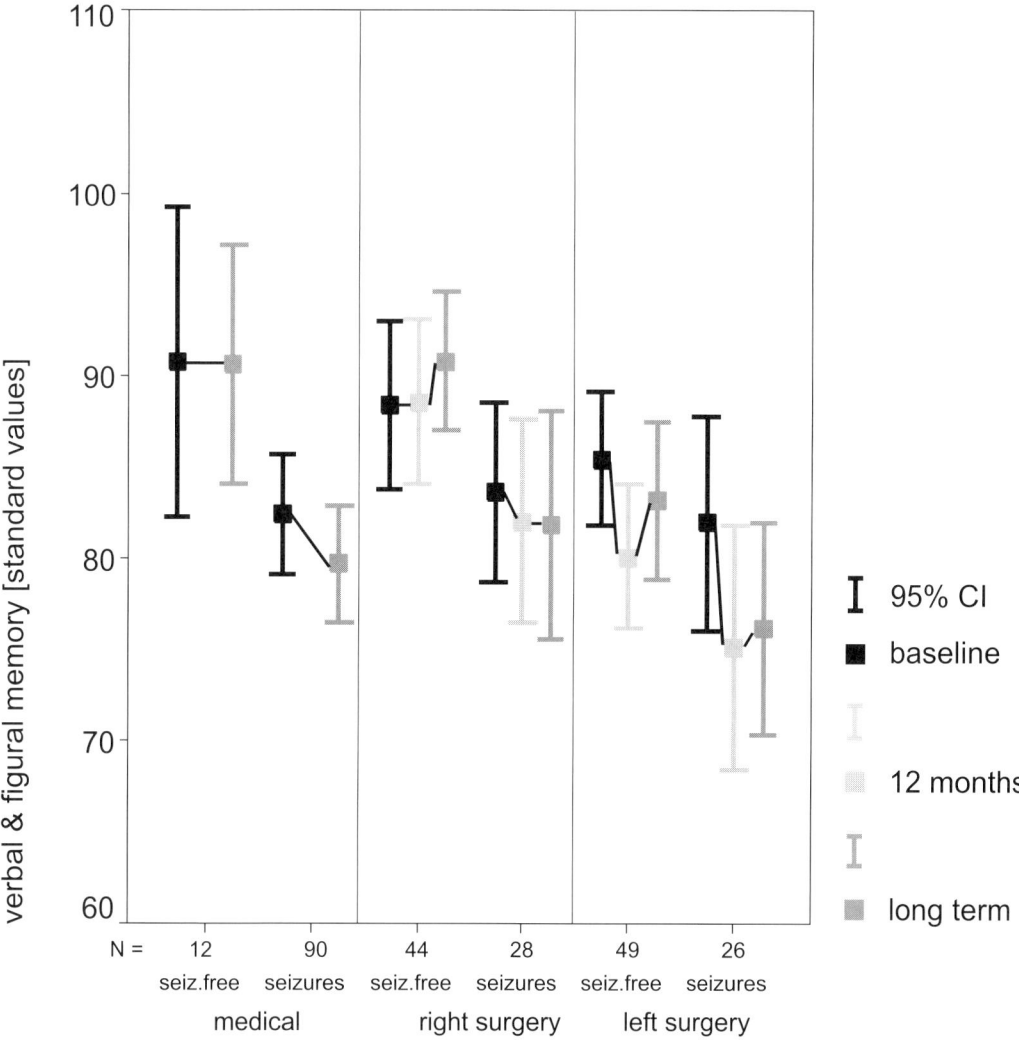

**Figure 7.** Longitudinal change in a composite (verbal/nonverbal) memory score in medically treated TLE patients (2-10 yrs), and early (1 yr) *versus* late (2-10 yrs) changes in patients after left or right temporal lobectomy. Note the losses particularly in medically treated and left temporal resected patients, and note the decisive effect of seizure control on the course of memory.

can hardly be differentiated from that observed with normal mental aging. However, because memory decline in patients starts from a significantly lower initial level than in healthy subjects, patients will end up at very poor performance levels earlier than neurologically intact individuals with further aging. Furthermore, acquired damage in the course of epilepsy can accelerate processes of mental aging, particularly in the presence of limited reserve capacities. As for memory, a principal differentiation must be taken into consideration with regards to the more cortical and more mesial aspects of memory, namely learning and short-term memory *versus* long-term consolidation. Similarly, episodic and semantic memory must be differentiated. Presumably because of its more neocortical and unilateral disposition, short term memory and learning are more coupled with intellectual development, material specificity, and aging. The more mesial function of long-term consolidation appears bilaterally disposed and thus more independent from this development. This difference is of importance also for the development of semantic memory.

As for the treatment of temporal lobe epilepsy, early and complete seizure control and the prevention of any additional damage appear mandatory for the prevention of developmental disablement in childhood and adolescence or accelerated cognitive decline with aging.

## References

Adab N, Kini U, Vinten J, Ayres J, Baker G, Clayton-Smith J, et al. The longer term outcome of children born to mothers with epilepsy. *J Neurol Neurosurg Psychiatry* 2004; 75 (11): 1575-83.

Aikia M, Salmenpera T, Partanen K, Kalviainen R. Verbal memory in newly diagnosed patients and patients with chronic left temporal lobe epilepsy. *Epilepsy Behav* 2001; 2: 20-7.

Aldenkamp AP, Arends J. Effects of epileptiform EEG discharges on cognitive function: is the concept of "transient cognitive impairment" still valid? *Epilepsy Behav* 2004; 5 (suppl 1): 25-34.

Arfanakis K, Hermann BP, Rogers BP, Carew JD, Seidenberg M, Meyerand ME. Diffusion tensor MRI in temporal lobe epilepsy. *Magn Reson Imaging* 2002; 20 (7): 511-9.

Austin JK, Dunn DW, Caffrey HM, et al. Recurrent seizures and behavior problems in children with first recognized seizures: a prospective study. *Epilepsia* 2002; 43: 1564-73.

Balota DA, Dolan PO, Ducheck JM. Memory changes in healthy older adults. In: Tulving E & Craik FIM, eds. *The Oxford handbook of memory*. Oxford: University Press, 2000: 395-408.

Baltes PB, Lindenberger U. Emergency of a powerful connection between sensory and cognitive functions across the adult life span: a new window to the study of cognitive aging. *Psychol. Aging* 1997; 12: 12-21.

Bjornaes H, Stabell K, Henriksen O, Loyning Y. The effects of refractory epilepsy on intellectual functioning in children and adults. A longitudinal study. *Seizure* 2001; 10: 250-9.

Bourgeois BF, Prensky AL, Palkes HS, Talent BK, Busch SG. Intelligence in epilepsy: a prospective study in children. *Ann Neurol* 1983; 14: 438-44.

Dietl T, Urbach H, Helmstaedter C, Staedtgen M, Szentkuti A, Grunwald T, Meyer B, Elger C, Kurthen M. Persistent severe amnesia due to seizure recurrence after unilateral temporal lobectomy. *Epilepsy Behav* 2004; 5 (3): 394-400.

Dodrill CB. Neuropsychological effects of seizures. *Epilepsy Behav* 2004; 5 (suppl 1): 21-4.

Eichenbaum H. A cortical hippocampal system for declarative memory. *Nature Reviews Neuroscience* 2000; 1: 41-50.

Elger CE, Helmstaedter C, Kurthen M. Epilepsy and cognition. *Lancet Neurology* 2004: 3 (11): 663-72.

Ellenberg JH, Hirtz DG, Nelson KB. Do seizures in children cause intellectual deterioration? *N Engl J Med* 1986; 24: 1085-8.

Farwell JR, Dodrill CB, Batzel LW. Neuropsychological abilities of children with epilepsy. *Epilepsia* 1985; 26: 395-400.

Gleissner U, Sassen R, Schramm J, Elger CE, Helmstaedter C. Greater functional recovery after temporal lobe epilepsy surgery in children. *Brain* 2005, in press.

Helmstaedter C. Prediction of memory reserve capacity. *Adv Neurol* 1999; 81: 271-9.

Helmstaedter C. Effects of chronic epilepsy on declarative memory systems. *Prog Brain Res* 2002; 135: 439-53.

Helmstaedter C, Elger CE. The phantom of progressive dementia in epilepsy. *Lancet* 1999; 354 (9196): 2133-4.

Helmstaedter C, Elger CE, Lendt M. Postictal courses of cognitive deficits in focal epilepsies. *Epilepsia* 1994a; 35 (5): 1073-8.

Helmstaedter C, Kurthen M. Memory and epilepsy: characteristics, course, and influence of drugs and surgery. *Curr Opin Neurol* 2001; 14 (2): 211-6.

Helmstaedter C, Kurthen M, Linke DB, Elger CE. Right hemisphere restitution of language and memory functions in right hemisphere language-dominant patients with left temporal lobe epilepsy. *Brain* 1994b; 117 (Pt 4): 729-37.

Helmstaedter C, Kurthen M, Linke DB, Elger CE. Patterns of language dominance in focal left and right hemisphere epilepsies: relation to MRI findings, EEG, sex, and age at onset of epilepsy. *Brain Cogn* 1997; 33 (2): 135-50.

Helmstaedter C, Pohl C, Elger CE. Relations between verbal and nonverbal memory performance: evidence of confounding effects particularly in patients with right temporal lobe epilepsy. *Cortex* 1995; 31 (2): 345-55.

Helmstaedter C, Kurthen M. Elger CE. Sex Differences in Material-specific Cognitive Functions Related to Language Dominance: An Intracarotid Amobarbital Study in Left Temporal Lobe Epilepsy. *Laterality* 1999; 4 (1): 51-63.

Helmstaedter C, Lendt M. Neuropsychological outcome of temporal end extratemporal lobe resection in children. In: Jambaque I, Lassond M, Dulac O, eds. *Neuropsychology of childhood epilepsy*. Advances in behavioral Biology, vol. 50. Boston: Kluwer Academic/Plenum Press, 2001: 215-27.

Helmstaedter C, Reuber M, Elger CC. Interaction of cognitive aging and memory deficits related to epilepsy surgery. *Ann Neurol* 2002; 52 (1): 89-94.

Helmstaedter C, Kurthen M, Lux S, Reuber M, Elger CE. Chronic epilepsy and cognition: a longitudinal study in temporal lobe epilepsy. *Ann Neurol* 2003; 54 (4): 425-32.

Helmstaedter C, Brosch T, Kurthen M, Elger CE. The impact of sex and language dominance on material-specific memory before and after left temporal lobe surgery. *Brain* 2004; 127 (Pt 7): 1518-25.

Helmstaedter C, Fritz N, Hoffmann J, Elger CE. The impact of newly diagnosed and untreated symptomatic/cryptogenic epilepsy on cognition. *Epilepsia* 2005 Abstract Suppl.

Hermann BP, Seidenberg M, Schoenfeld J, Davies K. Neuropsychological characteristics of the syndrome of mesial temporal lobe epilepsy. *Arch Neurol* 1997; 54 (4): 369-76.

Hermann BP, Seidenberg M, Bell B, Rutecki P, Sheth R, Ruggles K, Wendt G, O'Leary D, Magnotta V. The neurodevelopmental impact of childhood-onset temporal lobe epilepsy on brain structure and function. *Epilepsia* 2002; 43 (9): 1062-71.

Hermann BP, Hansen R, Seidenberg M, Magnotta V, O'Leary D. Neurodevelopmental vulnerability of the corpus callosum to childhood onset localization-related epilepsy. *Neuroimage* 2003; 18 (2): 284-92.

Hermann BP, Seidenberg M, Hansen R, Jones J, Bell B, Dow Ch, Rutecki P. Progression in temporal lobe epilepsy. *Epilepsia* 2004; 43 (suppl 7): 183.

Hirsch E, de Saint-Martin A, Arzimanoglou A. New insights into the clinical management of partial epilepsies. *Epilepsia* 2000; 41 (suppl 5): 13-17.

Jokeit H, Ebner A. Effects of chronic epilepsy on intellectual functions. *Prog Brain Res* 2002; 135: 455-63.

Kotloski R, Lynch M, Lauersdorf S, Sutula T. Repeated brief seizures induce progressive hippocampal neuron loss and memory deficits. *Prog Brain Res* 2002; 135: 95-110.

Lee TM, Yip JT, Jones-Gotman M. Memory deficits after resection from left or right anterior temporal lobe in humans: a meta-analytic review. *Epilepsia* 2002; 43 (3): 283-91.

Lendt M, Helmstaedter C, Kuczaty S, Schramm J, Elger CE. Behavioural disorders in children with epilepsy: early improvement after surgery. *J Neurol Neurosurg Psychiatry* 2000; 69 (6): 739-44.

Liu RS, Lemieux L, Bell GS, Sisodiya SM, Bartlett PA, Shorvon SD, Sander JW, Duncan JS. The structural consequences of newly diagnosed seizures. *Ann Neurol* 2002; 52 (5): 573-80.

Lutz MT, Elger CE, Helmstaedter C. Effects of age at onset and duration of Epilepsy on cognition in the framework of Cattell's theory of fluid and crystallized abilities. *Epilepsia* 2004; 45 (suppl 7): 346.

Oguni H, Mukahira K, Tanaka T, Awaya Y, Saito K, Shimizu H, et al. Surgical indication for refractory childhood epilepsy. *Epilepsia* 2000; 41 (suppl 9): 21-5.

Ogunrin O, Adamolekun B, Ogunniyi AO, Aldenkamp AP. Cognitive function in Nigerians with newly diagnosed epilepsy. *Can J Neurol Sci* 2000; 27: 148-51.

Oostrom KJ, Smeets-Schouten A, Kruitwagen CL, et al. Not only a matter of epilepsy: early problems of cognition and behavior in children with "epilepsy only" – a prospective, longitudinal, controlled study starting at diagnosis. *Pediatrics* 2003; 112: 1338-44.

Oyegbile TO, Dow C, Jones J, Bell B, Rutecki P, Sheth R, Seidenberg M, Hermann BP. The nature and course of neuropsychological morbidity in chronic temporal lobe epilepsy. *Neurology* 2004; 62 (10): 1736-42.

Pitkanen A, Nissinen J, Nairismagi J, Lukasiuk K, Grohn OH, Miettinen R, Kauppinen R. Progression of neuronal damage after status epilepticus and during spontaneous seizures in a rat model of temporal lobe epilepsy. *Prog Brain Res* 2002; 135: 67-83.

Pulliainen V, Kuikka P, Jokelainen M. Motor and cognitive functions in newly diagnosed adult seizure patients before antiepileptic medication. *Acta Neurol Scand* 2000; 101: 73-8.

Rausch R, Kraemer S, Pietras CJ, Le M, Vickrey BG, Passaro EA. Early and late cognitive changes following temporal lobe surgery for epilepsy. *Neurology* 2003; 60 (6): 951-9.

Robinson S, Park TS, Blackburn LB, Bourgeois BF, Arnold ST, Dodson WE. Transparahippocampal selective amygdalohippocampectomy in children and adolescents: efficacy of the procedure and cognitive morbidity in patients. *J Neurosurg* 2000; 93: 402-9.

Roeschl-Heils A, Bledowski C, Elger CE, Heils A, Helmstaedter C. Neuropsychological functioning among 32 patients with temporal lobe epilepsy and their discordant siblings. *Epilepsia* 2002; 43 (suppl 7): 185.

Salmenpera T, Kononen M, Roberts N, Vanninen R, Pitkanen A, Kalviainen R. Hippocampal damage in newly diagnosed focal epilepsy: a prospective MRI study. *Neurology* 2005; 64 (1): 62-8.

Strauss E, Loring D, Chelune G, Hunter M, Hermann BP, Perrine K, Westerveld M, Trenerry M, Barr W. Predicting cognitive impairment in epilepsy: findings from the Bozeman epilepsy consortium. *J Clin Exp Neuropsychol* 1995; 17 (6): 909-17.

Vargha-Khadem F, Gadian DG, Mishkin M. Dissociations in cognitive memory: the syndrome of developmental amnesia. *Philos Trans R Soc Lond B Biol Sci* 2001; 356 (1413): 1435-40.

Wieser HG, ILAE Commission on Neurosurgery of Epilepsy. ILAE Commission Report. Mesial temporal lobe epilepsy with hippocampal sclerosis. *Epilepsia* 2004; 45 (6): 695-714.

# Attention deficit hyperactivity disorder and attentional problems in children with temporal lobe epilepsy

D.W. Dunn, W. Kronenberger

*Departments of Psychiatry and Neurology, Divisions of Child and Adolescent Psychiatry and Child Psychology, Indiana University School of Medicine, Indianapolis Indiana, USA*

---

Children with epilepsy have an increased risk of cognitive difficulties. Some children with epilepsy suffer from severe cognitive problems characterized by learning disability or mental retardation. These children usually have central nervous system damage or symptomatic epilepsies as the etiology for both the epilepsy and cognitive dysfunction. The seizure disorder is seldom the single or main factor in the determination of the mental handicap. Other children with epilepsy have normal intelligence but academic difficulties. These children may have multiple factors contributing to the occurrence of learning difficulty, including underlying neurological dysfunction, seizure factors, adverse effects of antiepileptic drugs, or psychosocial dysfunction.

Neuropsychological deficits predict academic underachievement in children with normal intelligence and epilepsy. Specific cognitive deficits associated with underachievement include impairment of language, memory, executive function, and attention (Fastenau, Dunn, and Austin, 2004). Problems with attention may be particularly important. Williams et al. (2001) have shown that, after controlling for intelligence, attention is more significant in predicting academic problems than memory, self-esteem, or socioeconomic factors.

Though language deficits and memory problems are more often found in patients with temporal lobe epilepsy, in this chapter, we will focus on attentional and processing difficulties in children with seizures arising in the temporal lobes. We will ask the following questions.

1. Do children with epilepsy have more problems with attention or attention deficit hyperactivity disorder (ADHD) than other children?

2. Is ADHD more common in children with temporal lobe seizures than in children with other seizure types?
3. Are children with temporal lobe epilepsy at increased risk for problems with attention when compared to children with other seizure types?
4. Are children with benign focal epilepsy with centrotemporal spikes at any increased risk for difficulties with attention or other executive function skills?
5. If the child with temporal lobe epilepsy has problems with attention or ADHD, what is the most appropriate therapy?

## ■ Defining and measuring attention

Clinical assessment and research focusing on attention problems in children with epilepsy are complicated by the wide variety of definitions and assessment tools pertaining to the attention construct. One issue is the relationship between attention as a specific ability and attention as a disorder. Throughout this chapter we will be considering both attention and attention deficit hyperactivity disorder. Though there is considerable overlap, the two are not the same. *Attention* is a neuropsychological construct that defines the processes involved in perception, selection, and maintaining or detaching from stimuli. In a recent review of attention and epilepsy, Sanchez-Carpintero and Neville (2003) found that sustained attention, selective attention, and divided attention were most often assessed in studies of children with epilepsy. Sustained attention, usually defined by scores on a continuous performance task, was most consistently impaired in children with epilepsy.

In comparison, *attention deficit hyperactivity disorder* (ADHD) is a categorical disorder defined by symptoms and duration of illness. The diagnosis of ADHD is based on criteria from the Diagnostic and Statistical Manual-IV (DSM-IV). Symptoms must be present prior to 7 years of age, cause impairment in two or more settings, and not be better explained by another diagnosis or occur only during the course of autistic spectrum disorders or psychosis. The child must have six of nine symptoms of inattention and/or six of nine symptoms of hyperactivity and impulsivity present for at least 6 months. Symptoms of inattention include difficulty concentrating, careless mistakes on school work, daydreaming, incomplete work, procrastination, poor organization, distractibility, forgetfulness, and a tendency to lose things needed for home or school. Symptoms of hyperactivity and impulsivity include frequent or almost constant gross motor movements, fidgeting, inability to stay seated, excessive running, loud, noisy play, excessive talk, blurting out answers, interrupting, and inability to wait one's turn. The disorder is called ADHD, combined type if the child meets criteria for both inattention and hyperactivity/impulsivity, ADHD, predominantly inattentive type if only the inattention criteria are met, and ADHD, predominantly hyperactive/impulsive type if only hyperactive/impulsive criteria are met (American Psychiatric Association, 1994).

In addition to the issue of attention problems *vs* ADHD, there are different ways of measuring attention as a neuropsychological ability. In the broadest sense, formal psychological testing methods for attention may be divided into behavior questionnaire measures and office-based performance tests.

Behavior questionnaire measures consist of a series of questions that are rated by an observer, usually a teacher or parent (some self-report forms exist for adolescents and adults as well, but children are notoriously unreliable self-reporters of attention and impulsivity). It is important to note that the actual content of the questions may have some bearing on the result that is obtained. Questionnaires such as the ADHD-Rating Scale (DuPaul et al., 1998), Symptom Inventories – 4 (Gadow & Sprafkin, 1997), and NICHQ Vanderbilt Assessment Scale (Wolraich et al., 2003) use items that are direct rewordings of DSM-IV ADHD symptoms. Other questionnaires, such as the Child Behavior Checklist (Achenbach & Rescorla, 2001) and Behavior Assessment System for Children – 2 (Reynolds & Kamphaus, 2004) measure a broader set of behaviors, ranging from depression to aggression to attention. These questionnaires contain subscales with items that overlap somewhat with DSM-IV ADHD symptoms but that also capture other dimensions of attention and hyperactivity-impulsivity. Various forms of the Conners' Rating Scales (Conners, 1997) are based on DSM-IV ADHD symptoms, a collection of items that partially overlap with DSM-IV symptoms, or factor-derived scales that have only a moderate overlap with the DSM-IV conceptualization of attention problems. Other behavior questionnaires, such as the Behavior Rating Inventory of Executive Function (Gioia, Isquith, Guy & Kenworthy, 2000) aim to measure the behavioral manifestations of the underlying neuropsychological functions that may relate or contribute to attention. Although issues of respondent bias must be taken into account in interpreting results, behavior questionnaires are one of the most reliable and valid ways of measuring attention with a structured assessment tool (Kronenberger & Meyer, 2001).

Office-based performance tests for attention and concentration are psychological or neuropsychological tests that are usually individually administered and require the child to demonstrate attention through performance and problem-solving. These tests are numerous and vary substantially in administration, content, and interpretation. Among the most widely used of these performance tests are Continuous Performance Tests (CPTs). CPTs present the child with a long sequence of stimuli, and for each individual stimulus, the child gives or withholds a simple response (button press, single word response, etc.) based on a predefined rule. The Conners' CPT (Conners, 2000), for example, presents the child with letters from the English alphabet, one at a time, in the center of a computer screen. The child presses the space bar after every letter except "X". Measures are obtained for accurate responses, omission errors (letters other than X for which the child did not press the space bar), commission errors (pressing the space bar after the letter X), and speed of responding. Measures derived from accuracy, errors, and variability in response speed reflect attention, concentration, and impulsivity. Other CPT's include the Test of Variables of Attention (Leark, Dupuy, Greenberg, Corman & Kindschi, 1996), and the Intermediate Visual and Auditory Continuous Performance Test (Sandford & Turner, 1993).

In addition to CPT's, components of attention and related mental processing may be measured by tests of **working memory** (ability to remember rote, short-term information while simultaneously engaging in another mental task; see subtests from the Wechsler Intelligence Scale for Children – Fourth Edition [Wechsler, 2000] and Wide Range Assessment of Memory and Learning – Second Edition [Sheslow &

Adams, 2003] for examples), **ability to resist distraction/interference** (such as the Stroop Color-Word Test; Golden, Freshwater & Golden, 2003), **ability to flexibly shift response set** (such as the Trail-Making Test [Delis, Kaplan & Kramer, 2001] and Wisconsin Card Sorting Test [Heaton, Chelune, Talley, Kay & Curtiss, 1993]), **ability to inhibit responses during planning** (such as Maze tests and Tower problem-solving tests; Delis et al., 2001), and **ability to engage in fluent/rapid, sustained processing of information** (such as visual attention processing speed tests and creative fluency tests; Delis et al., 2001; Korkman, Kirk & Kemp, 1998). Many of these tests are considered measures of executive functioning, a broader neuropsychological area reflecting planning, inhibition, self-direction, organization, and self-monitoring. Executive functioning is often considered to include attention and concentration (Barkley, 1997).

Office-based measures of attention and concentration are useful for understanding the child's ability under the tightly controlled, structured environment of the testing room. Research indicates that these measures correlate moderately with each other and more modestly with measures of behavior in the "real-world" environment. Furthermore, different measures may evaluate different components of attention and executive functioning (Barkley, 1997). As a result, for both clinical and research purposes, use of a broad set of questionnaire and office-based measures is generally recommended, as opposed to use of a single measure alone (Kronenberger & Meyer, 2001). Additionally, no single test gives diagnostically specific information that could be used in isolation to make or confirm a diagnosis. Sensitivity and specificity of these tests for the ADHD diagnosis range from as low as 0.60 to as high as 0.90, depending on the test and sample composition (e.g., Doyle, Biederman, Seidman, Weber & Faraone, 2000; Leark et al., 1996; Perugini, Harvey, Lovejoy, Sandstrom & Webb, 2000; Power et al., 1998). As a result, psychological tests of attention and concentration are used as important benchmarks to quantify and understand attentional problems but not to make or confirm diagnoses.

## ■ ADHD and attention in children with epilepsy

Reviews of the prevalence of psychiatric disorders in children with epilepsy report an increased risk of behavioral problems. Some studies report an association between behavioral problems and seizure type. Several of these studies define seizure types as generalized or partial without defining partial seizures by the lobe of origin of epileptiform discharge. Other studies use the International League Against Epilepsy (1989) classification of epileptic syndromes, but list focal seizures as idiopathic, symptomatic, or cryptogenic localization-related epilepsy without separation into the lobar origin. In this chapter, we will assume that focal seizures most often arise in the temporal lobe and will review studies that report ADHD or problems with attention in children with focal or localization-related epilepsies.

## Symptoms of ADHD in children with epilepsy

Studies vary in the diagnostic criteria used for disorders of attention or ADHD. Several studies have reported symptoms of inattention, hyperactivity, or impulsivity consistent with a diagnosis of ADHD, but have not used specific DSM criteria. Most studies utilized parent or teacher questionnaires to define ADHD or enumerate symptoms consistent with ADHD. Bennett-Levy and Stores (1984) questioned teachers about student performance. Children with epilepsy had poor concentration and slow processing. The children with epilepsy also had significant difficulty with alertness that persisted after discontinuation of antiepileptic drugs. They found no differences by seizure type. Aman et al. (1992) found more attention problems and hyperactivity in children with epilepsy compared to a control group. There was no significant difference between children with generalized seizures compared to those with partial seizures. Sturniolo and Galletti (1994) asked for teachers' opinions of student behaviors. The teachers described inattention or hyperactivity in 58% of the children with seizures. Symptoms of ADHD were seen in 57% of children with partial seizures and 50% of those with generalized seizures. Austin et al. (2001), in a sample of children with new-onset epilepsy, noted attention problems as measured by the Child Behavior Checklist (CBCL: Achenbach, 1991) more frequently in children with seizures than in siblings. Children with partial seizures had more behavior problems than children with generalized seizures, though this measure only reflected total behavior problems and not just attention problems.

Other studies have used measures that allow a DSM diagnosis of ADHD. Hempel et al. (1995) found an increased risk of ADHD in children with seizures compared to the general population. They noted a higher prevalence of ADHD in children with generalized seizures (52%) compared to children with partial or indeterminate seizures (26%). Caplan et al. (1998), in a study of children 5-16 years of age, compared children with complex partial seizures (CPS) to a group with primary generalized epilepsy (PGE). They found disruptive behavior disorders (ADHD, oppositional defiant disorder, or conduct disorder) in 25% of the children with CPS and 26% of those with PGE. Comorbid disruptive disorders and affective/anxiety disorders were seen in 14% of the children with CPS and 16% of those with PGE. In a subsequent study, Caplan et al. (2004) showed that more children with complex partial seizures had disruptive behavior disorders (17%) than controls (6%). In the children with complex partial seizures, verbal IQ predicted psychiatric diagnosis with more disorders seen in children with lower intelligence. Seizure factors did not predict psychopathology. Sherman et al. (2000) reported symptoms of ADHD, predominantly inattentive type in 50% of patients with epilepsy and symptoms of hyperactivity and impulsivity in 21%. They noted that children with frontal lobe foci had more evidence of inattention than children with other seizure types, but found no difference in prevalence of hyperactivity and impulsivity by seizure type. Ott et al. (2001) described disruptive disorders in 21% of children with complex partial seizures, 23% of children with primary generalized epilepsy, and 7% of controls. There was no statistically significant difference in the prevalence of psychiatric disorder by seizure type. Dunn et al. (2003) found evidence of ADHD in 37.7% of children with epilepsy present for at least 6 months. They noted ADHD, combined type in 11.4%, ADHD, inattentive type in 24%, and ADHD, hyperactive/impulsive type in 2.3%. There was no statistically significant difference in rate of ADHD by seizure type or focus of epileptiform activity. Symptoms of ADHD were found in 36.4% of children with a frontal lobe focus, 34.6% of those with a temporal focus, 33.4% of central, and 38.2% of generalized focus. Hesdorffer et al. (2004) looked for a past history of ADHD in a population-based study of children with new-onset epilepsy. They found that ADHD, predominantly inattentive type was associated with new-onset seizures, but noted no association between either combined type or hyperactive/impulsive type ADHD and new-onset seizures. They found that seizure type had no effect. Thome-Souza et al. (2004) used a structured psychiatric history to assess behavioral problems and classified seizures as partial or generalized. They found that 29.1% of the 78 children and adolescents had ADHD. The prevalence of ADHD was higher in the patients with partial seizures (62.5%) than in patients with generalized seizures (37.5%).

*The studies that addressed symptoms of ADHD in children with epilepsy have consistently found a higher prevalence of problems in children with epilepsy as compared to controls or population based norms.* The prevalence figures range from 17% to 58% with studies on average reporting one in four to one in three children with epilepsy having symptoms of ADHD. Prevalence by seizure type has been more inconsistent, with no evidence that children with temporal lobe epilepsy are more likely to have symptoms of ADHD than children with generalized seizures.

## ■ Neuropsychological assessment of attention and processing speed in children with epilepsy

Neuropsychological assessments of children with epilepsy have often documented difficulties with attention. McCarthy et al. (1995) compared children with complex partial seizures, generalized tonic clonic seizures, and absence seizures on a measure of sustained attention and found no effect of seizure type on impairment. Williams et al. (1998) noted reduced attention in relation to general intelligence. There were no significant differences in cognitive or behavioral measures based on seizure type. In a subsequent test, this same group documented impaired attention in children with epilepsy compared to controls (Williams et al., 2001). Seizure type was not associated with academic performance. After controlling for intelligence, they found that attention, but not memory, self-esteem, or socioeconomic status, was associated with scores on academic achievement tests. In a longitudinal study, Bailet and Turk (2000) found impaired psychomotor speed at baseline and year one, but not year two, in children with epilepsy compared to controls. There was no significant difference in psychomotor speed by seizure type. Haverkamp et al. (2001) found selective attention deficits in patients with epilepsy regardless of seizure type. Oostrom et al. (2002) studied children with normal intelligence and idiopathic or cryptogenic new-onset seizures. They noted impaired sustained attention in children with seizures compared to controls but no difference in motor speed or execution time. There was no effect by seizure type.

Comparisons of frontal and temporal lobe epilepsy have given variable results. Snyder et al. (2003) found no difference in a measure of sustained attention, but Hernandez et al. (2003) noted both slower processing speed and impaired attention in children with frontal lobe foci compared to those with temporal lobe foci. Borgatti et al. (2004) described change over time in attention. Problems with attention were found in 21% at baseline and 42% on follow up one year later. They found no difference in prevalence of attention problems comparing focal to generalized seizures. Fastenau et al. (2004) found that children with chronic seizures had more difficulty with attention tests and slower processing speed. These difficulties were associated with lower achievement scores in math, reading, and writing. Family environment seemed to moderate the effect of neuropsychological deficits on writing and reading, but seizure-related variables had no effect.

Neuropsychological assessments obtained with simultaneous video EEG recording have been helpful in defining seizure factors important in problems with attention and processing speed. In a first study, Aldenkamp et al. evaluated 11 children with seizures during testing and 11 with epileptiform spike but no seizures. Partial seizures were most common in these groups. Slow reaction time was associated with number of seizures during testing, whereas memory performance was associated with duration of seizures. In a second study, they compared 121 children with epilepsy to 31 controls, again performing simultaneous neuropsychological testing and video EEG (Aldenkamp and Arends, 2004). There were 83 patients with partial seizures, 36 with generalized, and 3 with other types of seizures. They found that frequent epileptiform discharges were associated with slowing of processing speed, seizure number with slow processing and attentional deficits, and seizure duration with memory impairment.

*In summary*, the neuropsychological assessments show that children with epilepsy have more impairment in attention and slower processing speed than controls. As with symptoms of ADHD, neuropsychological dysfunction is found in children with a variety of seizure types. Deficits on neuropsychological tests of attention or processing speed do not seem to be more common in children with temporal lobe epilepsy *versus* children with generalized seizures.

## ADHD and attention in studies of children with temporal lobe epilepsy

Several studies have assessed the prevalence of behavioral problems and neuropsychological deficits in children with temporal lobe epilepsy. Within this group, some studies separate children with partial seizures into groups by origin of epileptiform discharge, but others utilize only diagnosis of complex partial epilepsy or partial seizures.

Several studies have emphasized the increased frequency of ADHD or symptoms consistent with ADHD in children with temporal lobe epilepsy. In their classical outcome study of 100 children with temporal lobe seizures, Lindsay, Ounsted, and Richards (1979) reported the hyperkinetic syndrome in 26 children. These children were more often male, had an earlier onset of seizures, and suffered from cerebral damage or prior status epilepticus. The presence of the hyperkinetic syndrome was also a strong predictor of poor psychosocial outcome in adulthood. Glaser (1967) noted hyperactivity in 70 of 120 children with limbic epilepsy. Stores (1977) described inattention and hyperactivity in children with left temporal lobe spikes, but inattention only in boys with right temporal lobe spikes. In a subsequent study, Stores (1978) found that boys with epilepsy had more inattention and hyperactivity than girls with epilepsy and boys without epilepsy. Harvey et al. (1997) noted that parents reported hyperactivity in 14 of 63 children with new-onset temporal lobe epilepsy. In a recent study, Schoenfeld et al. (1999) found that children with partial epilepsy had more attention problems than sibling controls as measured by the CBCL. Attention problems were significantly associated with the frequency of complex partial seizures but not age of onset or frequency of secondary generalized seizures. Baños et al. (2004) evaluated both adolescents and adults with temporal lobe seizures and noted problems with attention and concentration on a self-report questionnaire. There was a trend for patients with left temporal lobe epileptiform foci to have more problems.

In addition to symptoms of ADHD, attentional functions have been investigated in children with temporal lobe epilepsy. Stores, Hart, and Piran (1978) found that boys with temporal lobe epilepsy demonstrated more impairment on parent- and teacher-completed attention questionnaires as well as tests of sustained attention and activity level, compared to boys without epilepsy. However, girls with epilepsy did not differ from controls on those measures. Semrud-Clikeman and Wical (1999) used a continuous performance test to compare children with complex partial seizures and ADHD, children with epilepsy alone, children with ADHD, and controls. The children with the combination of ADHD and epilepsy did worse on measures of sustained attention. The children with epilepsy alone and the children with ADHD showed impairment similarly and both groups did worse than controls. Schoenfeld et al. (1999) compared children with partial epilepsy to sibling controls and found the children with epilepsy to perform worse on both mental efficiency and timed fine motor skills. Poorer performance on mental efficiency was associated with younger age of onset and longer duration of seizures. Shouten et al. (2000) studied set-shifting, one component of attention, in 10 children with epilepsy, 8 of whom had simple or complex partial seizures. They showed that the children with seizures had unstable set-shifting.

Neuropsychological studies of adults with temporal lobe seizures have also shown variable impairment. Researchers from Wisconsin have performed several studies of neuropsychological function in patients with temporal lobe epilepsy. They showed that patients with temporal lobe seizures had impairment in multiple areas including memory, language, executive function and motor speed (Oyegbile et al., 2004). The patients with temporal lobe epilepsy and reduced white matter volume had slower processing speed than those with normal white matter volumes and normal control subjects (Dow et al., 2004). Attention and processing speed was not related to age of onset or to the presence of hippocampal sclerosis (Hermann et al., 1997; Hermann et al., 2002). Partially consistent with the findings of inattention and slow processing speed, Fleck et al. (2002) reported decreased reaction time but normal accuracy in a continuous performance task attempted by adults with temporal lobe epilepsy. In contrast, Martin et al. (1999) found that adults with left temporal lobe epilepsy and either mesial temporal sclerosis (MTS) or MTS plus developmental malformations of the left temporal lobe were in the average to low average range on measures of attention and executive function. Similarly, Palmese and Hamberger (2004) noted slower processing speed in patients with MTS compared to patients without MTS. They found no difference between patients with left or right epileptiform discharges.

Just as was found in series of children with epilepsy, *the studies that focus on children with temporal lobe epilepsy show an increased risk of ADHD and problems with attention and slowing of processing speed.* Within the group of patients with temporal lobe epilepsy, boys seem to be at increased risk for problems. The laterality of epileptiform discharges and specific temporal lobe pathology do not consistently predict attention problems, though reduction in white matter in patients with long standing temporal lobe epilepsy may be a risk factor.

## ADHD and problems with attention in children with benign childhood epilepsy with centrotemporal spikes (BCECTS)

Benign childhood epilepsy with centrotemporal spikes (BCECTS) is a familial, idiopathic focal epilepsy that characteristically begins between 5-10 years of age and remits during adolescence. It often does not require antiepileptic drug treatment and, for most affected individuals, causes little reduction in quality of life. However, recent studies have found some cognitive and academic difficulties in these children.

Early studies described BCECTS as a disorder with little or no effect on intelligence or behavior. Heijbel and Bohman (1975) found no evidence of ADHD in a sample of 29 children with BCECTS. Subsequent neuropsychological studies have found inconsistent changes in attention and other executive functions. D'Alessandro et al. (1990), comparing 44 children with BCECTS to 9 controls, found significant impairment in all measures of attention. Piccirilli et al. (1994) used a figure cancellation task to evaluate attention in 43 children with BCECTS and 15 controls. The patients had worse scores on attention, dependent in part on focus of EEG discharges. Weglage et al. (1997) noted no difference between children with BCECTS and controls on a measure of motor reaction time. Croona et al. (1999) described a reduction in processing speed but no impairment in attention. Deonna et al. (2000) found problems with attention in only two of 22 children with benign partial epilepsy. In contrast, Baglietto et al. (2001), comparing 9 children with BCECTS to 9 controls, reported significant reductions in attention, cognitive flexibility, and fluency in patients.

Two studies specifically addressed variation in attention by focus of EEG discharge. D'Alessandro et al. (1990) noted a significant decrease in attention that was most pronounced for the BCECTS children with bilateral EEG foci with lesser impairment for those with a left sided focus. Piccirilli et al. (1994) also found significant impairment in attention in children with BCECTS and bilateral foci; however, children with a right-sided focus fared worse than controls whereas those with a left-sided focus performed as well as controls.

The long term outcome for children with BCECTS seems good. Two studies reported changes over time. D'Alessandro et al. (1990) were able to reassess 11 children with BCECTS that had been seizure free for 4 years and had normal EEGs during that time. At follow up, there was no difference between patients and controls on measures of attention. Lindgren et al. (2004) reevaluated 26 of the 32 patients originally studied by Croona et al. (1999) and compared them to a matched control group of 25 children. On tests of executive function, the children with BCECTS were not significantly different from controls, though patients fared worse on these measures. Baglietto et al. (2001) repeated neuropsychological evaluations after a follow up period of 2 years. When patients were retested, there was improvement in sustained attention and no difference between patients and controls on performance.

*In summary*, children with BCECTS appear to be at risk for problems with attention and processing speed, though results are not consistent. The children with bilateral foci on EEG have more problems than those with unilateral foci. The problems with attention are usually transient with little indication of persistent problems on assessment after two or more years.

## ■ Treatment for problems with attention and ADHD in children with temporal lobe epilepsy

Therapy for the children with temporal lobe epilepsy and problems with attention or ADHD should include both reassessment of seizure control and review of antiepileptic drug (AED) regime. If attention does not improve with reduction of seizure frequency or alteration in AEDs, then specific interventions for improving attention or reducing symptoms of ADHD should be made. Although there are no double-blind placebo-controlled trials of interventions for the child with temporal lobe epilepsy and problems with attention, there are recommendations that can be made based on studies of therapy for ADHD and attentional problems in children with epilepsy.

Re-evaluation of seizure control should be the initial step in assessment. Though there are no studies that show improvement in attention following reduction in seizure frequency, the association of inattention and frequent seizures, shown by Aldenkamp and Arends (2004), suggests that cognitive improvement should follow improved seizure control. In addition to assessment for recurrent seizures, evaluation for adverse effects of medication for seizures is essential. Phenobarbital, benzodiazepines, topiramate, and vigabatrin have been associated with inattention and/or hyperactivity (Schmitz, 2002; Aldenkamp, De Krom, and Reijs, 2003). A change in AED may lead to improvement in cognitive functioning. (A complete discussion of behavioral side effects of antiepileptic drugs can be found in the chapter by Aldenkamp and Bootsma in this book).

Temporal lobe resection for intractable complex partial seizures may be beneficial in improving cognitive function. Lendt et al. (2000) evaluated 20 children that underwent temporal lobe resection. The children with both left and right temporal lobe resection had significant ($p < 0.05$) improvement in measures of attention. In contrast, memory function did not change. Lendt et al. (2000) also used the CBCL to assess for symptoms of ADHD. Mean scores on the attention problem scale obtained prior to surgery dropped significantly by reassessment 6 months later. A control group had no change in attention problem scores over the same six-month period. Similarly, in an assessment of symptoms consistent with ADHD, Danielsson et al. (2002) described improvement in attention and reduction of hyperactivity following temporal lobe resection. In contrast to these studies, Smith et al. (2004) compared 51 children with seizure surgery to 21 controls. They found no change in cognitive or psychosocial function in either the surgery or the control group at follow up one year after initial assessment.

If seizure factors have been managed optimally and inattention continues to be problematic, specific therapy for problems with inattention should be tried. Behavior modification, parent training, and cognitive rehabilitation have been used. As one example, Engelberts et al. (2002) described cognitive rehabilitation for adult patients with focal seizures and attention deficits. They recruited 44 patients and treated one group using computerized tasks, trained a second group in ways to circumvent attention problems, and enrolled the third group as wait list controls. They found improvements in neuropsychological function and quality of life in both active treatment groups. The patients that received training in coping and adaptation were most improved, and patients with active seizures changed more than those with well controlled seizures.

Stimulant medication may be an option for those children with attention problems and temporal lobe epilepsy. A large scale, multisite, randomized study of treatments for ADHD in children without seizure disorders reported more improvement in the core symptoms of ADHD with both combined behavioral and medication treatment and methylphenidate therapy alone than seen with behavioral therapy alone or community controls (MTA Cooperative Group, 1999). Physicians and parents have been reluctant to use stimulant medications for the child with epilepsy because of worries about possible exacerbation of seizures. Several studies have suggested that stimulant drugs are not contraindicated. Feldman et al. (1989) treated 10 children with controlled seizures using methylphenidate 0.3 mg/kg/dose. They saw no recurrence of seizures and found significant improvement in attention and academic functioning. Gross-Tsur et al. (1997) evaluated 25 children with controlled seizures and five with active seizures. Children received methylphenidate 0.3 mg/kg. None of the children in the controlled seizure group had a breakthrough in their seizures. Three of the children with active seizures had an increase in seizure number and two a decrease in seizures. There was improvement in attention in 70% of the children. Semrud-Clikeman and Wical (1999) performed computerized performance tests before and after methylphenidate administration on two groups of children, one with complex partial seizures and ADHD and a second with ADHD alone. The children with ADHD alone had normalization of scores and the patients with both seizures and ADHD scores improved from 3.5 standard deviations below average to 1.5 standard deviations below average. Gucuyener et al. (2003) studied 57 children with ADHD and epilepsy and 62 children with ADHD and an abnormal EEG but no seizures. Children received methylphenidate 0.3-1 mg/kg/day. No seizures occurred in the children with ADHD and an abnormal EEG. There was no change in mean seizure frequency in the children with ADHD and epilepsy. In the epilepsy group, 5 of 57 children experienced an increase in seizure frequency. In both groups, there was a decrease in epileptiform activity over one year of follow up. In a recent abstract, Gonzalez-Heydrich et al. (2004) described 36 children, 17 with no seizures in the past 6 months and 19 with active seizures, who were treated with stimulant medication. They found that 63% of the children receiving methylphenidate responded to medication *versus* only 24% of children receiving dextroamphetamine. Three of the 19 patients with active seizures had an increase in seizure frequency that returned to baseline with a discontinuation of stimulant or a change in antiepileptic drug dose.

*In summary*, treatment of ADHD or attention problems in the child with temporal lobe epilepsy should include attempts to reduce seizure frequency and modification of antiepileptic drug therapy to avoid adverse effects. Improvement in attention probably follows a reduction in seizure frequency after temporal lobe resection for intractable seizures. Stimulant medication can be safely used for the child with ADHD and well controlled seizures. Stimulant medication may be used even with continuing seizures but a minority of patients may develop increased seizure frequency.

# References

Achenbach TM. *Manual for the Child Behavior Checklist/4-18 and 1991 Profile*. Burlington VT: University of Vermont Department of Psychiatry, 1991.

Achenbach TM, Rescorla LA. *Manual for the ASEBA School-Age Forms & Profiles*. Burlington, VT: University of Vermont, Research Center for Children, Youth & Families, 2001.

Aldenkamp AP, Arends J, Overweg-Plandsoen TCG, et al. Acute cognitive effects of nonconvulsive difficult-to-detect epileptic seizures and epileptiform electroencephalographic discharges. *J Child Neurol* 2001; 16: 119-23.

Aldenkamp AP, De Krom M, Reijs R. Newer antiepileptic drugs and cognitive issues *Epilepsia* 2003; 44 (suppl 4): 21-29.

Aldenkamp A, Arends J. The relative influence of epileptic EEG discharges, short nonconvulsive seizures, and type of epilepsy on cognitive function. *Epilepsia* 2004; 45: 54-63.

Aman MG, Werry JS, Turbott SH. Behavior of children with seizures: comparisons with norms and effect of seizure type. *J Nerv Ment Dis* 1992; 180: 124-9.

American Psychiatric Association. *Diagnostic and Statistical Manual of Mental Disorders*, Fourth Edition. Washington DC: American Psychiatric Association, 2004.

Austin JK, Harezlak J, Dunn DW, Huster GA, Rose DF, Ambrosius WT. Behavior problems in children before first recognized seizures. *Pediatrics* 2001; 107: 115-22.

Baglietto MG, Battaglia FM, Nobili L, et al. Neuropsychological disorders related to interictal epileptic discharges during sleep in benign epilepsy of childhood with centrotemporal or Rolandic spikes. *Dev Med Child Neurol* 2001; 43: 407-12.

Bailet LL, Turk WR. The impact of childhood epilepsy on neurocognitive and behavioral performance: a prospective longitudinal study. *Epilepsia* 2000; 41: 426-31.

Baños JH, LaGory J, Sawrie S, et al. Self-report of cognitive abilities in temporal lobe epilepsy: cognitive, psychosocial, and emotional factors. *Epilepsy Behav* 2004; 5: 575-9.

Barkley RA. *ADHD and the Nature of Self-control*. New York: Guilford, 1997.

Bennett-Levy J, Stores G. The nature of cognitive dysfunction in school-children with epilepsy. *Acta Neurol Scan* 1984; 69 (suppl 99): 79-82.

Borgatti R, Piccinelli P, Montirosso R, et al. Study of attentional processes in children with idiopathic epilepsy by Conners' continuous performance test. *J Child Neurol* 2004; 19: 509-15.

Caplan R, Arbelle S, Magharious W, et al. Psychopathology in pediatric complex partial and primary generalized epilepsy. *Dev Med Child Neurol* 1998; 40: 805-11.

Caplan R, Siddarth P, Gurbani S, Ott D, Sankar R, Shields WD. Psychopathology and pediatric complex partial seizures: seizure-related, cognitive, and linguistic variables. *Epilepsia* 2004; 45: 1273-81.

Committee on Classification and Terminology of the International League against Epilepsy. Proposal for revised classification of epilepsies and epileptic syndromes. *Epilepsia* 1989; 30: 389-99.

Conners CK. *Conners' Rating Scales – Revised.* North Tonawanda, NY: MHS, 1997.

Conners CK and MHS Staff. *Conners' Continuous Performance II computer program for Windows.* North Tonawanda, NY: MHS, 2000.

Croona C, Kihlgren M, Lundberg S, Eeg-Olofsson O, Eeg-Olofsson KE. Neuropsychological findings in children with benign childhood epilepsy with centrotemporal spikes. *Dev Med Child Neurol* 1999; 41: 813-8.

D'Alessandro P, Piccirilli M, Tiacci C, et al. Neuropsychological features of benign partial epilepsy in children. *Ital J Neurol Sci* 1990; 11: 265-9.

Danielsson S, Rydenhag B, Uvebrant P, Nordborg C, Olsson I. Temporal lobe resections in children with epilepsy: neuropsychiatric status in relation to neuropathology and seizure outcome. *Epilepsy Behav* 2002; 3: 76-81.

Delis DC, Kaplan E, Kramer JH. *Delis-Kaplan Executive Function System.* San Antonio, TX: Psychological Corporation, 2001.

Deonna T, Zesiger P, Davidoff V, Maeder M, Mayor C, Roulet E. Benign partial epilepsy of childhood: a longitudinal neuropsychological and EEG study of cognitive function. *Dev Med Child Neurol* 2000; 42: 595-603.

Dow C, Seidenberg M, Hermann B. Relationship between information processing speed in temporal lobe epilepsy and white matter volume. *Epilepsy Behav* 2004; 5: 919-25.

Doyle AE, Biederman J, Seidman LJ, Weber W, Faraone SV. Diagnostic efficiency of neuropsychological test scores for discriminating boys with and without attention deficit-hyperactivity disorder. *J Consult Clin Psychol* 2000; 68: 477-88.

DuPaul GJ, Power TJ, Anastopoulos AD, Reid R. *ADHD Rating Scale – IV: Checklists, norms, and clinical interpretation.* New York: Guilford, 1998.

Dunn DW, Austin JK, Harezlak J, Ambrosius WT. ADHD and epilepsy in childhood. *Dev Med Child Neurol* 2003; 45: 50-4.

Engelberts NH, Klein M, Ader HJ, Heimans JJ, Kasteleijn-Nolst Trenite DGA, van der Ploeg HM. The effectiveness of cognitive rehabilitation for attention deficits in focal seizures: a randomized controlled study. *Epilepsia* 2002; 43: 587-95.

Fastenau PS, Dunn DW, Austin JK. Pediatric epilepsy. In: Rizzo M, Eslinger PJ, eds. *Principles and Practice of Behavioral Neurology and Neuropsychology.* Philadelphia: W. B. Saunders Company, 2004: 965-82.

Fastenau PS, Shen J, Dunn DW, Perkins SM, Hermann BP, Austin JK. Neuropsychological predictors of academic underachievement in pediatric epilepsy: moderating roles of demographic, seizure, and psychosocial variables. *Epilepsia* 2004; 45: 1261-72.

Feddersen B, Herzer R, Hartmann U, Gaab MR, Runge U. On the psychopathology of unilateral temporal lobe epilepsy. *Epilepsy Behav* 2005; 6: 43-9.

Feldman H, Crumine P, Handen BL, et al. Methylphenidate in children with seizures and attention-deficit disorder. *Am J Dis Child* 1989; 143: 1081-6.

Fleck DE, Shear PK, Strakowski SM. A reevaluation of sustained attention performance in temporal lobe epilepsy. *Arch Clin Neuropsychol* 2002; 17: 399-405.

Gadow KD, Sprafkin J. *Child Symptom Inventory 4 norms manual.* Stonybrook, NY: Checkmate Plus, Ltd., 1997.

Gioia GA, Isquith PK, Guy SC, Kenworthy L. *Behavior Rating Inventory of Executive Function.* Odessa, FL: Psychological Assessment Resources, 2000.

Golden CJ, Freshwater SM, Golden Z. *Stroop Color and Word Test Children's Version for Ages 5-14.* Wood Dale, IL: Stoelting, 2003.

Glaser GH. Limbic epilepsy in childhood. *J Nerv Ment Dis* 1967; 144: 391-7.

Gonzalez-Heydrich J, Hsin O, Hickory M, et al. Comparisons of response to stimulant preparations in pediatric epilepsy. *AACAP Scientific Proceceedings* 2004; 31: 107-8.

Gross-Tsur V, Manor O, van der Meer J, et al. Epilepsy and attention deficit hyperactivity disorder: is methylphenidate safe and effective? *J Pediatric* 1997; 130: 670-4.

Gucuyener K, Erdemoglu AK, Senol S, Serdaroglu A, Soysal S, Kockar AI. Use of methylphenidate for attention-deficit hyperactivity disorder in patients with epilepsy or electroencephalographic abnormalities. *J Child Neurol* 2003; 18: 109-12.

Harvey AS, Berkovic SF, Wrennall JA, Hopkins IJ. Temporal lobe epilepsy in childhood: clinical, EEG, and neuroimaging findings and syndrome classification in a cohort with new-onset seizures. *Neurology* 1997; 49: 960-8.

Haverkamp F, Hanisch C, Mayer H, Noeker M. Evidence of a specific vulnerability for deficient sequential cognitive processing in epilepsy. *J Child Neurol* 2001; 16: 901-5.

Heaton RK, Chelune GJ, Talley JL, Kay GG, Curtiss G. *Wisconsin Card Sorting Test Manual: Revised and expanded.* Odessa, FL: Psychological Assessment Resources, 1993.

Heijbel J, Bohman M. Benign epilepsy of children with centrotemporal EEG foci: intelligence, behavior, and school adjustment. *Epilepsia* 1975; 16: 679-87.

Helmstaedter C. Neuropsychological aspects of epilepsy surgery. *Epilepsy Behav* 2004; 5 (suppl 1): S45-S55.

Hempel AM, Frost MD, Ritter FJ, Farnham S. Factors influencing the incidence of ADHD in pediatric epilepsy patients. *Epilepsia* 1995; 36 (suppl 4): 122.

Hermann BP, Seidenberg M, Schoenfeld J, Davies K. Neuropsychological characteristics of the syndrome of mesial temporal lobe epilepsy. *Arch Neurol* 1997; 54: 369-76.

Hermann B, Seidenberg M, Bell B, et al. The neurodevelopemental impact of childhood-onset temporal lobe epilepsy on brain structure and function. *Epilepsia* 2002; 43: 1062-71.

Hernandez MT, Sauerwein HC, Jambaque I, et al. Attention, memory, and behavioral adjustment in children with frontal lobe epilepsy. *Epilepsy Behav* 2003; 4: 522-36.

Hesdorffer DC, Ludvigsson P, Olafsson E, Gudmundsson G, Kjartansson O, Hauser WA. ADHD as a risk factor for incident unprovoked seizures and epilepsy in children. *Arch Gen Psychiatry* 2004; 61: 731-6.

Korkman M, Kirk U, Kemp S. *NEPSY: A developmental neuropsychological assessment.* San Antonio, TX: Psychological Corporation, 1998.

Kronenberger WG, Meyer RG. *The child clinician's handbook (2nd ed.).* Boston: Allyn & Bacon, 2001.

Leark RA, Dupuy TR, Greenberg LM, Corman, CL, Kindschi CL. *Test of Variables of Attention professional manual version 7.0.* Los Alamitos, CA: Universal Attention Disorders, Inc., 1996.

Lendt M, Helmstaedter C, Elger CE. Pre- and postoperative neuropsychological profiles in children and adolescents with temporal lobe epilepsy. *Epilepsia* 1999; 40: 1543-50.

Lendt M, Helmstaedter C, Kuczaty S, Schramm J, Elger CE. Behavioural disorders in children with epilepsy: early improvement after surgery. *J Neurol Neurosurg Psychiatry* 2000; 69: 739-44.

Lindgren A, Kihlgren M, Melin L, Croona C, Lundberg S, Eeg-Olofsson O. Development of cognitive functions in children with rolandic epilepsy. *Epilepsy Behav* 2004; 5: 903-10.

Lindsay J, Ounsted C, Richards P. Long-term outcome in children with temporal lobe seizures. III: Psychiatric aspects in childhood and adult life. *Dev Med Child Neurol* 1979; 21: 630-6.

Martin R, Dowler R, Ho S, *et al*. Cognitive consequences of coexisting temporal lobe developmental malformations and hippocampal sclerosis. *Neurology* 1999; 53: 709-15.

McCarthy AM, Richman LC, Yarbrough D. Memory, attention and school problems in children with seizure disorders. *Dev Neuropsychology* 1995; 11: 71-86.

MTA Cooperative Group. A 14-month randomized clinical trial of treatment strategies for attention-deficit hyperactivity disorder. *Arch Gen Psychiatry* 1999; 56: 1073-86.

Oostrom KJ, Schouten A, Kruitwagen CLJJ, Peters ACB, Jennekens-Schinkel A. Attention deficits are not characteristic of schoolchildren with newly diagnosed idiopathic or cryptogenic epilepsy. *Epilepsia* 2002; 43: 301-10.

Ott D, Caplan R, Guthrie D, *et al*. Measures of psychopathology in children with complex partial seizures and primary generalized epilepsy with absence. *J Am Acad Child Adolesc Psychiatry* 2001; 40: 907-14.

Oyegbile TO, Dow C, Jones J, *et al*. The nature and course of neuropsychological morbidity in chronic temporal lobe epilepsy. *Neurology* 2004; 62: 1736-42.

Palmese CA, Hamberger MJ. Attention and executive functioning in temporal lobe epilepsy patients with and without MTS. *Epilepsia* 2004; 45 (suppl 7): 181.

Perugini EM, Harvey EA, Lovejoy DW, Sandstrom K, Webb AH. The predictive power of combined neuropsychological measures for attention-deficit/hyperactivity disorder in children. *Child Neuropsych* 2000; 6: 101-14.

Piccirilli M, D'Alessandro P, Sciarma T, *et al*. Attention problems in epilepsy: possible significance of the epileptogenic focus. *Epilepsia* 1994; 35: 1091-6.

Power TJ, Andrews TJ, Eiraldi RB, Doherty BJ, Ikeda MJ, DuPaul GJ, Landau S. Evaluating attention deficit hyperactivity disorder using multiple informants: The incremental utility of combining teacher with parent reports. *Psychol Assessment* 1998; 10: 250-60.

Reynolds CR, Kamphaus RW. *Behavior Assessment System for Children, 2nd Edition manual*. Circle Pines, MN: AGS, 2004.

Sanchez-Carpintero R, Neville BGR. Attentional ability in children with epilepsy. *Epilepsia* 2003; 44: 1340-9.

Sandford JA, Turner A. *Intermediate Visual and Auditory Continuous Performance Test (IVA)*. Odessa, FL: Psychological Assessment Resources, 1993.

Schmitz B. The effects of antiepileptic drugs on behaviour. In: Trimble M, Schmitz B, eds. *The Neuropsychiatry of Epilepsy*. Cambridge UK: Cambridge University Press, 2002: 241-55.

Schoenfeld J, Seidenberg M, Woodard A, Hecox K, Inglese C, Mack K, Hermann B. Neuropsychological and behavioral status of children with complex partial seizures. *Dev Med Child Neurol* 1999; 41: 724-31.

Schouten A, Oostrom KJ, Peters ACB, Verloop D, Jennekens-Schinkel A. Set-shifting in health children and in children with idiopathic or cryptogenic epilepsy. *Dev Med Child Neurol* 2000; 42: 392-7.

Semrud-Clikeman M, Wical B. Components of attention in children with complex partial seizures with and without ADHD. *Epilepsia* 1999; 40: 211-5.

Sherman EMS, Armitage LL, Connolly MB, Wambera KM, Esther S. Behaviors symptomatic of ADHD in pediatric epilepsy: relationship to frontal lobe epileptiform abnormalities and other neurological predictors. *Epilepsia* 2000; 41 (suppl 7): 191.

Sheslow D, Adams W. *Wide Range Assessment of Memory and Learning Second Edition*. Wilmington, DE: Wide Range Inc., 2003.

Smith ML, Elliott IM, Lach L. Cognitive, psychosocial, and family function one year after pediatric epilepsy surgery. *Epilepsia* 2004; 45: 650-60.

Snyder TJ, Sinclair DB, McKean JD, Wheatley BM. The Boston qualitative scoring system (BQSS) for measuring executive function in children with frontal lobe epilepsy (FLE) *versus* temporal lobe epilepsy (TLE). *Epilepsia* 2003; 44 (suppl 9): 240.

Stores G. Behavior disturbance and type of epilepsy in children attending ordinary school. In: Penry JK, ed. *Epilepsy: Proceedings of the Eighth International Symposium*. New York: Raven Press, 1977: 245-9.

Stores G. School-children with epilepsy at risk for learning and behaviour problems. *Dev Med Child Neurol* 1978; 20: 502-9.

Stores G, Hart J, Piran N. Inattentiveness in schoolchildren with epilepsy. *Epilepsia* 1978; 19: 169-75.

Sturniolo MG, Galletti F. Idiopathic epilepsy and school achievement. *Arch Dis Child* 1994; 70: 424-8.

Thome-Souza S, Kuczynski E, Assumpção F, *et al*. Which factors may play a pivotal role on determining the type of psychiatric disorder in children and adolescents with epilepsy? *Epilepsy Behav* 2004; 5: 988-94.

Vercera SP, Rizzo M. Attention: normal and disordered processes. In: Rizzo M, Eslinger PJ. *Principles and Practice of Behavioral Neurology and Neuropsychology*. Philadelphia: W.B.Saunders Company, 2004: 223-45.

Weglage J, Demsky A, Pietsch M, Kurlemann G. Neuropsychological, intellectual, and behavioral findings in patients with centrotemporal spikes with and without seizures. *Dev Med Child Neurol* 1997; 39: 646-51.

Williams J, Griebel ML, Dykman RA. Neuropsychological patterns in pediatric epilepsy. *Seizure* 1998; 7: 223-8.

Williams J, Phillips T, Griebel ML, *et al*. Factors associated with academic achievement in children with controlled epilepsy. *Epilepsy Behav* 2001; 2: 217-23.

Wolraich ML, Lambert W, Doffing MA, Bickman L, Simmons T, Worley K. Psychometric properties of the Vanderbilt ADHD Diagnostic Parent Rating Scale in a referred population. *J Ped Psychol* 2003; 28: 559-68.

# Brain maturation and development of socio-cognitive perception and neural damaging process

A. Laurent[1,2], A. Arzimanoglou[2], S. de Schonen[1,2]

[1] Developmental Neurocognition Group, LCD,
CNRS and University Paris 5
[2] Epilepsy Unit, Dpt of Child Neurology and Metabolic Disorders,
University Hospital Robert-Debré (AP-HP), Paris, France

---

One of the crucial questions that developmental cognitive neuroscience has to answer is whether a mental competence can develop based on other neural cortical associative networks than those involved in normal development. Functional cortical plasticity is often described in adults after cortical damage. However the young child brain differs from the adult brain in many aspects that are probably crucial for functional plasticity. In a way, functional plasticity is most probably greater than it is in adult (for instance, production of growth factors is greater). However, greater neural plasticity does not necessarily imply adaptive plasticity. Because fewer networks are functionally specialised, the constraints between networks are weaker so that deviations from normal interactions between networks are more likely. The plasticity issue is crucial for our understanding of neural mechanisms of mental functions as well as for biological therapy or rehabilitation.

Studies on effects of brain damage in adult patients and functional brain imaging in healthy adults have revealed the role of neural networks within the temporal lobe in several visuo- and auditory-social competences (see review by M. Zilbovicius and I. Meresse, this volume). However, commitment of these neural networks in socio-cognitive perception results from a normal developmental trajectory of the brain in interaction with normal environmental input, according to a normal developmental timetable. Not only during infancy and early childhood localisation of competences might be more diffuse than they are later on, but also competences might be less differentiated one from another. An epileptic focus situated in a given site might delay or, even worse, disturb or preclude the normal development of some competencies or components of a competence, and generate abnormal behaviour.

Moreover, what is observed for a competence or a set of competences might not apply for another set of those. Cognitive competences differ from each other by the kinds of neural computation they involve (for instance neural computation involved in speech perception might be different from neural computation involved in face perception). Differences between neural computations rely, among other factors, on differences between characteristics of the neural cells on which computation is based. For instance the consequence of an anterior early brain damage on speech development might differ from consequences of a posterior early brain damage on visuospatial development, not because the brain regions are not localised identically and the neural afferences and efferences are not identical, but because the neural cells of the network involved in one or the other competence do not have the same characteristics.

Finally, the long-term effect of an early brain damage with loss of tissue without seizures might differ from the long-term effect of repeated seizures. Indeed the course of functional specialisation of preserved networks surrounding a loss of tissue might differ from the functional specialisation of networks whose functional firing patterns are repeatedly disorganized by seizures for years.

## ■ Early forms of visuo-social and auditory-social competences

Neonates a few minutes old, look at a schematic frontal view of a face longer than at a non-face pattern with the same signal amplitude (Goren et al., 1975; Johnson et al., 1991). It must be underscored, however, that this preference is not based on a specific preference for faces. Indeed, neonates look at patterns with horizontal contrast longer than to patterns with vertical contrasts; they look longer to patterns that display heavier horizontal contrasts in their upper part than in their lower part, independently of whether the pattern looks like a face or not (Turati et al., 2002; Cassia et al., 2004). This general perceptual visual mechanism insures that the neonates' visual attention is more frequently oriented towards faces compared to patterns of other kinds. But it remains that neonate brain has to acquire some representation of faces from its interactions with its environment. The neural substrate of the neonates "preferential looking" for pseudo-face-like patterns is unknown so far. It might be based on a subcortical network (Johnson et al., 1991) or a temporary state of maturation of the visual areas V1 and V2 (de Schonen, 2002).

Three-day-olds are also able to learn about some aspects of a face: they have been shown to recognize a familiar face (their care-taker face) or a familiarized face and discriminate it from a stranger or a novel face (Bushnell et al., 1989; Pascalis & de Schonen, 1994; Pascalis et al., 1995). However, it is not known whether this early short lasting "pre-episodic" recognition involves the hippocampal and peri-hippocampal networks. Nevertheless some kind of memory is at work at that time (Pascalis & de Schonen, 1994).

During the first few months of life infants also use cues from adult gaze direction (Hood, 1995; Hood et al., 1998). Three-day-olds have been shown to prefer to look at faces that look directly to them than at faces which are looking towards another direction (Farroni *et al.*, 2002). In 4-month-olds, cortical processing (as recorded with event-related potentials – ERPs) is enhanced when accompanied by direct gaze: the ERP component N240 which seems to be the equivalent of the face N170 component in adults, shows a greater amplitude with face stimuli that look at the observer than for faces looking away. This result suggests that eye gaze processing shares overlapping neural processing with face processing as is also the case in adults (Wicker *et al.*, 1998). Also 4-month-olds can use the adult's eye gaze shift to orient their own visual attention towards a visual target cued by the eye movement of the adult. The assumption according to which this early behaviour is based upon a domain-general system responsive to the lateral motion of stimuli regardless of whether or not eyes are involved has been rejected (Farroni *et al.*, 2003).

Early imitation of tongue protrusion and finger movements by neonates and 3-day-old infants might also be taken as an argument for a very early specific orientation towards human kind in infants (Meltzoff & Moore, 1983; Fontaine, 1984). However not all studies have replicated these results in neonates (Anisfeld *et al.*, 2001).

Between birth and the age of three months, visual capacities and ability to process faces, gaze and expressions increase. Visual preference of 3-month-old infants, contrary to orientation towards faces in neonates, is now directed to true face patterns showing that infants have developed face representations that are more adult-like (Turati *et al.*, 2005). At the age of 3 months, recognition of faces across several different points of view is emerging (Pascalis *et al.*, 1998). Also, the inversion effect (better recognition of individual faces in an upright than in an inverted position) is present (Turati *et al.*, 2004). Three-month-olds are sensitive to the characteristics shared by the various faces they have experienced in their environment. For instance, 3-month-old infants reared in a Caucasian environment are able to recognize and discriminate Caucasian faces much better than Asian faces (Sangrigoli & de Schonen, 2004). Therefore, two kinds of memory can be observed at the age of three months. A memory for individual faces as assessed by recognition of photographed faces after a 24-hour delay (Pascalis *et al.*, 1998) and the progressive modification of the processing tools by the specific and common characteristics shared by the faces of the environment.

It has been shown that from age of 4-5 months at least to 11 months, infants process faces better with their right hemisphere than with their left (de Schonen & Mathivet, 1990). Moreover the right and left hemispheres do not process the same visual information. The general schema of all faces is identical: an oval with two eyes above a nose, above a mouth. But the relative positions and distances between features are idiosyncratic characteristic of each individual face. Faces differ also by more "local" information, specifically by the shape of the features. So there are at least two kinds of visual information which can be used to characterize and differentiate two individual faces: configural and local information. In infants, the right hemisphere is more sensitive to differences in position and distances between features within a face than to shape of features ("configural" information), whereas the left hemisphere is more sensitive to the shape of features ("local" information) within faces as well as within geometrical patterns (Deruelle & de Schonen, 1991; Deruelle & de Schonen, 1995, 1998; de Schonen et Mathivet, 1990; Le Grand *et al.*, 2003). This lateralisation of different kinds of face processing is also observed in adults (Rossion *et al.*, 2000).

One study has shown that neonates are sensitive to expressions and react differently to positive and negative adults' expressions (Field et al., 1982). Three-month-old infants are very sensitive to changes in adult facial expressions. For instance, infants decrease attention and smiling when an adult female presents a neutral unresponsive face compared to normal face-to-face interactions (Muir & Hains, 1993). Facial emotional expressions are categorized and discriminated early in life but the age depends on the category of expressions. At the age of 7 months, infants categorise happy faces and discriminate them from fearful expressions (Nelson & de Haan, 1996). EEG studies with 10 month old infants show that activity on the left frontal sites is related to both perceived and expressed positive emotion; activity over the right frontal sites is related to both perceived and expressed negative emotions (Davidson & Fox, 1982). These asymmetries are also found in adults (Davidson et al., 2004).

The infants' ability to interpret gaze and emotional expression, to relate gaze and emotional expression to intentional action seems to emerge after the age of 8 months at least in the experimental conditions used so far. Twelve-month-olds but not 8-month-olds were shown to recognize that an actor is likely to grasp the object, which he had visually regarded with positive affect. The ability to use information about an adult's direction of gaze and emotional expression to predict action is present and also develops at the end of the first year (Phillips et al., 2002).

Neonates and two-month-olds also start learning speech sounds on the basis of early sensitivity to several aspects of speech sounds (Eimas et al., 1971; Eimas, 1974; Kuhl et al., 2001; Kuhl, 2004). Some voice intonations are also discriminated at birth: neonates show a mismatch negativity (MMN) showing a discrimination between the vowels [I] and [a], and also between a steady pitch contour of [a] versus a rising pitch contour (Kujala et al., 2004). Some characteristics of the mother voice are learned in the womb: a neonate, born at term without aerial experience of the mother voice, is able to recognize it (Kisilevsky et al., 2003).

## ■ When in the perinatal and postnatal development does the temporal cortex start to be specifically involved in processing socio-perceptual stimuli?

A brain imaging study on 2-month-old infants, with PET scan and $H^2O_{15}$ as markers, was performed when infants were presented with women faces photographed under a frontal view and with a neutral expression in one condition and with a double circle of coloured diodes that were lighted one after the other in the other condition (Tzourio-Mazoyer et al., 2002). The comparison between the two conditions revealed that faces stimuli activate the core system for face perception identified in adults (the right fusiform gyrus and bilateral infero-occipital cortex, Kanwisher et al., 1997). However, the superior temporal sulcus (STS) was not significantly activated. The putative role of the STS in adults is to process and respond to changeable aspects of faces, perception of gaze and lip expression (Haxby et al., 2000; see also Zilbovicius, this volume). The lack of significant activation of the STS in 2-month-olds might be related to the poor development of face processing at this age (for instance recognition of a face under different view points emerges at about the age of 3-months (Pascalis et al., 1998) or to the uniformity of view and gaze direction and neutrality of expression in the face stimuli in the PET study reported above. The right localisation of the fusiform gyrus activation is most probably related to the right hemisphere advantage in face processing observed in infants during their first year of life (de Schonen & Mathivet, 1990; Deruelle & de Schonen, 1998) and which is frequently observed in adults (McCarthy et al., 1997; Gauthier et al., 1999; Rossion et al., 2000). Event-related potentials studies have also confirmed the right hemisphere advantage in face processing versus visual noise processing in 3 month-olds infants (Halit et al., 2004).

A right inferior parietal activation nearby the intraparietal sulcus was also observed. This region belongs to the extended face processing system in adults (Haxby et al., 2000). Surprisingly, face processing in 2-month-olds was found to recruit what will become a language network, the left inferior frontal and superior temporal gyrus. This co-activation of a speech network under face presentation is not observed in adults when presented with faces. This is an example of a difference between infant and adult brain: during development, co-activation might be replaced in some networks by inhibition so as to differentiate, for instance, between face perception with speech from face perception without speech.

Similar data were found in 3-month-old infants for speech perception. Precursors of adult cortical language areas are already active in infants, well before the onset of speech production (Dehaene-Lambertz et al., 2002).

All in all these data show that despite a low level of metabolic activity and the low density of synapses in the associative temporal cortex at this age, the visual and auditory associative cortical areas show some relatively specialized functional activity. This demonstrates that functional maturation does not require metabolic and anatomical maturation completion of the involved area. Maturation might proceed simultaneously in several connected and active cortical regions, involving a functional maturation of networks rather than area by area. The co-activation of left speech regions suggests that certain networks that appear to be independent in adults become separately activated after a period of co-activation. "Parcellation" of functional activations does constitute a developmental progress. Here again seizures might interfere with this kind of developmental process.

Thus, as long as no abnormal or damaging neural process interferes with the normal developmental trajectory, functional specialisation of neural networks will be approximately similar from individual to individual if the relevant inputs are provided by the environment at the proper time. Of course this allows for individual and group differences like those shown between male and female brain development. The effect of a damaging neural process will depend on the state of maturation and specialization of the brain in which it occurs. In spite of their early emergence, visuo-, auditory- and cognitivo-social competences show a protracted development. Therefore depending on the date of occurrence of an abnormal or damaging neural process even years after birth, the neuropsychological outcome can differ.

## ■ Right or left localisation and functional plasticity

The competences under discussion here are based on temporal networks. However the right and left temporal lobes do not seem to play the same role. Anatomo-functional data reported above on speech and face perception in infancy show that the dissymmetric roles of the hemispheres start very early when the first relevant inputs become available in the environment. Does this early dissymmetric localisation mean that the other hemisphere does not shelter neural networks relevant for developing the same competence? The answer to this question may differ according to the kind of competences under study. In the next section, we shall first report data showing dissymmetric functioning of the temporal lobes. Then we shall comment on lateralisation and post-lesional plasticity in children.

### Brain imaging studies in healthy adults

According to functional brain imaging studies in adults, many visuo- and auditory-social cues seem to be processed more in the right than in the left temporal cortex. More activation is found during face presentations and tasks with faces in the right than in the left ventro-temporal cortex (Kanwisher et al., 1997; Haxby et al. 2000; Winston et al., 2004; Rama & Courtney, 2005). Perceptual categorisation of facial expressions is related to greater activation in the right than in the left STS and amygdala (Winston et al., 2004; Streit et al., 1999); perception of gaze direction activates more the right than the left posterior part of the STS (Hoffman & Haxby, 2000). Similarly, the right anterior portion of the STS is more activated than the left during voice discrimination (Rama et al., 2005; Belin & Zatorre, 2003); the right posterior and middle portion of the STS is more activated than the left during perceptual tasks dealing with emotional prosody (George et al., 1996; Wildgruber et al., 2002; Grandjean et al., 2005). Despite having a greater lateralization in the right hemisphere, these functions are represented and processed by networks that are different one from the other. Thus, voice and face identity are processed in clearly distinct networks (Rama et al., 2005). Similarly, perception of face identity and facial emotional expressions are processed by different neural networks (Winston et al., 2004) just as face identity and gaze direction are processed by different networks (Hoffman & Haxby, 2000). Moreover, networks involved in perception of voice identity are different from those involved in perception of voice emotions (Imaizumi et al., 1997).

A difference in lateralization of amygdala activation in response to fear versus positive expressions has been reported in several studies. The left amygdala has been found to be highly activated in response to dynamic facial expressions relative to dynamic non facial and to static expression in the case of fearful expressions, but not in the case of happy expressions (Sato et al., 2004).

The function of amygdala responses was also investigated by comparing the effect of angry expressions when the face is looking at the observer or looking away. The left amygdala showed the interaction between emotional expression and face direction, indicating higher activity for angry expressions looking toward the subjects than angry expressions looking away from them. Subjects reported experiencing greater emotion when the face looked at them than in the other case. The correlation between the left amygdala activity and experienced emotion was positive and significant. These results suggest that the amygdala is involved in emotional but not visuo-perceptual processing for emotional facial expressions, which specifically includes the decoding of emotional significance and elicitation of one's own emotions corresponding to that significance (Sato et al., 2004).

Another study suggested two interesting points that remain to be confirmed. Adults were presented with two angry faces, one of which was associated by conditioning with a burst of white noise. The angry faces were presented for less than 40 ms and were followed by an expressionless mask in half of the trials so that the subjects reported having seen nothing. Nevertheless the masked presentation of the conditioned face elicited significant activation in the right but not the left amygdala. Unmasked presentation of the same face produced enhanced neural activity in the left but not the right amygdala. These data show that the amygdala discriminate between stimuli solely on the basis of their acquired significance; secondly, lateralization of the amygdala response seems to depend on the subject's level of awareness of the stimuli (Morris et al., 1998). Another study showed that while orbitofrontal cortex exhibited rapid reversal of acquired fear responses, the right ventral amygdala showed a persistent, non-reversing "memory" for previous fear-related stimulus associations (Morris & Dolan, 2004).

## Unilateral temporal brain damage in adults

In studies of unilateral brain damage consequences in adults, it was also observed that right lesions impair visuo- and auditory-social cues processing more than do left lesions. Prosopagnosia was most often observed with bilateral lesions but unilateral right lesions are associated with prosopagnosia or with deficit in face recognition (Hecaen & Angelergues, 1962; de Renzi, 1986; McNeil & Warrington, 1993; Hadjikhani & de Gelder, 2002; Rossion et al., 2003) more often than left ones. Deficits in processing facial emotional expressions (with no deficit in face processing of any other kind) are reported in patients with right temporal damage (Adolphs et al., 2001; Kucharska-Pietura et al., 2003). Similarly, specific deficits in voice discrimination are observed with right damage (Assal et al., 1976; Thuillard & Assal, 1983). Labelling and recognition of facial expressions and recognition of emotions conveyed by prosody are impaired in patients with unilateral right damage but are much less or not at all impaired in patients with unilateral left lesions. However, on the prosody test the LHD patients showed significant impairment, performing mid-way between the right hemisphere patients and the healthy comparison group. Recognition of positive emotional expressions was performed at a higher level than negative expressions in all subjects. Recognition of individual emotions in one modality correlated weakly with recognition in another, in all three groups. These data confirm the primacy of the right hemisphere in processing all emotional expressions across modalities – both positive and negative – but suggest that the left hemisphere role in emotion processing is modality specific. It is possible that the left hemisphere has a particular role in the perception of emotion conveyed through meaningful speech (Kucharska-Pietura et al., 2003).

## Early unilateral brain lesions

Despite an early adult-like lateralisation of face perception (see above), the effect of an early brain lesion on development of these competences does not seem to depend on the side of the damage. Children aged between 5 and 17 years who suffered a right or left unilateral posterior (temporal or occipito-temporal) lesion before or around birth, show severe deficits in face and/or emotional expression processing (de Schonen et al., 2005). Similarly, early right as well as left brain lesions can result in delayed speech development (Bates et al., 1997). These data together with the data on early lateralisation of speech and face processing, show a close dependency between the functional specialisation processes of the two hemispheres during early development (de Schonen et al., 2005).

Now it should be noted that post lesional plasticity after a pre- or peri-natal unilateral brain lesion is not identical for speech and visuo-spatial competence in children. Several studies have shown that after a unilateral brain lesion, speech development is delayed but eventually catches up at least in what concerns speech use at school and in daily life (very abstract use of speech might not be so well developed) (Bates et al., 1997; Brizzolara et al., 2002; Reilly et al., 1998). fMRI studies using verb, name or sentence generation tasks showed that language develops in the controlateral right hemisphere or in left regions that are anterior or posterior to the lesion (Liegeois et al., 2004; Hertz-Pannier et al., 2002). The behavioral data obtained showed that speech perception, comprehension and production did develop in these children. No explanation has yet been uncovered to account for the fact that in these children speech is sometimes developed in the right hemisphere and sometimes in regions next to the lesion.

By contrast with plasticity for language development after early unilateral brain lesion, the visuo-spatial competences seem to be much less plastic. Several studies show that even after several years of daily practice with faces, children who underwent a right or left unilateral posterior lesion before birth, during or soon after birth, show severe deficits in these competence together with other visuo-spatial deficits (Mancini et al., 1994; de Schonen et al., 2005; Stiles et al, 2003; Stiles & Thal, 1993; Stiles et al., 1997).

It is quite difficult to compare performances in two different domains of competences, therefore it is difficult to compare speech and face processing development after early brain injury in children. Nevertheless, the level of performance in face processing and other visuo-spatial competences is so poor compared to the level of performance in speech competences that it is strongly suggested that plasticity differs in the two domains. This suggests a difference in sensitivity of cells to growth factors, a difference which in turn suggests that neurons involved in speech development might not be the same as those involved in face and visuo-spatial processing development. Neurons for speech development would be present in both hemispheres, statistically more dense in the anterior part than in the posterior part of the brain. These neurons might remain plastic for years. Neurons for face processing and other visuo-spatial competences might also be present in both hemispheres, statistically more dense in the posterior and ventral part of the brain; but these neurons would remain plastic for a short period after birth (additional argument for this point is given below). If this conclusion is correct, it means that the plasticity of mental competences should be investigated carefully within small domain of competences and also by looking separately at what can be called "low level components of competences". IQ tests are useful but cannot provide us with any information on these questions.

## ■ Deficits in social cues processing in adults and children with temporal lobe epilepsy

Most of the studies on social competences in patients with unilateral focal epilepsy have been conducted in adults after surgery. Studies in patients before surgery are scarce. Recognition of emotional expressions, and more specifically of fear expression, is impaired in adult patients with right temporal epilepsy and hippocampal sclerosis. Impairment is more frequent when patients had their first seizure before age 5 or when they experienced complex febrile convulsions in infancy (Meletti et al., 2003; Benuzzi et al., 2004). In an fMRI study, 8 patients with right and 5 with left temporal epilepsy and healthy individuals were compared on a task dealing with facial emotion expressions. Patients with right temporal epilepsy showed less or no activation of the networks that were found to be activated by the task in healthy controls and patients with left epilepsy. The two latter groups had bilateral activations whereas patients with right epilepsy had less activation specifically in the right hemisphere (Bennuzzi et al., 2004). Deficit in facial expression recognition might be less likely in patients with left temporal epilepsy than in patients with right epilepsy.

In a patient with left temporal epilepsy who presented with ictal fear, no deficit in emotional expression recognition was found. However this patient showed abnormal judgment of facial emotional expression intensity, in particular for negative emotional expressions (Yamada et al., 2005).

It would be interesting to investigate social processing of other kinds in these patients. Moreover the age at which onset of epilepsy occurred appears to be crucial. It would also be important to document more precisely the possible relationships between the deficit in social competences and memory competences. Finally, it is necessary to know whether only mesial damage can result in such a pattern of deficit.

To our knowledge, socio-perceptual competences in children with unilateral temporal lobe epilepsy have been reported in only one study (Cohen et al., 1990) and patients were shown to have deficits in emotional prosodic identification. The deficit was found in 4 patients out of 12 with right temporal epilepsy, and in 2 out of 11 patients with left temporal epilepsy. These results do not allow suggesting a greater risk for children with right than left focus. Moreover the sample showed large diversity of etiologies.

In a recent study we tested face recognition (FR) in children with focal non-idiopathic epilepsy implicating the temporal lobe (5 children with left TLE and 5 with right TLE). Diagnosis was based on seizure semiology (Arzimanoglou et al., 2004) clinical history, video-EEG screening and MRI findings. Clinical information pertaining to the patients is presented in *table I*. All children were born in a Caucasian environment. PET scan

(CEA Orsay; Drs Zilbovicius and Boddaert) during rest in 5 of these patients (2 with left and 3 with right epilepsy) revealed hypoperfusion in the temporal lobe corresponding to the identified anatomo-electro-clinical abnormalities.

We tested face recognition (FR) in a same/different paradigm without any delay between the two stimuli presentation (unpublished pilot study). In this FR task only six photographs, each representing a different face in frontal view, were used. The hair was masked but the outer contour of the faces differed from one face to the other. Children learned the 6 photographs before performing the same/different task. Each of the 6 photographs was presented 3 times during 5 seconds (total: 15 seconds per face) for learning. After this learning phase, same/different trials consisted in two faces of the learned set being presented successively. The child was asked to tell whether the second was the same person as the first. The first stimulus was presented 250 ms and the second was presented 120 ms, with an inter-stimulus interval of 500 ms.

Moreover, two tasks were used to evaluate separately configural and local processing. One task evaluated the two processing modes within faces (these stimuli called "JANE" were given to us by D. Maurer, Hamilton, Ontario). Only black and white photographs of a frontal view of faces were used. An original face was transformed into two different ways. In the configural condition, faces were generated from the original face by modifying the distances only between the eyes, or/and between nose and mouth, and/or mouth and chin. Except for those modifications, all other features were kept unchanged. In the local condition, the eyes and mouth of other women were substituted to the eyes and mouth of the original face; no other features were modified. In all photographs the same surgeon cap covered the hair. The task was a same/different task. A face was presented for 200 ms followed by a blank screen for 300 ms, followed by another face for an unlimited duration. The child had to say whether the second face was the same or different from the first. In principle this task can be correctly performed even by a prosopagnosic patient as far as the observer can focus only on the distances between features (configural differences) or on the shape of the eyes or mouth (local differences) without processing the whole face. However a patient unable to process configural or local information within faces will fail in this task.

The other task evaluated configural and local processing in a geometrical pattern recognition task (GP). The pattern was made of 9 small geometrical elements situated symmetrically on each side of a vertical axis. In a number of patterns, the 9 elements were all identical; in other patterns, the elements were of two or three different kinds. A target pattern was shown for 500 ms followed by a forced choice between two patterns which remain on the screen until the child gave a response. In the forced choice, one pattern was identical to the target while the other differed from the target either by the position of a subset of elements (configural change) or by the shape of the elements (local change). The child had to say which of the two patterns was identical to the target.

Performances of each patient in each task were compared to the performances of a group of 8 control children, matched for age (patients' age ranged from 13 to 17 years whereas the 8 control children were aged 14 years). A patient was said to have a

Table I. Clinical information on patients, calibrated scores in tasks and neuropsychological information.

| PATIENTS | GENDER | AGE (Yrs; mths) | SEIZURE ONSET (Yrs; mths) | DURATION (Yrs; mths) | SIDE OF FOCUS | "FR" | "JANE" Configural | "JANE" Local | "GP" Configural | "GP" Local | IQ Verbal | IQ Performance | MEMORY (BEM) (immediat recall)* List of words | MEMORY (BEM) (immediat recall)* Story | MEMORY (BEM) (immediat recall)* List of shapes | MEMORY (BEM) (immediat recall)* Geometrical shape |
|---|---|---|---|---|---|---|---|---|---|---|---|---|---|---|---|---|
| FRI | M | 7;11 | 1 | 6;11 | L | −0,54 | – | – | −1,46 | −1,10 | 106 | 99 | 0,62 | −0,86 | 0,27 | −0,29 |
| NAV | F | 5;6 | 2;6 | 3;00 | L | −0,72 | 4,13 | 2,16 | 1,49 | 1,51 | 75 | 107 | −3,67 | −3,24 | −3,36 | −2,67 |
| DEL | M | 8;4 | 4 | 4;4 | L | 2,47 | −0,54 | 1,21 | −0,35 | 0,67 | 92 | 83 | 0,36 | 1,15 | −1,38 | 1,64 |
| FRA | M | 7;10 | 5 | 2;10 | L | −0,54 | – | – | 1,27 | −1,07 | 80 | 93 | −1,05 | −2,52 | −0,18 | 1,86 |
| MAD | M | 17;7 | 10;11 | 6;8 | L | 5,07 | 2,71 | −1,05 | 2,05 | −0,10 | 74 | 62 | −0,04 | 3,89 | −0,46 | 2,58 |
| ARA | M | 14;3 | 1 | 13;2 | R | −0,72 | 1,74 | 2,10 | – | – | 60 | 60 | −3,44 | −3,78 | −2,82 | −1,08 |
| ROB | F | 10;11 | 5;6 | 5;5 | R | −0,35 | – | – | 0,04 | 0,39 | 132 | 132 | – | – | – | – |
| AUS | F | 13;1 | 8;4 | 4;7 | R | 2,50 | 1,63 | 3,16 | – | – | 88 | 82 | −2,33 | −3,78 | −3,27 | −3,00 |
| CAR | M | 14;3 | 10,4 | 3;11 | R | 2,50 | – | – | −0,02 | −1,55 | 101 | 113 | −0,11 | −2,39 | – | – |
| BUR | M | 15;10 | 12;5 | 3;5 | R | 2,49 | 1,74 | 4,21 | 1,02 | −0,01 | 102 | 93 | 1,26 | −2,37 | 0,19 | 0,87 |

Calibrated scores showing a deficit are underlined.
* Calibrated scores in memory tas<s reach the deficit level if † −2.
[FR = face recognition; "JANE" and "GP" tasks: see text for details]

deficit when the difference between his/her score ($x_p$) and the mean score $m_c$ of his/her control group divided by the $SD_c$ of the control group was greater than 2 ($x_p - m_c / SD_c$). IQ and memory were also investigated with standardized tests.

Five of our patients showed a deficit in face processing. In four of them, this deficit could be accounted neither by a memory deficit, nor by a low level visual integration deficit. Among these four patients two had left TLE: one (DEL) had an hypersignal in the temporal hippocampo-polar region and a weak hypersignal in the insular region (Flair MRI), and hypoperfusion of the left temporal insular and polar region (PET scan) (Figure 1a and b); the other patient (MAD) had a globular left hippocampus and hypoperfusion of the left temporal pole (PET scan with $H^2O_{15}$). In the two other patients, with right TLE, one (BUR) showed a right hippocampus with an abnormal shape and a small hypersignal (T2, MRI); the other (CAR) had a normal MRI. The fifth patient (AUS) with right TLE had a severe deficit in memory. She had a right hippocampal sclerosis with a poor white/grey matter differentiation in the temporo-polar region; the PET scan ($H^2O_{15}$) showed a hypoperfusion of the mesial, and ventral (including the fusiform gyrus and the inferior temporal gyrus) and lateral (including the middle temporal gyrus) regions.

Among the children without face deficit, three had left TLE and two right TLE. One child (FRI) had a mesial left temporal lesion (DNET) and an hypoperfusion in a region slightly larger than the visible lesion; another (NAV) had a tumour in the left temporo-mesial region with hypoperfursion of the mesial and polar region; the third child (FRA) had a tumour situated in the temporo-mesial region; this child also showed a hypoperfusion of the mesial and polar temporal regions. Among the two children with a right epilepsy, one (ARA) had a cortical dysplasia in the right temporo-occipital region and hypoperfusion in the same region involving the fusiform gyrus, the middle gyrus, and middle occipital gyrus. The last child (ROB) showed an abnormal shape of the hippocampic region without atrophy; the PET scan revealed a hypoperfusion of the pole and the mesial temporal regions.

Patients with a right epilepsy did not display more deficits in configural processing of faces than patients with a left epilepsy. Conversely, patients with a left epilepsy had not more local face processing impairments than patients with a right TLE. Face recognition deficits were neither associated with a deficit in configural, nor in local processing of faces or geometrical patterns. It should be noted that the face recognition (FR) task was performed with very few errors by the control groups without any differences across age. In contrast, the controls' performances increased with age in the JANE and GP tasks, these two tasks appearing to be more difficult for control children than the FR task. Therefore the deficit observed in some patients in the FR task, cannot be explained by a greater difficulty of the FR task compared to the other tasks. The difficulty seen in the patients indicates that the observed deficit in face processing does not emerge from a deficit in lower level visual processing, but rather from impairment in higher levels of integration.

Surprisingly, the older the children were at first seizure, the greater was the deficit in face processing (Spearman rank correlation, $p = .002$). The older were the children at test, the greater was the deficit in face processing (Spearman rank correlation, $p = .02$). There are three possible interpretations of the correlation with the age of

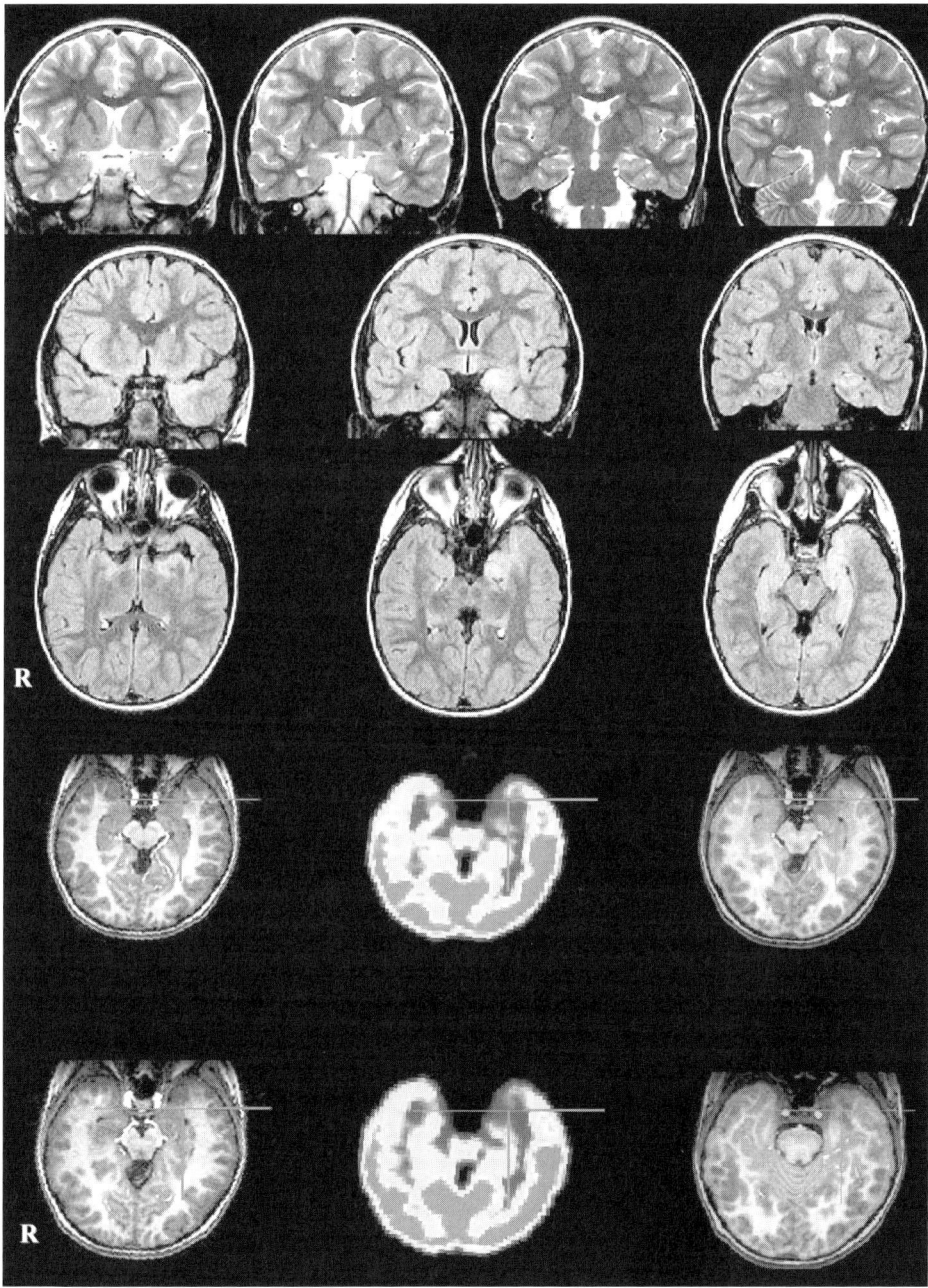

**Figure 1a and 1b.** FLAIR MRI sequences revealed a hypersignal of the left hippocampal and temporal pole regions. PET studies (FDG and $H^2O_{15}$) showed hypoperfusion and left temporal hypermetabolism mainly concerning the mesial and polar regions (from H. Zilbovicius & N. Boddaert).

the first seizure. First it might be that seizures occurring before age 5, allow better functional reorganization than seizures occurring later. Second, seizures occurring after age 5 might affect networks of a different kind than those affected by seizures occurring before age 5. Third, our results might be due to the accidental specificity of our sample.

Meletti et al. (2003) found very different results in their study of facial expression perception. They found that the deficit was greater the younger was the age of the first seizure in patients with a right epilepsy; no deficit was observed in patients with a left epilepsy. However for those patients with an early onset, it is not the age of the first seizures but the age of the first febrile seizure which was taken into consideration. Therefore it is impossible to compare the two samples. The fact that only patients with a right epilepsy showed a deficit in emotional expression perception, specifically with fear, sadness and disgust (but not, or much less frequently, for happiness and anger) might be related to connectivity with the right amygdala. Other experimental data reveal dissociation in the neural substrates of emotional expressions as well as between emotional expression and face processing. It should be reminded that perceptual categorization of emotional facial expression does not develop within the same period of time as face processing and does not rely on the same neural networks. Moreover, negative expressions do not have the same developmental timetable as positive expressions. Happiness is the expression which is perceived, discriminated and categorized the most early in life, but it is also an emotion which does not yield deficits in Meletti et al. (2003) study.

In summary, these small sets of data show that unilateral temporal epilepsy can generate deficits in a very early developing social competence, face processing, while preserving other visual competences. Given also the early development of social competences during the first years of life, it is worth investigating deficits in these domains in children with focal non-idiopathic epilepsy. It must be taken into account that the developmental timetables differ from one competence to another. Moreover plasticity might not be identical according to different kinds of competence. In this context, we are currently comparing in the same patients performances in face identity, facial emotion, gaze direction, lip reading tasks and in voice identity, emotional and prosody tasks.

Ictal and interictal activity constitute both an aggression of the neural cells and an input to the neural networks affected by these activities. Ictal and interictal activities might have an effect on the development of the social competences that rely on temporal cortex and its relationships with the limbic system. A unilateral epileptic focus might impair normal social development or at least preclude expertise acquisition in this domain.

## ■ Autism, socio-perceptual and low level visual competences

As mentionned in Zilbovicius & Meresse's chapter (this volume), recent results converge with earlier data implicating the temporal lobes in autism. Moreover socio-perceptual competences, not only theory of mind competences, are impaired in children with autism. For instance, face recognition across varying points of view was found to be more impaired than in children with Down syndrome, and control children matched for speech level, or matched for visuo-spatial performance in Ravenne Matrix (Gepner et al., 1996) showing that this normally early emerging visual capacity (see above) was impaired relatively to other abilities such as lip reading.

It is however difficult to exclude that these impairments develop from lower level processing deficits. Particularities of visual perception have been described (Shah & Frith, 1993; Jambaque et al., 1998; Bertone et al., 2003). For instance gestalt grouping principles are not used by autistic children in visual tasks (Brosnan et al., 2004). Severe insensitivity of posture to visual motion was revealed in 7 year-old autistic children compared to normal children (Gepner et al., 1995). Higher threshold for high coherence motion was also observed (Milne et al., 2002). In a recent study, autistic children had to match faces on either high- (i.e., local facial features) or low-spatial frequency information (i.e., global configuration of faces) (Deruelle et al., 2004). Contrary to the control subjects, children with autism showed better performance when using high rather than low spatial frequency, confirming low-level face-processing peculiarities in this population.

These findings suggest that perceptual particularities in children with autism are not exclusively related to temporal cortex dysfunction in biological motion and social objects perception. Some of their specificities might originate in lower level processing in occipito-temporal or/and occipito-parietal pathways. Gepner (2002) proposed that autistic children are impaired only in rapid visual-motion integration. However things might be more complex. The motion-sensitive area (V5) might not be a bottle neck for visual motion sensitivity, at least in adults. According to observation of patient LM (McLeod et al. 1996, Schenk. & Zihl, 1997; see Zilbovicius et al., this volume), perception of biological motion is possible in LM even though her sensitivity to low-level motion coherence is impaired. However, LM's ability to perceive biological motion was only partially preserved. The ventral dynamic form system might depend only partially on the dorsal motion processing in V5 (the area which is tested with task of detection of non-biological motion coherence). V5 might modulate the motion input to the ventral stream without being its sole source. As suggested by McLeod et al. (1996) and Schenk and Zihl (1997) the role of V5 might be required only when there are a number of objects with different movement characteristics in the display, so that segmentation of those elements that belong together becomes necessary. Now, it is plausible that once extracted, represented and perceptually categorised, these forms can be recognized with very poor sensitivity to non-biological motion and poor V5 activity. During development and acquisition of forms from motion, V5 might however be a necessary node. Extracting forms from motion might still require good sensitivity to non biological visual motion and modulation by V5. Therefore, if a young child has a deficit in sensitivity to visual motion, it might not be excluded that this deficit generates difficulties in extracting forms from biological visual motion. As a consequence deficit in visuo-social competences in autistic children might be due to abnormal high level integration functions of the temporal lobe as well as from abnormal low level integration functioning of V5. Nevertheless it remains that abnormalities in attention control can also be a source of abnormal sensitivity to visual displays in autistic children.

Studies of visuo- and auditory-social competences in unilateral epilepsy might help to dissociate several aspects of autistic patterns of behavior and competences.

**Acknowledgments: Supported by ACI grant from the CNRS, a grant from the French Foundation for Epilepsy Research (FFRE) and a bursary from the French League Against Epilepsy.**

# References

Adolphs R, Tranel D, Damasio H. Emotion recognition from faces and prosody following temporal lobectomy. *Neuropsychology* 2001; 15 (3): 396-404.

Anisfeld M, Turkewitz G, Rose SA, Rosenberg FR, Sheiber FJ, Couturier-Fagan DA, Ger JS, Sommer I. No compelling evidence that newborns imitate oral gestures. *Infancy* 2001; 2: 111-22.

Arzimanoglou A, Guerrini R, Aicardi J. Aicardi's *Epilepsy in Children*, 3rd edition. Philadelphia: LWW, 2004: 137-42.

Assal G, Zander E, Kremin H, Buttet J. Discrimination des voix lors des lesions du cortex cerebral. *Arch Suis Neurol Neurochir Psychiat* 1976; 119: 307-15.

Bates E, Thal D, Trauner D, Fenson J, Aram D, Eisele J, Nass R. From first words to Grammar in children with focal brain injury. *Dev Neuropsychol* 1997; 13: 275-344.

Belin P, Zatorre RJ. Adaptation to speaker's voice in right anterior temporal lobe. *Neuroreport* 2003; 14 (16): 2105-9.

Benuzzi F, Meletti S, Zamboni G, Calandra-Buonaura G, Serafini M, Lui F, et al. Impaired fear processing in right mesial temporal sclerosis: a fMRI study. *Brain Res Bull* 2004; 63 (4): 269-81.

Bertone A, Mottron L, Jelenic P, Faubert J. Motion perception in autism: a "complex" issue. *J Cogn Neurosci* 2003; 15 (2): 218-25.

Brizzolara D, Pecini C, Brovedani P, Ferretti G, Cipriani P, Cioni G. Timing and type of congenital brain lesion determine different patterns of language lateralization in hemiplegic children. *Neuropsychologia* 2002; 40: 620-32.

Brosnan MJ, Scott FJ, Fox S, Pye J. Gestalt processing in autism: failure to process perceptual relationships and the implications for contextual understanding. *J Child Psychol Psychiatry* 2004; 45 (3): 459-69.

Bushnell IWR, Sai F, Mullin JT. Neonatal recognition of the mother's face. *Brit J Dev Psychology* 1989; 7: 3-15.

Cassia VM, Turati C, Simion F. Can a nonspecific bias toward top-heavy patterns explain newborns' face preference? *Psychol Sci* 2004; 15 (6): 379-83.

Cohen M, Prather A, Town P, Hynd G. Neurodevelopmental differences in emotional prosody in normal children and children with left and right temporal lobe epilepsy. *Brain Lang* 1990; 38 (1): 122-34.

Davidson RJ, Maxwell JS, Shackman AJ. The privileged status of emotion in the brain. *Proc Natl Acad Sci USA* 2004; 101 (26): 9827-32.

Davidson RJ, Fox NA. Asymmetrical brain activity discriminates between positive and negative affective stimuli in human infants. *Science* 1982; 218 (4578): 1235-7.

Dehaene-Lambertz G, Dehaene S, Hertz-Pannier L. Functional neuroimaging of speech perception in infants. *Science* 2002; 298 (5600): 2013-5.

de Renzi E. Prosopagnosia in two patients with CT scan evidence of damage confined to the right hemisphere. *Neuropsychologia* 1986; 24 (3): 385-9.

Deruelle C, Rondan C, Gepner B, Tardif C. Spatial frequency and face processing in children with autism and Asperger syndrome. *J Autism Dev Disord* 2004; 34 (2): 199-210.

Deruelle C, de Schonen S. Hemispheric asymmetries in visual pattern processing in infancy. *Brain Cogn* 1991; 16 (2): 151-79.

Deruelle C, de Schonen S. Pattern processing in infancy: hemispheric differences in the processing of shape and location of visual components. *Inf Behav Dev* 1995; 18 (2): 123-32.

Deruelle C, de Schonen S. Do the right and the left hemispheres attend to the same visuo-spatial information within a face in infancy? *Dev Neuropsy* 1998; 14: 535-54.

Eimas PD. Auditory and linguistic processing of cues for place of articulation by infants. *Percept Psychophys* 1974; 16 (3): 513-21.

Eimas PD, Siqueland ER, Jusczyk P, Vigorito J. Speech perception in infants. *Science* 1971; 171: 303-6.

Farroni T, Csibra G, Simion F, Johnson MH. Eye contact detection in humans from birth. *Proc Natl Acad Sci* 2002; 99 (14): 9602-5.

Farroni T, Mansfield EM, Lai C, Johnson MH. Infants perceiving and acting on the eyes: tests of an evolutionary hypothesis. *J Exp Child Psychol* 2003; 85 (3): 199-212.

Field TM, Woodson R, Greenberg R, Cohen D. Discrimination and imitation of facial expression by neonates. *Science* 1982; 218 (4568): 179-81.

Fontaine, R. Imitative skills between birth and 6 months. *Inf Beha Dev* 1984; 7: 323-33.

Gauthier I, Tarr MJ, Anderson AW, Skudlarski P, Gore JC. Activation of the middle fusiform "face area" increases with expertise in recognizing novel objects. *Nat Neurosci* 1999; 2 (6): 568-73.

George MS, Parekh PI, Rosinsky N, Ketter TA, Kimbrell TA, Heilman KM, Herscovitch P, Post RM. Understanding emotional prosody activates right hemisphere regions. *Arch Neurol* 1996; 53: 665-70.

Gepner B, de Gelder B, de Schonen S. Face processing in autistic children: a generalized deficit? *Child Neuropsychology* 1996; 2: 1-17.

Gepner B, Masson G. Rapid visual-motion integration deficit in autism. *Trends Cogn Sci* 2002; 6 (11): 455.

Gepner B, Mestre D, Masson G, de Schonen S. Postural effects of motion vision in young autistic children. *Neuroreport* 1995; 6 (8): 1211-4.

Grandjean D, Sander D, Pourtois G, Schwartz S, Seghier ML, Scherer KR, Vuilleumier P. The voices of wrath: brain responses to angry prosody in meaningless speech. *Nat Neurosci* 2005; 8 (2): 145-6.

Goren CC, Sarty M, Wu PY. Visual following and pattern discrimination of face-like stimuli by newborn infants. *Pediatrics* 1975; 56 (4): 544-9.

Hadjikhani N, de Gelder B. Neural basis of prosopagnosia: an fMRI study. *Hum Brain Mapp* 2002; 16 (3): 176-82.

Halit H, Csibra G, Volein A, Johnson MH. Face-sensitive cortical processing in early infancy. *J Child Psychol Psychiatry* 2004; 45 (7): 1228-34.

Haxby JV, Hoffman EA, Gobbini MI. The distributed human neural system for face perception. *Trends Cogn Sci* 2000; 4 (6): 223-33.

Hecaen H, Angelergues R. Agnosia for faces (prosopagnosia). *Arch Neurol* 1962; 7: 92-100.

Hertz-Pannier L, Chiron C, Jambaque I, Renaux-Kieffer V, Van de Moortele PF, Delalande O, Fohlen M, Brunelle F, Le Bihan D. Late plasticity for language in a child's non-dominant hemisphere: a pre- and post-surgery fMRI study. *Brain* 2002; 125: 361-72.

Hoffman EA, Haxby JV. Distinct representations of eye gaze and identity in the distributed human neural system for face perception. *Nat Neurosci* 2000; 3 (1): 80-4.

Hood B. Shifts of visual attention in the human infant: A neuroscientific approach. In: Rovee-Collier C, Lipsitt L, ed. *Advances in infancy research 9*. Ablex: Norwood NJ, 1995: 000.

Hood BM, Willen JD, Driver J. Adult's eyes trigger shifts of visual attention in human infants. *Psychol Sci* 1998; 9: 53-6.

Imaizumi S, Mori K, Kiritani S, Kawashima R, Sugiura M, Fukuda H, et al. Vocal identification of speaker and emotion activates different brain regions. *Neuroreport* 1997; 8 (12): 2809-12.

Jambaque I, Mottron L, Ponsot G, Chiron C. Autism and visual agnosia in a child with right occipital lobectomy. *J Neurol Neurosurg Psychiatry* 1998; 65 (4): 555-60.

Johnson MH, Dziurawiec S, Ellis H, Morton J. Newborns' preferential tracking of face-like stimuli and its subsequent decline. *Cognition* 1991; 40 (1-2): 1-19.

Kanwisher N, Mc Dermott J, Chun MM. The fusiform face area: a module in human extrastriate cortex specialized for face perception. *J Neurosci* 1997; 17 (11): 4302-11.

Kisilevsky BS, Hains SM, Lee K, Xie X, Huang H, Ye HH, Zhang K, Wang Z. Effects of experience on fetal voice recognition. *Psychol sci* 2003; 14 (3): 220-4.

Kucharska-Pietura K, Phillips ML, Gernand W, David AS. Perception of emotions from faces and voices following unilateral brain damage. *Neuropsychologia* 2003; 41 (8): 1082-90.

Kuhl PK. Early language acquisition: cracking the speech code. *Nat Rev Neurosci* 2004; 5 (11): 831-43

Kuhl PK, Tsao FM, Liu HM, Zhang Y, De Boer B. Language/culture/mind/brain. Progress at the margins between disciplines. *Ann N Y Acad Sci* 2001; 935: 136-74.

Kujala A, Huotilainen M, Hotakainen M, Lennes M, Parkkonen L, Fellman V, Naatanen R. Speech-sound discrimination in neonates as measured with MEG. *Neuroreport* 2004; 15 (13): 2089-92.

Le Grand R, Mondloch CJ, Maurer D, Brent HP. Expert face processing requires visual input to the right hemisphere during infancy. *Nat Neurosci* 2003; 6 (12): 1329.

Liegeois F, Connelly A, Cross JH, Boyd SG, Gadian DG, Vargha-Khadem F, Baldeweg T. Language reorganization in children with early-onset lesions of the left hemisphere: an fMRI study. *Brain* 2004; 127: 1229-36.

McCarthy G, Puce A, Gore JC, Allison T. Face specific processing in the human fusiform gyrus. *J Cogn Neurosci* 1997; 9: 605-10.

McLeod P, Dittrich W, Driver J, Perrett D, Zihl J. Preserved and impaired detection of structure from motion by "motion-blind" patient. *Vis Cog* 1996; (4): 363-91.

McNeil JE, Warrington EK. Prosopagnosia: a face-specific disorder. *Q J Exp Psychol A* 1993; A46 (1): 1-10.

Mancini J, de Schonen S, Deruelle C, Massoulier A. Face recognition in children with early right or left brain damage. *Dev Med Child Neurol* 1994; 36 (2): 156-66.

Meletti S, Benuzzi F, Rubboli G, Cantalupo G, Stanzani Maserati M, Nichelli P, Tassinari CA. Impaired facial emotion recognition in early-onset right mesial temporal lobe epilepsy. *Neurology* 2003; 60 (3): 426-31.

Meltzoff AN, Moore MK. Newborn infants imitate adult facial gestures. *Child Dev* 1983; 54 (3): 702-9.

Milne E, Swettenham J, Hansen P, Campbell R, Jeffries H, Plaisted K. High motion coherence thresholds in children with autism. *J Child Psychol Psychiatry* 2002; 43 (2): 255-63.

Morris JS, Dolan RJ. Dissociable amygdala and orbitofrontal responses during reversal fear conditioning. *Neuroimage* 2004; 22 (1): 372-80.

Morris JS, Ohman A, Dolan RJ. Conscious and unconscious emotional learning in the human amygdala. *Nature* 1998; 393 (6684): 467-70.

Muir DW, Hains SMJ. Infant sensititivity to perturbations in adult facial, vocal, tactile and contingent stimulation during face-to-face interactions. In: de Boysson-Bardies B, de Schonen S, Juszyk P, Mac-Neilage P, Morton J, ed. *Developmental neurocognition: Speech and face processing in the first year of life.* Dordrecht: Kluwer, 1993: 171-85.

Nelson CA, De Haan M. Neural correlates of infants' visual responsiveness to facial expressions of emotion. *Dev Psychobiol* 1996; 29 (7): 577-95.

Pascalis O, de Haan M, Nelson CA, de Schonen S. Long-term recognition memory for faces assessed by visual paired comparison in 3- and 6-month-old infants. *J Exp Psychol Learn Mem Cogn* 1998; 24 (1): 249-60.

Pascalis O, de Schonen S. Recognition memory in 3-4-day old human infants. *Neuroreport* 1994; 5: 1721-4.

Pascalis O, de Schonen S, Morton J, Deruelle C, Fabre-Grenet M. Mother's face recognition by neonates: a replication and an extension. *Inf Behav Dev* 1995; 18: 79-85.

Phillips AT, Wellman HM & Spelke ES. Infants' ability to connect gaze and emotional expression to intentional action. *Cognition* 2002; 85 (1): 53-78.

Rama P, Courtney SM. Functional topography of working memory for face or voice identity. *Neuroimage* 2005; 24 (1): 224-34.

Reilly J, Bates EA, Marchman VA. Narative discourse in children with early focal brain injury. *Brain Lang* 1998; 61: 335-75.

Rossion B, Caldara R, Seghier M, Schuller AM, Lazeyras F, Mayer E. A network of occipito-temporal face-sensitive areas besides the right middle fusiform gyrus is necessary for normal face processing. *Brain* 2003; 126: 81-95.

Rossion B, Dricot L, Devolder A, Bodart JM, Crommelinck M, De Gelder B, Zoontjes R. Hemispheric asymmetries for whole-based and part-based face processing in the human fusiform gyrus. *J Cogn Neurosci* 2000; 12: 793-802.

Sangrigoli S, de Schonen S. Recognition of own-race and other-race faces by three-month-old infants. *J Child Psychol Psychiatry* 2004; 45 (7): 1219-27.

Sato W, Kochiyama T, Yoshikawa S, Naito E, Matsumura M. Enhanced neural activity in response to dynamic facial expressions of emotion: an fMRI study. *Brain Res Cogn Brain Res* 2004; 20 (1): 81-91.

Sato W, Yoshikawa S, Kochiyama T, Matsumura M. The amygdala processes the emotional significance of facial expressions: an fMRI investigation using the interaction between expression and face direction. *Neuroimage* 2004; 22 (2): 1006-13.

Schenk T, Zihl, J. Visual motion perception after brain damage: II. Deficits in form-from perception. *Neuropsychologia* 1997; 35: 1299-310.

de Schonen S. Epigenesis of the Cognitive Brain: a task for the XXI century. In: Bäckman L, von Hofsten C, eds. *Psychology at the term of the millenium*, vol. 1. Hove: Psychology Press, 2002: 55-89.

de Schonen S, Mancini J, Camps R, Maes E, Laurent A. Early brain lesions and face processing development. *Developmental Psychobio* 2005; 46 (3): 184-208

de Schonen S, Mancini J, Liegeois F. About functional cortical specialization: The development of face recognition. In: Simion F, Butterworth G, ed. *The development of sensory, motor and cognitive capacities in early infancy*: Hove, UK: Psychology Press, 1998: 103-16.

de Schonen S, Mathivet E. Hemispheric asymmetry in a face discrimination task in infants. *Child Dev* 1990; 61 (4): 1192-205.

Shah A, Frith U. Why do autistic individuals show superior performance on the block disgn task? *J Ch Psychol Psych* 1993; 34: 1351-64.

Stiles J, Mose P, Roe K, Akshoomoff NA, Trauner D, Hesselink J, *et al*. Alternative brain organization after prenatal cerebral injury: convergent fMRI and cognitive data. *J Int Neuropsychol Soc* 2003; 9: 604-22.

Stiles J, Thal D. Linguistic and spatial cognitive development following early focal brain injury: Patterns of deficit and recovery. In: Johnson M, ed. *Brain Development and Cognition Cambridge*. MA: Blackwell, 1993: 643-64.

Stiles J, Trauner D, Engel M, Nass R. The development of drawing in children with congenital focal brain injury: evidence for limited functional recovery. *Neuropsychologia* 1997; 35: 299-312.

Streit M, Ioannides AA, Liu L, Wolwer W, Dammers J, Gross J, *et al*. Neurophysiological correlates of the recognition of facial expressions of emotion as revealed by magnetoencephalography. *Brain Res Cogn Brain Res* 1999; 7: 481-91.

Thuillard F, Assal G. The relationship of the right hemisphere in voice recognition. *Rev Med Suisse Romande* 1983; 103 (4): 311-3.

Tincoff R, Hauser M, Tsao F, Spaepen G, Ramus F, Mehler J. The role of speech rhythm in language discrimination: further tests with a non-human primate. *Dev Sci* 2005; 8 (1): 26-35.

Turati C, Sangrigoli S, Ruel J, de Schonen S. Is the face-inversion effect present at 4 months of age? *Infancy* 2004; 6: 2.

Turati C, Simion F, Milani I, Umilta C. Newborns' preference for faces: what is crucial? *Dev Psychol* 2002; 38 (6): 875-82.

Turati C, Valenza E, Leo I, Simion F. Three-month-olds' visual preference for faces and its underlying visual processing mechanisms. *J Exp Child Psychol* 2005; 90 (3): 255-73.

Tzourio-Mazoyer N, de Schonen S, Crivello F, Quinton O, Reutter B, Aujard Y, Mazoyer B. Neural correlates of woman face processing by 2-month-olds infants. *Neuroimage* 2002; 15 (2): 454-61.

Wicker B, Michel F, Henaff MA, Decety J. Brain regions involved in the perception of gaze: a PET study. *Neuroimage* 1998; 8 (2): 221-7.

Wildgruber D, Pihan H, Ackermann H, Erb M, Grodd W. Dynamic brain activation during processing of emotional intonation: influence of acoustic parameters, emotional valence, and sex. *Neuroimage* 2002; 15 (4): 856-69.

Winston JS, Henson RN, Fine-Goulden MR, Dolan RJ. fMRI-adaptation reveals dissociable neural representations of identity and expression in face perception. *J Neurophysiol* 2004; 92 (3): 1830-9.

Yamada M, Murai T, Sato W, Namiki C, Miyamoto T, Ohigashi Y. Emotion recognition from facial expressions in temporal lobe epileptic patient with ictal fear. *Neuropsychologia* 2005; 43: 434-41.

# Autism spectrum disorder in children with temporal lobe epilepsy

**J.H. Cross, A. McLellan, S. Davies, I. Heyman**

*Institute of Child Health & Great Ormond Street Hospital for Children NHS Trust, London, UK*

---

Children with epilepsy have high rates of emotional and behavioural difficulty, when compared with healthy controls and children with other chronic disorders. This comorbidity is important for a variety of reasons, not least because the additional disability conferred by mental health problems contributes significantly to the impairment experienced by the child with epilepsy and their family. In many patients these behavioural difficulties go unrecognised in the standard clinic setting (Davies et al., 2003; Rutter et al., 1970). Children with temporal lobe epilepsy appear to be particularly at risk. However it is difficult to determine whether this is because of specific brain behaviour links or whether they simply present for study more frequently.

## ■ Evidence of behaviour disorder in epilepsy

In the Isle of Wight study, Rutter, Graham and Yule (1970) reported that 29% of the 63 children with uncomplicated epilepsy had a psychiatric disorder relative to 12% of the 138 children with chronic but non-neurological disorders (Rutter et al., 1970). A more recent study has followed up children with either epilepsy or asthma, over a four year period (Austin et al., 2000). Children with epilepsy had approximately twice the risk of children with asthma of obtaining behavioural problems in the "at-risk" range, both at baseline (57% vs 32%; p = 0.001) and follow-up (49% vs 24%; p = 0.001). Data from the 1999 British Child Mental Health Survey (reviewing rates of psychiatric disorder in 5-15 year olds) not only confirmed the high prevalence rates of behaviour disorder in children with epilepsy relative to other chronic conditions (27.9% vs 10.6% with diabetes) but also showed a higher prevalence in children with epilepsy with additional neurological disorder compared to less complex epilepsy, with higher rates of ADHD, pervasive developmental disorder as well as severe learning difficulty (Davies et al., 2003).

There are clinical reports suggesting that children with focal seizures are more prone to mental health problems; perhaps particularly so in temporal lobe epilepsy (TLE) although direct comparative studies with extratemporal epilepsy are not available. In the Oxford longitudinal study of 100 children with TLE only 15% were free of psychological problems with 50% experiencing catastrophic rage attacks, hyperkinesis or a combination of the two (Ounsted et al., 1995) Interestingly, in a direct comparative study of children with complex partial seizures and primary generalised epilepsy (exact focus not defined – temporal or frontal), high rates of mental health problems were found in both groups with no significant difference between the two – but the rates were significantly higher than the control group (Ott et al., 2003). For a detailed review see also the chapter by Dunn and Kronenberger.

## Understanding brain-behaviour links

Study of psychopathology in the child with epilepsy may also help explain mechanisms that link brain abnormalities with behavioural change. At the most general level, there is evidence that the high rates of psychopathology in epilepsy are linked to the brain disorder itself and are not simply a function of a chronic disorder. Evidence for this includes higher rates in those children with more severe brain disorders (structural abnormalities) and average rates of psychiatric disorder in children who have other chronic illness which does not primarily affect the brain, such as diabetes. If studied, it can be demonstrated that psychopathology may be seen at onset of the epilepsy (Austin et al., 2001; Oostrom et al., 2003). However, brain-behaviour relationships in epilepsy have multiple interacting variables. For example type/location/lateralisation of any brain lesion, timing of seizure onset developmentally, ongoing seizure type/severity, may all be related to the type and severity of psychopathology. When epilepsy arises as the result of a focal structural lesion it might be presumed that removal of the lesion and consequent seizure control should lead to improvement in any associated behavioural comorbidity. Studies increasingly reveal that such assumptions cannot be made.

## ■ Temporal lobe lesions in epilepsy and psychopathology

Individuals with temporal lobe epilepsy have been central to the study of brain-behaviour links in epilepsy. These patients present unique opportunities for the study of psychopathology, as temporal lobe epilepsy in adulthood is the most common form of epilepsy that comes to resective surgery. Both seizure localisation and underlying pathology have been well characterised, with seizures arising from the mesial temporal lobe being most common, and mesial temporal sclerosis being the most likely pathology. Postoperative psychiatric disturbance in a small but significant proportion is well described (Stevens, 1990; Taylor, 1972). In children with temporal lobe epilepsy, the underlying pathology may be more variable. Mesial temporal sclerosis causes a proportion of cases, but malformations of cortical development and developmental tumours are more common and may be associated with more variable clinical manifestations. Not only may it be difficult to determine the existence of focal seizures, but also their lobe of origin. However, detecting and characterising behaviour disorder in childhood temporal lobe epilepsy is important both for surgical and non surgical candidates, both for consideration of aetiology, treatment options and prognosis.

Adult studies reveal that between 29-89% of individuals with epilepsy considered for temporal lobe resection have a history of psychiatric disorder (Stevens, 1990; Taylor, 1972). The most common diagnoses in this group are emotional disorders (Glosser et al., 2000; Victoroff, 1994). Postoperatively some improve but others deteriorate with the emergence of new psychiatric diagnoses in some. Some studies suggest that acquisition of seizure freedom post-operatively is associated with favourable psychiatric outcome (Blumer et al., 1998). Prospective long term outcome data however are lacking; cross-sectional data are often used and direct comparative studies are not appropriate over time.

In many described paediatric surgical series, temporal lobe resections, particularly for mesial temporal sclerosis are in the minority, with hemispherectomies and multilobar/extratemporal resections being more common (Mathern et al., 1999; Morrison et al., 1992). More recently it has become apparent that mesial temporal sclerosis is not exclusively an adult disease; community based and surgical series reveal a similar prevalence in children and adults (Cascino et al., 1992; Cross et al., 1993; Grattan Smith et al., 1993; Kuzniecky et al., 1993). However, psychiatric comorbidity has remained under- reported; indeed in one series of 17 children coming to surgery for hippocampal sclerosis under the age of 12 years, no child was reported to have developmental delay or mental retardation (Mohamed et al., 2001). This would be inconsistent with more recent studies where child-specific developmental and psychiatric assessments have been used as part of the pre-surgical evaluation, and reveal high rates of both developmental and psychiatric difficulty.

Not all children with temporal lobe epilepsy undergo surgery. Psychiatric disorder has been less studied in non-surgical series so the prevalence of psychopathology with idiopathic forms is unknown – we are only aware that continuing epilepsy per se is associated with a higher likelihood of behaviour disorder (Austin et al., 1992). As indicated above, the Oxford longitudinal study of 100 children with TLE reported high rates of behaviour disorder (Ounsted et al., 1995). It has to be considered, though that in this study the range of associated pathology/comorbidities was wide, and it is unclear how many of the idiopathic syndromes were included as opposed to the symptomatic epilepsies. Nonetheless this study gives a useful insight into the range of psychiatric comorbidities seen in paediatric TLE.

Attempts to look more specifically at sub-types of psychiatric disorder in relation to lesion/seizure localisation, include a recent study of five children undergoing epilepsy surgery (Szabo et al., 1999). These children all had temporal lobe lesions, four of which were on the right-side of the brain, and all children had pervasive developmental disorder. The aim of the paper was to report on the outcome of PDD in a surgical series; four children were seizure free at follow-up, one child had a deterioration in her PDD. Neville et al. (1997) also reported two children who had focal epilepsy associated with social and language regression and who showed partial recovery after surgical treatment (Neville et al., 1997). Daniellsson and colleagues (2002) subsequently reviewed the psychopathology in 16 children undergoing surgery for temporal lobe epilepsy; 12 had a psychiatric diagnosis, 5 of whom had autistic spectrum disorder (ASD). Of the 5 with ASD, only one became seizure free, and all remained autistic postoperatively, but a positive change in behaviour was noted in 3; they became calmer, less aggressive and less hyperactive.

A retrospective case note review of 60 children who underwent temporal lobe resection for epilepsy, revealed DSM-IV psychiatric diagnoses in 83% of the cases at some time pre or postoperatively (McLellan et al., 2005). This was a group of children that had undergone surgery at a mean age of 10 year and 5 months (range 1-18 year) and had a mean length of follow up of 5 year and 2 months; 53% had a cognitive ability within the normal range. The type of underlying pathology varied: 33 patients with hippocampal sclerosis; 22 with foreign tissue lesion; 7 with malformation of cortical development; 5 with other pathology. At follow up 60% were seizure free and a further 5% had rare seizures. In this group of children one or more psychiatric diagnoses were present in 72% children preoperatively and 72% children postoperatively. In 16% mental health problems completely resolved following surgery, but in 12%, who had been free of a diagnosis preoperatively, psychopathology emerged post-operatively. Diagnoses included pervasive developmental disorder (38% preop, 37% postop), Attention Deficit-Hyperactivity Disorder (23% preoperatively and postoperatively), oppositional defiant disorder/conduct disorder (22% preop, 21% postop), emotional disorder (8% preop and 21% postop), disruptive behaviour disorder (40% preoperatively, 42% postoperatively), eating disorder 4%, conversion disorder 4% and psychosis in 2%. Many had two or more diagnoses; 45% preoperatively and 57% postoperatively. There was no clear relationship between seizure freedom postoperatively and any psychiatric disorder, though children who were seizure free were more likely to lose a diagnosis (24%) than those who continued to have seizures (4%). No relationship was seen with type of pathology or medication. The only possible relationship to cognitive ability was seen in those with emotional disorders, which were more common in children with a normal-range IQ.

## Pervasive developmental disorder and epilepsy – associations or causal links?

The striking aspect of the group reported as a whole (McLellan et al., 2005) was the relatively high number of children with a diagnosis of pervasive developmental disorder (23/60) nine of whom had autistic disorder, two Asperger's syndrome and 11 PDD not otherwise specified (PDD-NOS). When compared to the group of children who did not have this diagnosis, PDD was significantly associated with younger age at seizure onset (1.75 years in PDD; 0.75 yr in AD) compared with 4.49 years in non-PDD) and right sided lesions ($p < 0.05$), confirming findings from previous studies (Neville et al., 1997; Szabo et al., 1999). There was no clear association with underlying pathology; autism spectrum disorders occurred equally frequently in children with either hippocampal sclerosis (HS) or foreign tissue lesions. In children with HS and PDD however, seizure outcome was significantly worse than in HS without PDD (43% vs 70% seizure free). One of the features of this sample of children with epilepsy and autistic spectrum disorders, was the large proportion which could only be classified PDD-NOS. By definition these children did not meet full criteria for classical or core autism, usually because they lacked one of the three core features of delayed/deviant language, social aloofness and repetitive/stereotyped behaviours. It was not established whether there was a relationship between the presence or absence of PDD and seizure semiology, the presence or absence of secondary generalisation, (suggesting wider spread outside the temporal lobe) or differences in areas of involvement on EEG between PDD and non-PDD groups. There was no difference in sleep recordings between the two groups.

The relationship between pervasive developmental disorder and epilepsy remains a subject of research and debate. In "idiopathic" autism, 30% of children are reported to develop epilepsy, and a further 30% have epileptiform activity on the EEG. Usually the diagnosis of autism precedes the diagnosis of epilepsy, but it remains unknown whether seizures or underlying EEG abnormalities might contribute to the development of the autistic phenotype, or whether treatment may improve autistic symptoms. Is it ever the case that the onset of epilepsy triggers autistic regression? Does epilepsy have a role in those who present with autistic spectrum disorder? And if there is any relationship, particularly in those children presenting with lesional epilepsy, is it reversible or even preventable?

The possibility of a link between autism and epilepsy arises from apparent clinical presentation of some of the epileptic encephalopathies, which may present with cognitive and/or language regression in association with the onset of catastrophic epilepsy. The term implies that the functional deficits seen are potentially reversible as they are presumed attributable to epileptiform activity. Examples of this include the syndrome of Continuous Spike Wave of Slow Sleep, Llandau Kleffner syndrome and infantile spasms. "Autistic regression" may be defined as a regression in social and communication skills with the emergence of stereotyped behaviours; such regression however is only seen in about one third of children diagnosed as "classic" autism (Tuchman and Rapin, 1997). On the other hand individuals with autism may present with epilepsy. There is a bimodal distribution of presentation; under the age of five (Volkmar and Nelson, 1990) and in adolescence (Gionvanardi-Rossi et al., 2000). With a higher the proportion of older children included in the sample an increasing prevalence of epilepsy is seen in populations or children with autism (Gionvanardi-Rossi et al., 2000; Wong, 1993). A larger proportion of such individuals may have epileptiform activity in the EEG (up to 46%). Nonetheless, the role of aetiology of autism remains unclear in many of the children (Tuchman et al., 1997). It is likely however that although features of autistic spectrum disorder are seen in the epileptic encephalopathies, the relationship is complex and the specific phenotypes nonidentical. The presence of autism with epilepsy as a cause without antecedant definitive seizures appears unlikely. The group of children with PDD within the surgical temporal lobe series showed a high rate of learning difficulty, and lower rate of seizure freedom following surgery than children without PDD (McLellan et al., 2005). This may suggest more widespread pathology, although a more pervasive effect of the seizure disorder at a time of early development cannot be excluded.

It is difficult to separate the effect of mental retardation, and whether this is related to the PDD or cause of the epilepsy. A recent meta-analysis of studies demonstrated no difference in prevalence of epilepsy between the normal population and groups with high-functioning autism (normal range IQ), whereas children with lower IQs and autism had higher rates of epilepsy (L Mottron, personal communication). This suggests that epilepsy may not be specifically associated with the autistic phenotype, but rather may be linked to the underlying aetiology, and subsequent brain disorder which results in both mental retardation, epilepsy and autism. Delong (1999) and others suggest that there may be different routes into autism, and propose that two groups of children might be defined. One group acquires autism in association with temporal lobe pathology, and tends to have more mental retardation, the other group are proposed to be more genetically determined to develop autism and are higher-functioning. There is some support from other studies of temporal lobe pathology being associated with the risk for autism. Bolton and colleagues have examined the possible risk factors for the development of autism in the context of tuberous sclerosis (Bolton et al., 2002). In this prospective study of 19 children with tuberous sclerosis an association between autistic spectrum disorder and tubers was demonstrated in the temporal lobe associated also with temporal lobe epileptiform activity on the EEG, and early onset seizures (< 3 years) (Bolton et al., 2002) However, tubers in the temporal neocortex in isolation did not support the association. Neither the number of tubers present or location within the superior temporal gyrus predicted outcome.

## PDD in TLE – aetiology and the possible effect of surgery

We have reported that children with temporal lobe epilepsy who undergo surgical resection have high rates of PDD when assessed in the preoperative period. These rates are much higher than general population rates of autistic disorder, but causal mechanisms remain unclear. Attempts at defining specific associations point to a a relationship between PDD and right temporal pathology, and also with early onset epilepsy. What is cause and what is effect are more difficult questions to answer. There is no evidence that children with the combination of surgically amenable temporal lobe epilepsy, and PDD have any additional surgical risks, and indeed many will benefit from improved seizure control. The autistic symptoms in this group are often a source of significant impairment and distress to children and families, but it remains unclear whether successful epilepsy surgery has the potential to alter the course of the autistic disorder, or reverse it. The assumption is that the development of the psychopathology is related to the development of the epilepsy in association with the brain pathology.

Current knowledge can only emphasise the high rates of psychopathology in children with TLE undergoing epilepsy surgery, the need to identify this, counsel children and families, and provide management for emotional and behavioural problems along side epilepsy treatments. Study of specific psychiatric subgroups, and their response to surgery may help establish associations between age of onset of seizures, lateralisation of pathology, and specific phenotypes of psychiatric disorder. The relatively small numbers of children studied in epilepsy surgery programs, the lack of prospective psychiatric evaluation and the heterogeneity of samples all make it difficult to predict the effects of surgery on psychiatric outcome. Further study is required to determine directions of effect, and likely predictors of longer term benefit.

## References

Commission on Classification and Terminology of the International League Against Epilepsy. Proposal for revised classification of epilepsies and epileptic syndromes. *Epilepsia* 1989; 30: 389-99.

Austin JK, Dunn DW, HusterGA. Childhood Epilepsy and Asthma: Changes in behaviour problems related to gender and change in condition severity. *Epilepsia* 2000; 41: 615-23.

Austin JK, Harezlak J, Dunn DW. Behavior problems in children befor recognized seizures. *Pediatrics* 2001; 107: 115-22.

Austin JK, Risinger MW, Beckett LA. Correlates of behavior problems in children with epilepsy. *Epilepsia* 1992; 33: 1115-22.

Blumer D, Wakhlu S, Davies K, Hermann B. Psychiatric outcome of temporal lobectomy for epilepsy:incidence and treatment of psychiatric complications. *Epilepsia* 1998; 39: 478-80.

Bolton PF, Park RJ, Higgins NP, Griffiths PD, Pickles A. Neuroepileptic determinants of autistic spectrum disorder in tuberous sclerosis complex. *Brain* 2002; 125: 1247-55.

Cascino GD, Jack CR, Jr, Parisi JE, Marsh WR, Kelly PJ, Sharbrough FW, Hirschorn KA, Trenerry MR. MRI in the presurgical evaluation of patients with frontal lobe epilepsy and children with temporal lobe epilepsy: pathologic correlation and prognostic importance. *Epilepsy Res* 1992; 11: 51-9.

Cross JH, Jackson GD, Neville BGR, Connelly A, Kirkham FJ, Boyd SG, et al. Early detection of abnormalities in partial epilepsy using magnetic resonance. *Arch Dis Child* 1993; 69: 104-9.

Danielsson S, Rydenhag B, Uvebrant P, Nordborg C, Olsson I. Temporal lobe resections in children with epilepsy: neuropsychiatric status in relation to neuropathology and seizure outcome. *Epilepsy and Behaviour* 2002; 3: 76-81.

Davies S, Heyman I, Goodman R. A population survey of mental health problems in children with epilepsy. *Dev Med Child Neurol* 2003; 4: 292-5.

DeLong GR. Autism: New data suggest a new hypothesis. *Neurology* 1999; 52: 911-6.

Gionvanardi-Rossi P, Posar A, Parmeggiani A. Epilepsy in adolescents and young adults with autistic disorder. *Brain Dev* 2000; 2229: 102-6.

Glosser G, Zwil AS, Glosser DS, O'Conner MJ, Sperling M. Psychiatric aspects of temporal lobe epilepsy before and after anterior lobectomy. *J Neurol Neurosurg Psychiatry* 2000; 68: 53-8.

Grattan Smith JD, Harvey AS, Desmond PM, Chow CW. Hippocampal sclerosis in children with intractable temporal lobe epilepsy: detection with MR imaging. *AJR Am J Roentgenol* 1993; 161: 1045-8.

Kuzniecky R, Murro A, King D, Morawetz R, Smith J, Powers R, et al. Magnetic resonance imaging in childhood intractable partial epilepsies: pathologic correlations. *Neurology* 1993; 43: 681-7.

Mathern GW, Giza CC, Yudovin S, Vinters H, Peacock WJ, Shewmon A, Shields WD. Postoperative seizure control and antiepileptic drug use in pediatric epilepsy surgery patients: The UCLA experience, 1986-1997. *Epilepsia* 1999; 40: 1740-9.

McLellan A, Davies S, Heyman I, Harding B, Harkness W, Taylor D, et al. Psychopathology in children undergoing temporal lobe resection for the treatment of epilepsy – a pre and post-operative assessment. *Dev Med Child Neurol* 2005 In press.

Mohamed A, Wyllie E, Ruggieri PM, Kotagal P, Babb T, Hilbig A., et al. Temporal lobe epilepsy due to hippocampal sclerosis in pediatric cnadidates for epilepsy surgery. *Neurology* 2001; 56: 1643-9.

Morrison G, Duchowny M, Resnick T, Alvarez L, Jayakar P, Prats AR, Dean P, Penate M. Epilepsy surgery in childhood. A report of 79 patients. *Pediatr Neurosurg* 1992; 18: 291-7.

Neville BGR, Harkness WF, Cross JH, et al. Surgical treatment of severe autistic regression in childhood. *Pediatr Neurol* 1997; 16: 137-40.

Oostrom KJ, Schouten A, Kruitwagen CL, Peters AC, Jennekens-Schinkel A. Behavoral problems in children with newly diagnosed idiopathic or cryptogenic epilepsy attending normal schools are in majority not persistent. *Epilepsia* 2003; 44: 97-106.

Ott D, Siddarth P, Gurbani S, Koh S, Tournay A, Shields WD, Caplan R. Behavioral Disorders in Pediatric Epilepsy: Unmet Psychiatric Need. *Epilepsia* 2003; 44: 591-7.

Ounsted C, Lindsay J, Richards P. *Temporal Lobe Epilepsy 1948-1986: A Biographical Study*. Oxford: MacKeith Press, 1995: 1-129.

Rutter M, Graham P, Yule W. *A neuropsychiatric study in childhood. Clinics in Developmental Medicine*. 35 ed. Heinemann Medical, London, 1970.

Stevens JR. Psychiatric consequences of temporal lobectomy for intractable seizures: a 20-30-year follow-up of 14 cases. *Psychol Med* 1990; 20: 529-45.

Szabo CA, Wyllie E, Dolske M, Stanford L, Kotagal P, Comair Y. Epilepsy Surgery in Children With Pervasive Developmental Disorder. *Pediatr Neurol* 1999; 20: 349-53.

Taylor DC. Mental state and temporal lobe epilepsy. A correlative account of 100 patients treated surgically. *Epilepsia* 1972; 13: 727-65.

Tuchman RF, Jayakar P, Yayali I, Villalobos R. Seizures and EEG findings in children with autism spectrum disorders. *CNS Spectrums* 1997; 3: 61-70.

Tuchman RF, Rapin I. Regression in pervasive developmental disorders: seizures and epileptiform electroencephalogram correlates. *Pediatrics* 1997; 99: 560-6.

Victoroff JI. DSM-III-R psychiatric diagnosies in candidates for epilepsy surgery: lifetime prevalence. Neuropsychiatry, Neuropsychology and Behavioural. *Neurology* 1994; 7: 87-97.

Volkmar FR, Nelson DS. Seizure disorders in autism. *J Am Acad Child Adolesc Psychiatry* 1990; 29: 127-9.

Wong V. Epilepsy in children with autistic spectrum disorder. *J Child Neurol* 1993; 8: 316-22.

# Temporal lobe and social abilities

M. Zilbovicius, I. Meresse

*ERM0205, INSERM-CEA, Service hospitalier Fréderic-Joliot, Orsay, France*

## ■ Temporal lobe and social interactions. An introduction

The temporal lobe has been implicated in both object and face perception as well as social behavior. The picture that is emerging from human and monkey studies is that representations of features of the outside social world are first assembled in the temporal lobe cortices of the primate brain (for a review see Allison et al., 2000).

Meaningful social events are registered when a host of signals and relevant contextual information are integrated. For example, the movements of the faces and bodies provide stimuli of considerable interest to the social primate. Studies of single cells, field potential recordings and functional neuroimaging data indicate that specialized visual mechanisms exist in the superior temporal sulcus (STS) of both human and non-human primates that produce selective neural responses to moving natural images of faces and bodies. These seem to have developed out of a necessity to differentiate between someone approaching with friendly or hostile intent. The visual features of a face have to be assembled into an image of a particular individual so that past interactions with this individual can be recalled. Next, movements of the eyes and mouth indicate the person's disposition. Information about head position and body movement tells where the person is looking or going, thus providing the raw material for the representation of a mental state with regard to the person's goal or desire. As these processes are taking place, the neural representation of the social intentions of others must be linked to an appropriate responsive behaviour in the perceiver. Response dispositions should be activated "downstream" from the temporal cortices, where face-responsive neurons have been found in limbic structures such as the amygdala. The amygdala, together with several others interconnected structures, receives sensory information and in turn projects directly to somatic effector structures such as the hypothalamus, brainstem, and primitive motor centers, thus making the amygdala a candidate for the link between social perception and response. Evidence suggests that our brains are specially equipped for social interaction, and that the temporal lobes are a key structure for such crucial function.

## Temporal lobe and social capacities. An evolutionary perspective

Human evolution can be viewed in terms of the species' increasing ability to function effectively within a social context. By consequence, our brain has evolved a specialized ability for social cognition (Brothers *et al.*, 1990). Brothers *et al.* (1990) proposed that the amygdala, the orbitofrontal cortex (OFC), inferotemporal face-responsive regions and superior temporal sulcus (STS) represent areas primarily involved in the processing of socially relevant information. Adolphs (2003) extended this proposal by differentiating between higher-order sensory cortices such as fusiform gyrus and superior temporal sulcus which are involved in detailed perceptual processing and amygdala, ventral striatum, and orbitofrontal cortex which link sensory representations of stimuli to their motivational value.

The ability of recognizing a specific individual within a social context is one of the foundations of social behavior. In less evolved mammals, the recognition of specific individual is largely based on smell. By contrast, monkeys and humans recognize individuals mostly by their facial features and the intonation of their voice.

The brain structures that detect these social signs are located in temporal isocortex in the case of primates and olfactory allocortex in the case of macrosmatic mammals. Both are highly connected with the amygdala, which in primates also contains face-sensitive neurons.

In humans, the information is thus predominantly conveyed by the visual and auditory modalities and their isocortical projection and associations areas in the temporal lobes. Evidently, any dysfunction in these areas may have negative consequences for the individuals' social interaction and interpersonal relationships.

## Studies in the monkey-face recognition cells in temporal lobe

A particularly interesting group of neurons in the temporal visual association cortex of monkeys are those cells that respond selectively to the sight of faces (monkey and human) or to that of a hand (Gross *et al.*, 1972; Gross and Sergent, 1992). Some cells respond preferentially to the individuality of the face; others to facial expression. Again others respond only to moving faces or to expressive emotional movements. Some cells are maximally stimulated by the direction of gaze. There thus exists an astonishing variety of perceptual features to which face neurons can respond differentially. Detecting all these facial perceptual features is important to socially living animals such as monkeys in which social signalling is realized by means of facial movements and the direction of gaze as well as vocalizations. Evidently, such facial signals are also very important for social interactions in humans. By being able to read the social significance of facial expression, gestures, body postures, movements, gaze direction and vocalization, monkeys become adept at integrating themselves successfully into their social nexus.

In monkeys, gaze direction is an important component of facial expressions, particularly those related to dominance and submission (Hinde and Rowell, 1962; Mendelson, 1982; Mistlin and Perrett, 1990; Brothers et al., 1990). Given the importance of these facial signals, it is not surprising that some neurons in monkey temporal visual cortex (primarily in the STS) are sensitive to eye and head direction (Hasselmo et al., 1989; Perrett et al., 1985, 1992). These neurons may play a role in what Perrett et al. (Perrett et al., 1992) have called "social attention", referring to cells that signal the direction of another individual's attention. In the monkey temporal lobe, cells responsive to direction of gaze tend to be located within the STS, whereas cells responsive to face identity tend to be located in adjacent inferior temporal cortex (Hasselmo et al., 1989; Perrett et al., 1992; Yamane et al., 1988; Mistlin and Perrett, 1990). Hence, monkey studies have indicated that there are cells in monkey temporal cortex that respond differentially to facial features and gaze orientation (Perrett et al., 1982; Perrett et al., 1985). These studies have further shown that cells with preference for a specific face direction also prefer the corresponding gaze direction (*i.e.*, cells that respond to face forward also show greatest response to forward direction of gaze) (Perrett et al., 1985). Furthermore, Perrett et al. found that sensitivity to gaze direction could override sensitivity to head orientation, which provides support for a model in which gaze direction may affect perception of head orientation, but not vice versa.

In addition to face-specific cells, the cortex of the superior temporal sulcus has other complex response properties. It has been shown that visual information about the shape and posture of the fingers, hands, arms, legs and torso all impact on STS cell tuning in addition to facial details such as the shape of the mouth and the direction of gaze (Desimone et al., 1984; Jellema et al., 2000; Wachsmuth et al., 1994; Perrett et al., 1984; Perrett et al., 1985).

Motion information from dorsal stream projections arrives in the STS some 20 ms ahead of form information from the ventral stream. However, despite this asynchrony, STS processing overcomes the "binding problem", and only form and motion arising from the same biological object are integrated within 100 ms of the moving form becoming visible (Oram and Perrett, 1996). Indeed, STS cell integration of form and motion is widespread, and there are numerous cell types specializing in the processing of different types of face, limb and whole body motion (Perrett et al., 1985; Carey et al., 1997; Jellema et al., 2000; Perrett et al., 2002). Responses to purposeful hand object actions such as reaching, picking, tearing and manipulating objects have also been found in the STS (Jellema et al., 2000; Mistlin and Perrett, 1990; Perrett et al., 1989). These STS cells are sensitive to the form of the hand performing an action, but unresponsive to the sight of tools manipulating objects in the same manner as hands. Furthermore, the cells code the spatio-temporal interaction between the agent performing the action and the object of the action. For example, cells tuned to hands manipulating an object cease to respond if the hands and object move appropriately but are spatially separated. This selectivity ensures that the cells are more responsive in situations where the agent's motion is causally related to the object's motion. Thus, as is evident from single cell responses, the STS region contains neural populations representing multiple aspects of the face (including gaze) and body and their movements. These same regions of superior temporal cortex also responded to mouth movement.

Mouth movements are another important component of facial gesture. For example, mouth opening and teeth baring are gestures of threat or fear for many species, whereas "smiling" denotes submission or positive affect (Chevalier-Skolnikoff, 1973; Redican, 1982).

*In summary, studies in nonhuman primates have suggested a functional differentiation of regions responsive to faces.* Face-sensitive neurons are found within monkey inferior temporal (IT) cortex and within the superior temporal sulcus (STS) (Baizer et al., 1991; Gross and Sergent, 1992; Perrett et al., 1992; Rolls, 1992). Some neurons within the STS are also sensitive to gaze and head direction and facial parts (Hasselmo et al., 1989; Perrett et al., 1985; Perrett et al., 1992; Yamane et al., 1988). Furthermore there are cells in the STS that respond specifically to moving views of the head and body (Perrett et al., 1989) as well as to "biological motion" (Oram and Perrett, 1996).

## ■ Lesion studies in the monkey. The Klüver-Bucy syndrome

The importance of the temporal lobes for visual perception and social skills received only scant attention until the 1930s when Klüver and Bucy reported "psychic blindness" in monkeys after bilateral removal of the temporal lobes including the temporal isocortex and mesially located limbic structures. The lesioned monkeys approached inanimate and animate objects without hesitation or fear and explored them orally or olfactory as if they could no longer rely on their visual sense.

In monkeys, bilateral lesions limited of the upper bank of the superior temporal sulcus produces an exacerbated Klüver-Bucy syndrome. Monkeys with such lesions show an increased tendency to approach and touch objects, a decrease in emotional responses to aversive visual stimuli as well as a deficit in object discrimination. This phenomenon suggests that the superior temporal sulcus normally provides the amygdala with visual information that contributes to the identification of the affective or motivational significance of visually perceived objects.

## ■ Lesion studies in humans

In humans, bilateral total or partial loss of the temporal isocortex is rare. The most dramatic case of almost total loss of the temporal lobes is that of a young epileptic patient in whom a bilateral temporal lobectomy was carried out to control his seizures. The surgery produced the closest human facsimile of the classical Klüver-Bucy syndrome observed in monkeys. The patient displayed a loss of affective behaviour as well as abnormal sexual and eating behaviour associated with severe visual social agnosia; he was unable to recognize people, including his mother, in the absence of severe object agnosia. Patients with herpes encephalitis and subsequent bilateral temporal lobe destruction present similar clinical signs.

Evidence for the existence of specialized brain systems that analyze biological motion (motion of humans and non-humans) stems from neuropsychological lesion studies. Dissociations between the ability to perceive biological motion and other types of motion have been demonstrated. Some patients who to all intents and purposes are "motion blind" are still able to discriminate biological motion stimuli (Vaina et al., 1990; McLeod et al., 1996). The opposite pattern, i.e. an inability to perceive biological motion in the presence of normal general motion perception, has also been reported (Schenk and Zihl, 1997).

## ■ Anatomical considerations. Temporal lobe connections in a social perspective

Temporal isocortex is interposed between "lower order" sensory systems on the one hand and the frontal and the limbic systems on the other. Much of the temporal isocortex can in fact be regarded as "higher order" sensory cortex, particularly for the visual and the auditory modalities. The pathways through the temporal isocortex within these two sensory systems have branching outputs to other isocortical association areas in the parietal and frontal lobes and to the premotor frontal cortex. The STS brain region is known to be an area of convergence for the dorsal and ventral visual streams. Most of the input to the STS is derived from third-order sensory association areas and others polymodal areas (parietal, prefrontal cortex, limbic, and paralimbic regions) (Barnes and Pandya, 1992; Seltzer and Pandya, 1994), suggesting that multimodal STS areas are involved in the highest level of cortical integration of both sensory and limbic information. Superior temporal areas would therefore be primordial in the construction of coherent internal representations since these areas are central to the integration of complex perceptual multimodal information (Gloor, 1997).

The STP area derives its input from the MST area in the dorsal pathway and the anterior inferiortemporal area in the ventral pathway (Boussaoud et al., 1990; Felleman and Van Essen, 1991). The cortex of the STS has connections with the amygdala (Aggleton et al., 1980) as well as with the orbitofrontal cortex (Barbas, 1988) regions implicated in the processing of stimuli of social and emotional significance in both human and non-human primates (reviewed in Baron-Cohen 1995; Brothers, 1997; Adolphs, 1999).

## ■ Human neuroimaging and electrophysiological studies. Towards a better understanding of the social role of the temporal lobes

Prior to the advent of functional brain imaging nothing was known about specific functions of the superior temporal sulcus in humans. The first suggestion that humans may possess specialized biological motion perception mechanisms came from a study using a point light display depicting a moving body to investigate the response properties of medial temporal/V5, a region of occipito-temporal cortex known to respond to motion. In this fMRI study, activation was observed in MT/V5 and areas of superior temporal cortex. At the time, this was regarded as surprising, since the activation appeared to involve brain regions traditionally thought to be dedicated to auditory processing of speech sounds (Howard et al., 1996). Localization of primary auditory cortex was not performed in this visual stimulation study. In a PET study published in the same year, Bonda et al. (1996) demonstrated that human motion stimuli selectively activated the inferior parietal region and the STS. Specifically, body motion stimuli selectively activated the right posterior STS, whereas movement of the hand activated the left intraparietal sulcus and the posterior STS.

## ■ From static to moving face – eye gaze studies

From the earliest stages of postnatal development, faces are salient for the developing child. Faces derive their significance, in part, from the wealth of social information they convey. This information includes the bearer's identity as well as his emotional state, intentions and focus of attention. The capacity to extract socially relevant information from faces is fundamental to normal reciprocal social interaction and interpersonal communication. Among the core facial features (*i.e.* eyes, nose, and mouth), the eyes are thought to provide the most critical information and preferentially attract a viewer's attention. Adult viewers devote 70% or more of their fixation to the eyes. This pattern of face scanning emerges as early as the second month of postnatal life and is disturbed in schizophrenia and autism.

Information regarding the direction of gaze is thought to be particularly important in guiding social interactions. Gaze can provide information regarding the mental states of others, facilitate social control, regulate turn taking, direct attention, and communicate intimacy. Sensitivity to gaze direction emerges early in ontogeny. For example, infants detect direction of perceived gaze and modulate their own attention accordingly. Recent neurofunctional models of the human face processing system distinguish cortical regions involved in processing invariant characteristics of faces (*i.e.* those carrying information about identity) from regions involved in processing dynamic aspects of faces (*i.e.* those facilitating communication).

McCarthy identified four nodes of the human face processing system, all located in the temporal lobe. Two of these nodes, the lateral posterior fusiform gyrus and the anterior ventral temporal cortex are involved in structural encoding and face memory, respectively. A third node, centered in the superior temporal sulcus (STS), is implicated in the analysis of face motion such as eye and mouth movements. The remaining node, located in the amygdala, is involved in the analysis of facial expression (McCarthy, 1999).

Research on automatic processing of low-level facial features has provided consistent evidence of the role of the fusiform gyrus (FG) in the representation of fixed facial features. This research was prompted by the discovery that prosopagnosic patients who display specific deficits in identifying faces almost always have lesions in the ventral temporal lobe (De Renzi et al., 1991; Meadows, 1974; Sergent and Signoret, 1992b). Neuroimaging, surface and intracranial EEG and MEG studies of face perception have provided supportive evidence of the role of the FG in face processing

(Clark et al., 1996; Eimer and McCarthy, 1999; George et al., 1996; Halgren et al., 2000; Halgren et al., 1994; Kanwisher et al., 1997; McCarthy et al., 1999; Puce et al., 1995; Sergent et al., 1992; Sergent and Signoret, 1992a; McCarthy et al., 1997).

Several studies have demonstrated STS activation during viewing of static faces (Halgren et al., 1999; Kanwisher et al., 1997). More recently, the posterior superior temporal sulcus (STS) has been implicated in the processing of more changeable facial features like gaze direction. The eyes move not only in the service of visual perception but also to support communication by indicating direction of attention, intention or emotion. Using functional magnetic resonance imaging (fMRI), Puce et al. (1998) identified a bilateral region of activation centered in the posterior STS in response to observed eye or mouth movements This activation was not attributable to movement per se. Nonfacial, non biological movement in the same part of the visual field as occupied by the eyes or mouth, or movement of a radial background preferentially activated area MT/V5.

In the monkey, neurons have been found in the STS that respond selectively to face and gaze direction (Perrett et al., 1985). Using event-related potential (ERP) recordings, Bentin et al. (1996) demonstrated that an N170 ERP recorded from scalp electrodes overlying the STS was larger when evoked by isolated eyes than by whole faces or other facial components, and Puce et al. (2000) showed that the N170 ERP was larger in response to the movement of eyes averting their gaze away from the viewer than to movement of the eyes directing their gaze at the observer. In a PET study, Wicker et al. (1998) identified several regions of activation in response to mutual and averted gaze including portions of the STS. Finally, using fMRI, Hoffman and Haxby (2000) found that attention to gaze elicited a stronger response in STS than attention to identity. It should however be noted that some of these studies used static stimuli that varied in direction of gaze while others used dynamic stimuli in which the eyes moved.

The differential roles of FG and STS in face processing are not known. Hoffman and Haxby (2000) have attempted to differentiate the functions of these regions by looking at variations in task instructions. They found that the STS is more strongly activated during judgment of gaze direction than during judgment of identity, whereas fusiform and inferior occipito-temporal activation is stronger during judgment of identity than gaze direction. In addition, intracranial ERP recordings indicate that the STS responds to facial motion whereas the ventral-temporal cortex responds more strongly to static facial images (Puce & Allison, 1999). This is not surprising if one considers that eye gaze direction changes are transient and that their detection might require motion processing systems, whereas identity judgments can be made independently of facial movements. Indeed, the processing of dynamic information about facial expression and the processing of static information about facial identity appear to be neuropsychologically dissociable (Campbell, 1992; Humphreys et al., 1993).

Finally, there is evidence that the amygdala is also centrally involved in gaze processing. Patients with bilateral amygdala damage experience difficulty identifying gaze direction. PET studies of passive viewing of direct and averted gaze have shown bilateral amygdala activation to detection of eye contact and left amygdala activation to averted gaze (Kawashima et al., 1999). These results illustrate that the amygdala is instrumental in the perception of direct gaze.

Direct eye contact is also an important aspect of gaze behavior. Unlike averted gaze, direct gaze indicates that the attention is focused on the viewer. Perceiving eye contact directs and fixes attention on the observed face. In visual search paradigms, direct eye contact is detected faster than averted gaze. Eye contact has been shown to increase physiological response in social interactions. The amount and quality of eye contact are considered important indicators of social and emotional functioning. Poor eye contact is a specific diagnostic feature of autism and a key component of the negative symptom syndrome in schizophrenia. Thus, investigating neural mechanisms of gaze may provide key insights for the understanding of the neurobiological factors mediating social development and social interactions. Furthermore, it may provide information about how dysfunctions in these mechanisms might be related to symptoms observed in disorders such as autism and schizophrenia.

*In conclusion*, there is mounting evidence to suggest that specific regions of the temporal lobe, such as the fusiform gyrus, the superior temporal sulcus and the amygdala, are involved in gaze processing. Gaze is usually perceived in the context of a face, and faces are known to activate both the fusiform gyrus and the STS. However, the fusiform gyrus responds more readily to whole faces and the STS responds more strongly to facial features, particularly the eyes. Face identity judgments generate relatively stronger activation in fusiform gyrus whereas gaze direction judgment of the same visual stimuli produce stronger activation in STS (Haxby et al., 2000; Hoffman and Haxby, 2000).

Furthermore, lesions in the region of the fusiform gyrus can interfere with the ability to recognize familiar faces (Farah et al., 1995; Kanwisher, 2000; Young et al., 1993). Deficits in gaze direction discrimination are generally not found after damage of the fusiform gyrus but can be observed after STS damage (Campbell et al., 1990).

## ■ Emotion effects

Angry faces in gaze tasks are known to elicit more activity in the STS region than happy faces, and this activation extends from the STS dorsally through the intraparietal sulcus (Hooker et al., 2003). The influence of facial expression on STS activity adds support to the interpretation that the STS is responsive to gaze cues that are meaningful to social interaction. Gaze providing information about the direction of attention of an angry person may be more meaningful than the same information coming from a happy person. Understanding where an angry person is attending to and what they might be angry about has immediate relevance to the viewer's ability to successfully navigate a potentially threatening or aversive environment.

## ■ Mouth perception. Lip reading

One prominently active region to viewing eye movements (gaze aversion and gaze directed at the observer) is the cortex surounding the STS, particularly in the right hemisphere. This same region also responds to the perception of opening and closing movements of the mouth (Puce et al., 1998).

Lip reading, which is an important function for both hearing and deaf individuals, can be neuropsychologically dissociated from face recognition (Campbell, 1986) in a somewhat similar manner to gaze perception. Normal lip reading uses cortex of the STG in addition to other brain regions such as the angular gyrus, the posterior cingulate, medial frontal cortex and the frontal pole (Calvert et al., 1997). The STG and surrounding cortex are activated bilaterally when subjects view facial movements that could be interpreted as speech (Puce et al., 1998; Campbell et al., 2001), whereas some regions of the posterior right STS are activated by the sight of speech and non-speech mouth movements (Campbell et al., 2001). Centers of activation to visually perceived speech appear to overlap with those associated with auditory perception of speech (Calvert et al., 1997), indicating that these regions receive multimodal input during speech analysis (Kawashima et al., 1999; Calvert et al., 2000). These results suggest that a discrete region of cortex centred on the STS is involved in the perception of eye and mouth movements. That such a region may be lateralized is suggested by Campbell et al. (1986), who reported that a prosopagnosic patient with a right occipitotemporal lesion was deficient in determining the direction of gaze but could lip-read, whereas a patient with a left occipitotemporal lesion who was alexic could not lip-read but was able to recognize familiar faces and to determine the direction of gaze. The authors found that changes in direction of gaze activated the right STS more strongly than the left. Furthermore, Calvert et al. (1997) reported that silent lip-reading of words activated a bilateral region of the superior temporal gyrus (presumedly including cortex within the STS).

## ■ Hands and body movement

The STS may also participate in the perception of biological motion. When subjects viewed point-light simulations of hand action, body movement, object motion and random motion, a region of the STS was activated by hand and body movement but not by other movements (Bonda et al., 1996). Using PET, Rizzolatti et al. found that observation of grasping movements activated the left middle temporal gyrus and STS (Rizzolatti et al., 1996). This region is considerably more anteriorly located than the region activated by hand action in the study by Bonda et al. (1996) for reasons that remain unclear. However, taken together these studies strongly implicate the human STS and adjacent cortex in the perception of body movements of other individuals.

This notion is supported by several studies that have compared meaningful and non-meaningful human movements. When videos of American Sign Language were viewed, the STS was more strongly activated in viewers who understood the signals than in those who did not (Neville et al., 1998). STS activation has also been reported in response to possible *versus* impossible human movements (Stevens et al., 2000) and to meaningful *vs* non-meaningful hand movements (Decety et al., 1997). The data indicate that STS processing is concerned with more than just the perceptual aspects of moving or movable body parts. Rather, networks in this brain region may analyze gaze and other movements to the extent that these cues meaningfully contribute to social communication. These findings suggest that joint attention, which constitutes a pivotal skill in social cognition, is facilitated by the analysis of sensory cues in the STS.

## ■ Voice perception. A social perception in the auditory world

The human voice is probably the most important sound category of our auditory environment. Evidently, it carries speech, which makes man a unique species. However, the voice is also an "auditory face", rich in information concerning the identity and affective state of the speaker. We are all able to extract this information – to a sometimes surprising degree – and to form representations in long-term memory that will allow us to recognize peoples' voices on the telephone, for example. Although these "vocal cognition" skills play a fundamental role in social interactions, little is known about the underlying cerebral mechanisms.

Research suggests that vocal cognition involves voice-selective regions of auditory cortex located along the superior temporal sulcus (STS), analogous to the "face areas" of visual cortex, and possibly organized in functionally distinct cortical pathways (Belin et al., 2000a). Dedicated neural territories that selectively respond to voices rather than to other natural sounds are located along both superior temporal sulci (STS) (Belin et al., 2000a). Preferential responses to voices have been observed in regions along both STS with a right hemispheric predominance (Belin et al., 2000b; Belin et al., 2002; Belin and Zatorre, 2003). Recognition of both familiar and non-familiar voices has also been found to activate the posterior STS (Kriegstein and Giraud, 2004). In this voice recognition study, Kriegstein and Giraud (2004) delineated three distinct areas involved in different aspects of voice processing along the right STS. Like in the visual system, these areas include an anteroventral pathway which would subserve object recognition (the "what" system), a posterodorsal pathway which would integrate acoustic signals into complex auditory scenes based on the spatial location of sound (the "where" system) (Rauschecker and Tian (Rauschecker and Tian, 2000) and an area devoted to spectral auditory motion (the "how" system) (Belin and Zatorre, 2000). The properties of the three areas in the right STS are compatible with such a scheme in that recognition of a voice belonging to a specific person involves predominantly an anteroventral STS region whereas recognition of voices as target acoustic stimuli that are not associated with other person-related features involves predominantly a posterodorsal STS region.

## ■ More abstract representations of intentional action

Two sets of recent neuroimaging data suggest that the role of the posterior superior temporal sulcus (pSTS) may extend beyond a response to biological motion to more abstract representations of intentional acts. In this context, Castelli et al. (2000) and

Schultz et al. (2003) reported that a region of the pSTS showed a significantly higher response to animations of moving geometric shapes depicting complex social interactions than to animations depicting inanimate motion. Furthermore, using movies of human actors engaged in structured goal-directed activities (e.g. cleaning the kitchen), Zacks et al. (2001) found that activation in the pSTS was enhanced when the actors switched from one activity to another, suggesting that this region encodes the goal-structure of actions. Both of these results are consistent with a role for a region of pSTS cortex in representing intentional actions, not just biological motion.

Activations in the posterior STS have also been consistently reported in social cognition or so-called "theory of mind" tasks (Castelli et al., 2000; Calder et al., 2002; Gallagher et al., 2000; Winston et al., 2002) and in moral judgment tasks (Greene et al., 2001; Heekeren et al., 2003). The cognitive process underlying the ability to attribute intentions to self and others has variously been termed "theory of mind" (ToM) (Premack and Woodruff, 1978), "intentional stance" (Dennett, 1987), or "mentalizing" (Frith et al., 1991). Far from being a complex process of conscious inferences, mentalizing is thought to be an automatic cognitive process (Leslie, 1987; Scholl and Leslie, 1999) which does not require a deliberate decision to attend. The three cortical regions most consistently activated during mentalizing are the paracingulate cortex, the temporal poles, and the superior temporal sulcus at the temporoparietal junction (Frith, 2001). Posterior STS activation has been reported during mentalizing or "theory of mind" tasks requiring the understanding of intentions, feelings and goals of others, be it persons or moving objects (e.g., geometric shapes) engaged in complex interactions (Castelli et al., 2000; Gallagher et al., 2000; Schultz et al., 2003: for a review, see also Frith and Frith, 2003). Recent evidence suggests that activity in STS may be mediated by explicit attention to socially salient features (see also Schultz et al., 2003), and that, in contrast to the amygdala, right posterior STS activation is greater when subjects make explicit judgments about trustworthiness compared to age judgments of facial stimuli (e.g., Winston et al., 2002).

There is a great overlap between the posterior temporal regions identified by ToM and gaze studies. It is clear that the region of posterior temporal cortex (i.e. STS) that Haxby et al. (2000) associated with the visual analysis of changeable aspects of the face (i.e. gaze, emotional expressions, mouth movements, etc.), is very similar to the regions engaged by ToM tasks. Moreover, it is noteworthy that none of the ToM studies included gaze or face processing tasks.

One possibility is that the posterior temporal region, identified by the gaze experiments, forms part of a more general post-perceptual system involved in the processing of the actions of external agents. For example, Frith and Frith (2003) have proposed that this area is involved in the detection of the behaviour of agents, and the analysis of the goals and outcomes of this behaviour. In addition, it is consistent with Hikosaka's (1993) work showing that the posterior STS in the macaque brain constitutes a polysensory area involved in the direction of global attention to sensory cues from multiple modalities.

The temporal poles were also consistently found to be involved in mentalizing tasks. Five different mentalizing tasks studying familiar faces and voices (Nakamura et al., 2000; Nakamura et al., 2001), coherence (Maguire et al., 1999), semantics (Vandenberghe et al., 1996; Noppeney and Price, 2002), sentences (Bottini et al., 1994; Vandenberghe et al., 2002) and autobiographical memory (Fink et al., 1996; Maguire and Mummery, 1999; Maguire et al., 2000) have been found to elicit activity in both temporal poles, predominantly on the left side. This region of the anterior temporal cortex is a site for potential convergence of all sensory modalities and limbic inputs (Moran et al., 1987). Humans spontaneously imbue the world with social meaning: we not only perceive emotions and intentional behaviors in humans and other animals, we also attribute these behaviors to inanimate objects (e.g., by perceiving anger in thunderstorms or willful sabotage in crashing computers).

Converging evidence supports the role of the amygdala in the processing of emotionally and socially relevant information. Patients with bilateral amygdala damage describe a film of animated shapes (normally seen as full of social content) in entirely asocial, geometric terms, despite normal visual perception.

## ■ Some developmental issues. Studies in neonates

Making eye contact is the most powerful mode of establishing a communicative link between humans. During their first year of life, infants learn rapidly that the looking behavior of others conveys significant information. Two experiments were carried to demonstrate special sensitivity to direct eye contact from birth (Farroni et al., 2002). The first experiment tested the ability of 2- to 5-day-old newborns to discriminate between direct and averted gaze. The second experiment measured the brain electric activity of 4-month-old infants' during the processing of faces involved in direct (as opposed to averted) eye gaze. The results show that, from birth, human infants prefer faces that engage them in mutual gaze and that from an early age on, healthy babies show enhanced neural responses to direct gaze. The exceptionally early sensitivity to mutual gaze, demonstrated in these studies, is arguably the major foundation for the later development of social skills (Farroni et al., 2002).

The perception of faces and the understanding that faces can reflect internal states of social partners, are vital skills for the typical development of humans. Processing information about eyes and eye-gaze direction is particularly important. Although the perception of averted gaze can elicit an automatic shift of attention in the same direction, allowing the establishment of "joint attention", mutual gaze (eye contact) provides the main mode of establishing a communicative link between humans. It is known that, from at least 4 months of age, human infants will shift their spatial attention toward the direction of a gaze shift when viewing a face, and there is general agreement that such skills are vital for subsequent social development (for review see Farroni et al., 2002). Furthermore, it has been shown that human newborns have a visual preference for face-like stimuli; they prefer faces with eyes open and tend to imitate facial gestures. Preferential attention to perceived faces with direct gaze provide the most compelling evidence to date for the notion that neonates are born prepared to detect socially relevant information.

## Evidence from clinical data – autism

Autism is a complex, severe, and lifelong developmental disorder. Its main symptom is a deficit in social interaction and communication (Kanner, 1943; Rapin, 1997). Autistic children have difficulties processing emotional expressions. They tend to have narrow interests and poor imagination (Gillberg and Coleman, 1992). Recently, two independent high-resolution PET and SPECT studies have revealed localized bilateral temporal hypoperfusion at rest in children with primary autism. These abnormalities were centered in the superior temporal sulcus and the superior temporal gyrus (Ohnishi et al., 2000 and Zilbovicius et al., 2000). This finding is congruent with the observation of a bilateral grey matter decrease in the superior temporal lobes of children with primary autism (Boddaert et al., 2004). The superior temporal sulcus is increasingly recognized as a key component of the "social brain" (Allison et al., 2000). Autistic children have deficits in the perception of gaze, make poor eye contact during communication, and have difficulties accessing information allowing them to infer the mental state of others (Howard et al., 2000). "I had no idea that other people communicated through subtle eye movements", remarked an adult with autism, "until I read it in a magazine five years ago". Thus, the capacity to perceive subtle social cues communicated through the eyes may be a prerequisite for "theory of mind" or social cognition, which is severely impaired in autism (Baron-Cohen et al., 1999; Frith, 2001 and Happe et al., 1996). There is also evidence that the STS is implicated in successful imitation (Rizzolatti et al., 2001) and human voice perception (Belin et al., 2000), both of which are essential skills for interpersonal communication. In this context, an fMRI study has shown that individuals with autism fail to activate the voice-selective regions of the superior temporal sulcus in response to vocal sounds, while showing normal activation to non-vocal sounds (Gervais et al., 2004). These findings are in line with earlier data implicating the temporal lobes in acquired clinical models of autism (Bolton and Griffiths, 1997; Chugani et al., 1996 and Gillberg, 1991). For instance autistic behavior has been observed in temporal lobe pathology, such as epilepsy and herpes simplex encephalitis (Gillberg, 1991). Furthermore, neuropathological studies have revealed temporal lobe abnormalities in patients with autism (Bauman and Kemper, 1985 and Casanova et al., 2002). Finally, recent neuroimaging studies point to an association between temporal lobe abnormalities and the occurrence of secondary autism (Bolton and Griffiths, 1997 and Chugani et al., 1996).

## Summary and concluding remarks

Despite the popularity of technical means of communication, face-to-face contact is still favored when unambiguity is necessary. What causes us to prefer face-to-face interaction over other methods of communication? Face-to-face interaction enables us to deduct from nonverbal signals sent by the other person if our message is being received. We then use these intended and unintended nonverbal clues to make judgments about the emotional state and the potential course of action of others. Physiological studies in humans and monkeys suggest that the interpretation of the movements and actions of others recruit neural pathways specialized in the perception of social signals (Allison et al., 2000; Blakemore and Decety, 2001). The perception of motion of animate objects preferentially activates the cortex of the superior temporal sulcus (STS) in humans (Bonda et al., 1996; Puce et al., 1998) and monkeys (Perrett et al., 1985; Oram and Perrett, 1994). In monkeys, it has been proposed that the STS response is a result of the integration of form and motion information in the anterior superior temporal polysensory area (STPa) (Oram and Perrett, 1996). Human neuroimaging studies using point-light displays of human motion have shown activation in motion sensitive regions in posterior temporal/inferior parietal cortex (Bonda et al., 1996; Grossman et al., 2000). These regions have been shown to respond to motion involving natural images of faces (Puce et al., 1998), as well as to natural images of implied motion (Kourtzi and Kanwisher et al., 2000).

Humans have the remarkable ability to extract information regarding direction of attention, mental state and intentions from facial expression and direction of gaze. These abilities are critical components of normal social interaction. The extraction of information from faces presumably requires several hierarchical processing stages such as recognizing the constellation of facial features, identifying the face, determining the facial expression and the direction of gaze and placing this information into a social context. The processing of non-verbal messages in the form of face and hand gestures, is crucial for social primates to interact with one another, and there are considerable similarities in the higher-level biological motion processing systems of human and nonhuman primates.

STS activity may reflect the analysis of biological cues that provide meaningful social signals. More specifically, the STS may analyze meaningful biological motion, where "meaning" depends on the social situation in which the movement occurs. Furthermore, given that gaze provides a highly informative window into mental state, the STS appears to be part of a larger neural network mediating "theory of mind" or social cognition. This region probably acts as a high-level perceptual processor, sending vital information to the other structures in the network, which enables them to evaluate and interpret affective and social information. Indeed, fMRI data indicate that activation in these regions can occur when social meaning is gleaned from stimuli that do not involve human (or animal) form (Weisberg and Martin, 2001; Castelli et al., 2000, 2002). Earlier studies in monkeys have identified neurons within the STS, in area STPa, that integrate form and motion (Oram and Perrett, 1994, 1996). In addition, neurons in the amygdala have been reported to respond to complex body motion within a social context (Brothers et al., 1990).

However, the STS/orbitofrontal/amygdala circuit is not the only cortical network that is active during the interpretation of the actions of others. A "mirror" system (Rizzolatti et al., 2001) has been found in the premotor cortex of monkeys which is activated irrespective of whether the animals perform or observe acts of grasping (Gallese et al., 1996; Rizzolatti et al., 1996a). A similar parallel activation system has recently been observed in human imaging studies.

Using PET (Rizzolatti et al., 1996b), fMRI (Iacoboni et al., 1999) and MEG (Nishitani and Hari, 2000) activation in response to both observation and imitation of grasping movements was detected in or close to the Broca area. Interestingly, scalp

ERP recordings have indicated that observation of not only hand movements but also movements of the body produces neural activity in centrofrontal regions (Wheaton et al., 2001). In sum, there appear to be multiple cortical networks in the primate brain that are specialized for the processing of information regarding the actions of others. One network, involving the STS (in monkey the STPa) and the amygdala seem to be primarily involved in the processing of social and emotional cues. The other network, centered on the prefrontal cortex (area F5 in the monkey) may be biased for the interpretation of actions, including object manipulation of other primates and actions such as grasping behaviors of the hand and mouth.

Other behaviors, perceived as potential threats, may activate more than one of these networks. It is still unknown how these systems relate to one another and what, if any, other structures are involved in monitoring or coordinating their activity. The importance of understanding the actions of others is evident in clinical disorders such as autism and Asperger syndrome in which comprehension of social cues is impaired. These individuals cannot adequately process incoming social messages communicated by body and facial movements of others and react appropriately to such signals (e.g. Williams et al., 2001). Further neuroimaging and neurophysiological studies of healthy subjects and individuals with impaired motion processing may shed new light on the interactions between the various components of these higher-level biological motion processing systems.

# References

Adolphs R. Social cognition and the human brain. *Trends Cogn Sci* 1999; 3: 469-79.

Adolphs R. Cognitive neuroscience of human social behaviour. *Nat Rev Neurosci* 2003; 4: 165-78.

Aggleton JP, Burton MJ, Passingham RE. Cortical and subcortical afferents to the amygdala of the rhesus monkey (Macaca mulatta). *Brain Res* 1980; 190: 347-68.

Allison T, Puce A, McCarthy G. Social perception from visual cues: role of the STS region. *Trends Cogn Sci* 2000; 4: 267-78.

Baizer JS, Ungerleider LG, Desimone R. Organization of visual inputs to the inferior temporal and posterior parietal cortex in macaques. *J Neurosci* 1991; 11: 168-90.

Barbas H. Anatomic organization of basoventral and mediodorsal visual recipient prefrontal regions in the rhesus monkey. *J Comp Neurol* 1988; 276: 313-42.

Barnes CL, Pandya DN. Efferent cortical connections of multimodal cortex of the superior temporal sulcus in the rhesus monkey. *J Comp Neurol* 1992; 318: 222-44.

Belin P, McAdams S, Thivard L, Smith B, Savel S, Zilbovicius M, Samson S, Samson Y. The neuroanatomical substrate of sound duration discrimination. *Neuropsychologia* 2002; 40: 1956-64.

Belin P, Zatorre RJ. "What", "where" and "how" in auditory cortex. *Nat Neurosci* 2000; 3: 965-6.

Belin P, Zatorre RJ. Adaptation to speaker's voice in right anterior temporal lobe. *Neuroreport* 2003; 14: 2105-9.

Belin P, Zatorre RJ, Lafaille P, Ahad P, Pike B. Voice-selective areas in human auditory cortex. *Nature* 2000; 403: 309-12.

Bentin S, Allison T, Puce A, Perez E, McCarthy G. Electrophysiological studies in human face perception in humans. *J Cogn Neurosci* 1996; 8: 551-65.

Boddaert N, Chabane N, Gervais H, Good CD, Bourgeois M, Plumet MH, Barthelemy C, et al. Superior temporal sulcus anatomical abnormalities in childhood autism: a voxel-based morphometry MRI study. *Neuroimage* 2004; 23: 364-9.

Bolton PF, Griffiths PD. Association of tuberous sclerosis of temporal lobes with autism and atypical autism. *Lancet* 1997; 349: 392-5.

Bonda E, Petrides M, Ostry D, Evans A. Specific involvement of human parietal systems and the amygdala in the perception of biological motion. *J Neurosci* 1996; 16: 3737-44.

Bottini G, Corcoran R, Sterzi R, Paulesu E, Schenone P, Scarpa P, Frackowiak RS, Frith CD. The role of the right hemisphere in the interpretation of figurative aspects of language. A positron emission tomography activation study. *Brain* 1994; 117 (Pt 6): 1241-53.

Boussaoud D, Ungerleider LG, Desimone R. Pathways for motion analysis: cortical connections of the medial superior temporal and fundus of the superior temporal visual areas in the macaque. *J Comp Neurol* 1990; 296: 462-95.

Brothers L. *Friday's footprint: How society shapes the human mind.* Oxford, England: Oxford University Press, 1997.

Brothers L, Ring B, Kling A. Response of neurons in the macaque amygdala to complex social stimuli. *Behav Brain Res* 1990; 41: 199-213.

Calder AJ, Lawrence AD, Keane J, Scott SK, Owen AM, Christoffels I, Young AW. Reading the mind from eye gaze. *Neuropsychologia* 2002; 40: 1129-38.

Calvert GA, Bullmore ET, Brammer MJ, Campbell R, Williams SC, McGuire PK, Woodruff PW, Iversen SD, David AS. Activation of auditory cortex during silent lipreading. *Science* 1997; 276: 593-6.

Calvert GA, Campbell R, Brammer MJ. Evidence from functional magnetic resonance imaging of crossmodal binding in the human heteromodal cortex. *Curr Biol* 2000; 10: 649-57.

Campbell R. The lateralization of lip-read sounds: a first look. *Brain Cogn* 5: 1-21.

Campbell R. The neuropsychology of lipreading. *Philos Trans R Soc Lond B Biol Sci* 1986; 335: 39-44.

Campbell R, Heywood C, Cowey A, Regard M, Landis T. Sensitivity to eye gaze in prosopagnosia patients and monkeys with temporal sulcus ablation. *Neuropsychologia* 1990; 28: 1123-42.

Campbell R, Landis T, Regard M. Face recognition and lipreading. A neurological dissociation. *Brain* 1986; 109 (Pt 3): 509-21.

Campbell R, MacSweeney M, Surguladze S, Calvert G, McGuire P, Suckling J, Brammer MJ, David AS. Cortical substrates for the perception of face actions: an fMRI study of the specificity of activation for seen speech and for meaningless lower-face acts (gurning). *Brain Res Cogn Brain Res* 2001; 12: 233-43.

Carey DP, Perrett DI, Oram MW. Recognizing, understanding and reproducing action. In: Boller F, Grafman J, ed. *Handbook of neuropsychology.* Holland: Elsevier, 1997: 111-29.

Casanova MF, Buxhoeveden DP, Switala AE, Roy E. Minicolumnar pathology in autism. *Neurology* 2002; 58: 428-32.

Castelli F, Happe F, Frith U, Frith C. Movement and mind: a functional imaging study of perception and interpretation of complex intentional movement patterns. *Neuroimage* 2000; 12: 314-25.

Chevalier-Skolnikoff S. Visual and tactile communication in Macaca arctoides and its ontogenetic development. *Am J Phys Anthropol* 1973; 38: 515-8.

Chugani HT, Da SE, Chugani DC. Infantile spasms: III. Prognostic implications of bitemporal hypometabolism on positron emission tomography. *Ann Neurol* 1996; 39: 643-9.

Clark VP, Keil K, Maisog JM, Courtney S, Ungerleider LG, Haxby JV. Functional magnetic resonance imaging of human visual cortex during face matching: a comparison with positron emission tomography. *Neuroimage* 1996; 4: 1-15.

De Renzi E, Faglioni P, Grossi D, Nichelli P. Apperceptive and associative forms of prosopagnosia. *Cortex* 1991; 27: 213-21.

Decety J, Grezes J, Costes N, Perani D, Jeannerod M, Procyk E, Grassi F, Fazio F. Brain activity during observation of actions. Influence of action content and subject's strategy. *Brain* 1997; 120 (Pt 10): 1763-77.

Dennett DC. *The intentional stance*. Cambridge: Bradford Books/MIT Press, 1987.

Desimone R, Albright TD, Gross CG, Bruce C. Stimulus-selective properties of inferior temporal neurons in the macaque. *J Neurosci* 1984; 4: 2051-62.

Eimer M, McCarthy RA. Prosopagnosia and structural encoding of faces: evidence from event-related potentials. *Neuroreport* 1999; 10: 255-9.

Farah MJ, Wilson KD, Drain HM, Tanaka JR. The inverted face inversion effect in prosopagnosia: evidence for mandatory, face-specific perceptual mechanisms. *Vision Res* 1995; 35: 2089-93.

Farroni T, Csibra G, Simion F, Johnson MH. Eye contact detection in humans from birth. *Proc Natl Acad Sci USA* 2002; 99: 9602-5.

Felleman DJ, Van Essen DC. Distributed hierarchical processing in the primate cerebral cortex. *Cereb Cortex* 1991; 1: 1-47.

Fink GR, Markowitsch HJ, Reinkemeier M, Bruckbauer T, Kessler J, Heiss WD. Cerebral representation of one's own past: neural networks involved in autobiographical memory. *J Neurosci* 1996; 16: 4275-82.

Frith U. Mind blindness and the brain in autism. *Neuron* 2001; 32: 969-79.

Frith U, Frith CD. Development and neurophysiology of mentalizing. *Philos Trans R Soc Lond B Biol Sci* 2003; 358: 459-73.

Frith U, Morton J, Leslie AM. The cognitive basis of a biological disorder: autism. *Trends Neurosci* 1991; 14: 433-8.

Gallagher HL, Happe F, Brunswick N, Fletcher PC, Frith U, Frith CD. Reading the mind in cartoons and stories: an fMRI study of "theory of mind" in verbal and nonverbal tasks. *Neuropsychologia* 2000; 38: 11-21.

George N, Evans J, Fiori N, Davidoff J, Renault B. Brain events related to normal and moderately scrambled faces. *Brain Res Cogn Brain Res* 1996; 4: 65-76.

Gervais H, Belin P, Boddaert N, Leboyer M, Coez A, Sfaello I, Barthelemy C, Brunelle F, Samson Y, Zilbovicius M. Abnormal cortical voice processing in autism. *Nat Neurosci* 2004; 7: 801-2.

Gillberg C, Coleman M. *The biology of autistic syndromes*. London: Mac Keith, 2000.

Gloor P. *The temporal lobe and limbic system*. New York: Oxford University Press, 1997.

Grafton ST, Arbib MA, Fadiga L, Rizzolatti G. Localization of grasp representations in humans by positron emission tomography. 2. Observation compared with imagination. *Exp Brain Res* 1996; 112: 103-11.

Greene JD, Sommerville RB, Nystrom LE, Darley JM, Cohen JD. An fMRI investigation of emotional engagement in moral judgment. *Science* 2001; 293: 2105-8.

Gross CG, Rocha-Miranda CE, Bender DB. Visual properties of neurons in inferotemporal cortex of the Macaque. *J Neurophysiol* 1972; 35: 96-111.

Gross CG, Sergent J. Face recognition. *Curr Opin Neurobiol* 1992; 2: 156-61.

Halgren E, Baudena P, Heit G, Clarke JM, Marinkovic K, Clarke M. Spatiotemporal stages in face and word processing. I. Depth-recorded potentials in the human occipital, temporal and parietal lobes [corrected]. *J Physiol Paris* 1994; 88: 1-50.

Halgren E, Dale AM, Sereno MI, Tootell RB, Marinkovic K, Rosen BR. Location of human face-selective cortex with respect to retinotopic areas. *Hum Brain Mapp* 1999; 7: 29-37.

Halgren E, Raij T, Marinkovic K, Jousmaki V, Hari R. Cognitive response profile of the human fusiform face area as determined by MEG. *Cereb Cortex* 2000; 10: 69-81.

Hasselmo ME, Rolls ET, Baylis GC. The role of expression and identity in the face-selective responses of neurons in the temporal visual cortex of the monkey. *Behav Brain Res* 1989; 32: 203-18.

Haxby JV, Hoffman EA, Gobbini MI. The distributed human neural system for face perception. *Trends Cogn Sci* 2000; 4: 223-33.

Heekeren HR, Wartenburger I, Schmidt H, Schwintowski HP, Villringer A. An fMRI study of simple ethical decision-making. *Neuroreport* 2003; 14: 1215-9.

Hikosaka O, Miyauchi S, Shimojo S. Visual attention revealed by an illusion of motion. *Neurosci Res* 1993; 18: 11-8.

Hinde RA, Rowell TE. Communication by postures and facial expressions in the rhesus monkey (Macaca mulata). *Proc Zool Soc London* 1962; 1-21.

Hoffman EA, Haxby JV. Distinct representations of eye gaze and identity in the distributed human neural system for face perception. *Nat Neurosci* 2000; 3: 80-4.

Hooker CI, Paller KA, Gitelman DR, Parrish TB, Mesulam MM, Reber PJ. Brain networks for analyzing eye gaze. *Brain Res Cogn Brain Res* 2003; 17: 406-18.

Howard RJ, Brammer M, Wright I, Woodruff PW, Bullmore ET, Zeki S. A direct demonstration of functional specialization within motion-related visual and auditory cortex of the human brain. *Curr Biol* 1996; 6: 1015-9.

Howard MA, Cowell PE, Boucher J, Broks P, Mayes A, Farrant A, Roberts N. Convergent neuroanatomical and behavioural evidence of an amygdala hypothesis of autism. *Neuroreport* 2000; 11: 2931-5.

Humphreys GW, Donnelly N, Riddoch MJ. Expression is computed separately from facial identity, and it is computed separately for moving and static faces: neuropsychological evidence. *Neuropsychologia* 1993; 31: 173-81.

Jellema T, Baker CI, Wicker B, Perrett DI. Neural representation for the perception of the intentionality of actions. *Brain Cogn* 2000; 44: 280-302.

Kanner L. Autistic disturbances of affective contact. *Nervous Child* 1943; 2: 217-50.

Kanwisher N. Domain specificity in face perception. *Nat Neurosci* 2000; 3: 759-63.

Kanwisher N, McDermott J, Chun MM. The fusiform face area: a module in human extrastriate cortex specialized for face perception. *J Neurosci* 1997; 17: 4302-11.

Kawashima R, Imaizumi S, Mori K, Okada K, Goto R, Kiritani S, Ogawa A, Fukuda H. Selective visual and auditory attention toward utterances-a PET study. *Neuroimage* 1999a; 10: 209-15.

Kawashima R, Sugiura M, Kato T, Nakamura A, Hatano K, Ito K, Fukuda H, Kojima S, Nakamura K. The human amygdala plays an important role in gaze monitoring. A PET study. *Brain* 1999b; 122 (Pt 4): 779-83.

Kriegstein KV, Giraud AL. Distinct functional substrates along the right superior temporal sulcus for the processing of voices. *Neuroimage* 2004; 22: 948-55.

Leslie AM. Pretense and representation: The origins of " theory of mind". *Psychol Rev* 1987; 94: 412-26.

Maguire EA, Frith CD, Morris RG. The functional neuroanatomy of comprehension and memory: the importance of prior knowledge. *Brain* 1999; 122 (Pt 10): 1839-50.

Maguire EA, Mummery CJ. Differential modulation of a common memory retrieval network revealed by positron emission tomography. *Hippocampus* 1999; 9: 54-61.

Maguire EA, Mummery CJ, Buchel C. Patterns of hippocampal-cortical interaction dissociate temporal lobe memory subsystems. *Hippocampus* 2000; 10: 475-82.

McCarthy G. Physiological studies of face processing in humans. In: Gazzaniga M, eds. *The new cognitive neurosciences*. Cambridge, England: MIT Press, 1999: 393-410.

McCarthy G, Puce A, Belger A, Allison T. Electrophysiological studies of human face perception. II: Response properties of face-specific potentials generated in occipitotemporal cortex. *Cereb Cortex* 1999; 9: 431-44.

McCarthy G, Puce A, Gore JC, Allison T. Face-specific processing in the human fusiform gyrus. *J Cogn Neurosci* 1999; 9: 605-10.

McLeod P, Dittrich W, Driver J, Perrett D, Zihl J. Preserved and impaired detection of structure from motion from a "motion-blind" patient. *Vis Cogn* 1996; 3: 363-91.

Meadows JC. The anatomical basis of prosopagnosia. *J Neurol Neurosurg Psychiatry* 1974; 37: 489-501.

Mendelson MJ. Visual and social responses in infant rhesus monkeys. *Am J Primatol* 1982; 3: 333-40.

Mistlin AJ, Perrett DI. Visual and somatosensory processing in the macaque temporal cortex: the role of "expectation". *Exp Brain Res* 1990; 82: 437-50.

Moran MA, Mufson EJ, Mesulam MM. Neural inputs into the temporopolar cortex of the rhesus monkey. *J Comp Neurol* 1987; 256: 88-103.

Nakamura K, Kawashima R, Sato N, Nakamura A, Sugiura M, Kato T, Hatano K, Ito K, Fukuda H, Schormann T, Zilles K. Functional delineation of the human occipito-temporal areas related to face and scene processing. A PET study. *Brain* 2000; 123 (Pt 9): 1903-12.

Nakamura K, Kawashima R, Sugiura M, Kato T, Nakamura A, Hatano K, Nagumo S, Kubota K, Fukuda H, Ito K, Kojima S. Neural substrates for recognition of familiar voices: a PET study. *Neuropsychologia* 2001; 39: 1047-54.

Neville HJ, Bavelier D, Corina D, Rauschecker J, Karni A, Lalwani A, Braun A, Clark V, Jezzard P, Turner R. Cerebral organization for language in deaf and hearing subjects: biological constraints and effects of experience. *Proc Natl Acad Sci USA* 1998; 95: 922-9.

Noppeney U, Price CJ. A PET study of stimulus- and task-induced semantic processing. *Neuroimage* 2002; 15: 927-35.

Ohnishi T, Matsuda H, Hashimoto T, Kunihiro T, Nishikawa M, Uema T, Sasaki M. Abnormal regional cerebral blood flow in childhood autism. *Brain* 2000; 123: 1838-44.

Oram MW, Perrett DI. Integration of form and motion in the anterior superior temporal polysensory area (STPa) of the macaque monkey. *J Neurophysiol* 1996; 76: 109-29.

Perrett DI, Harries MH, Bevan R, Thomas S, Benson PJ, Mistlin AJ, Chitty AJ, Hietanen JK, Ortega JE. Frameworks of analysis for the neural representation of animate objects and actions. *J Exp Biol* 1989; 146: 87-113.

Perrett DI, Hietanen JK, Oram MW, Benson PJ. Organization and functions of cells responsive to faces in the temporal cortex. *Philos Trans R Soc Lond B Biol Sci* 1992; 335: 23-30.

Perrett DI, Penton-Voak IS, Little AC, Tiddeman BP, Burt DM, Schmidt N, Oxley R, Kinloch N, Barrett L. Facial attractiveness judgements reflect learning of parental age characteristics. *Proc R Soc Lond B Biol Sci* 2002; 269: 873-80.

Perrett DI, Rolls ET, Caan W. Visual neurones responsive to faces in the monkey temporal cortex. *Exp Brain Res* 1982; 47: 329-42.

Perrett DI, Smith PA, Mistlin AJ, Chitty AJ, Head AS, Potter DD, Broennimann R, Milner AD, Jeeves MA. Visual analysis of body movements by neurones in the temporal cortex of the macaque monkey: a preliminary report. *Behav Brain Res* 1985a; 16: 153-70.

Perrett DI, Smith PA, Potter DD, Mistlin AJ, Head AS, Milner AD, Jeeves MA. Neurones responsive to faces in the temporal cortex: studies of functional organization, sensitivity to identity and relation to perception. *Hum Neurobiol* 1984; 3: 197-208.

Perrett DI, Smith PA, Potter DD, Mistlin AJ, Head AS, Milner AD, Jeeves MA. Visual cells in the temporal cortex sensitive to face view and gaze direction. *Proc R Soc Lond B Biol Sci* 1985b; 223: 293-317.

Premack D, Woodruff G. Does the chimpanzee have a theory of mind? *Behav Brain Sci* 1978; 1: 515-26.

Puce A, Allison T, Bentin S, Gore JC, McCarthy G. Temporal cortex activation in humans viewing eye and mouth movements. *J Neurosci* 1998; 18: 2188-99.

Puce A, Allison T, Gore JC, McCarthy G. Face-sensitive regions in human extrastriate cortex studied by functional MRI. *J Neurophysiol* 1995; 74: 1192-9.

Puce A, Smith A, Allison T. ERPs evoked by viewing facial movements. *Cogn Neuropsychol* 2000; 17: 221-39.

Rauschecker JP, Tian B. Mechanisms and streams for processing of "what" and "where" in auditory cortex. *Proc Natl Acad Sci USA* 2000; 97: 11800-6.

Redican WK. An evolutionary perspective on human facial displays. In: Ekman P, ed. *Emotion in the human face*. Cambridge.: Cambridge Univ. Press, 1982: 212-80.

Rizzolatti G, Fadiga L, Matelli M, Bettinardi V, Paulesu E, Perani D, Fazio F. Localization of grasp representations in humans by PET: 1. Observation *versus* execution. *Exp Brain Res* 1996; 111: 246-52.

Rolls ET. Neurophysiological mechanisms underlying face processing within and beyond the temporal cortical visual areas. *Philos Trans R Soc Lond B Biol Sci* 1992; 335: 11-20.

Schenk T, Zihl J. Visual motion perception after brain damage: II. Deficits in form-from-motion perception. *Neuropsychologia* 1997; 35: 1299-310.

Scholl BJ, Leslie AM (1999) Modularity, development and "theory of mind". *Mind Language* 1999; 14: 131-53.

Seltzer B, Pandya DN. Parietal, temporal, and occipital projections to cortex of the superior temporal sulcus in the rhesus monkey: a retrograde tracer study. *J Comp Neurol* 1994; 343: 445-63.

Sergent J, Ohta S, MacDonald B. Functional neuroanatomy of face and object processing. A positron emission tomography study. *Brain* 1992; 115 (Pt 1): 15-36.

Sergent J, Signoret JL. Functional and anatomical decomposition of face processing: evidence from prosopagnosia and PET study of normal subjects. *Philos Trans R Soc Lond B Biol Sci* 1992a; 335: 55-61.

Sergent J, Signoret JL. Varieties of functional deficits in prosopagnosia. *Cereb Cortex* 1992b; 2: 375-88.

Stevens JA, Fonlupt P, Shiffrar M, Decety J. New aspects of motion perception: selective neural encoding of apparent human movements. *Neuroreport* 2000; 11: 109-15.

Vaina LM, Lemay M, Bienfang DC, Choi AY, Nakayama K. Intact "biological motion" and "structure from motion" perception in a patient with impaired motion mechanisms: a case study. *Vis Neurosci* 1990; 5: 353-69.

Vandenberghe R, Nobre AC, Price CJ. The response of left temporal cortex to sentences. *J Cogn Neurosci* 2002; 14: 550-60.

Vandenberghe R, Price C, Wise R, Josephs O, Frackowiak RS. Functional anatomy of a common semantic system for words and pictures. *Nature* 1996; 383: 254-6.

Wachsmuth E, Oram MW, Perrett DI. Recognition of objects and their component parts: responses of single units in the temporal cortex of the macaque. *Cereb Cortex* 1994; 4: 509-22.

Wicker B, Michel F, Henaff MA, Decety J. Brain regions involved in the perception of gaze: a PET study. *Neuroimage* 1998; 8: 221-7.

Winston JS, Strange BA, O'Doherty J, Dolan RJ. Automatic and intentional brain responses during evaluation of trustworthiness of faces. *Nat Neurosci* 5: 277-83.

Yamane S, Kaji S, Kawano K. What facial features activate face neurons in the inferotemporal cortex of the monkey? *Exp Brain Res* 1988; 73: 209-14.

Young AW, Newcombe F, de Haan EH, Small M, Hay DC. Face perception after brain injury. Selective impairments affecting identity and expression. *Brain* 1993; 116 (Pt 4): 941-59.

Zacks JM, Braver TS, Sheridan MA, Donaldson DI, Snyder AZ, Ollinger JM, Buckner RL, Raichle ME. Human brain activity time-locked to perceptual event boundaries. *Nat Neurosci* 2001; 4: 651-5.

Zilbovicius M, Boddaert N, Belin P, Poline JB, Remy P, Mangin JF, Thivard L, Barthelemy C, Samson Y. Temporal lobe dysfunction in childhood autism: A PET study. *Am J Psychiatry* 2000; 157: 1988-93.

# Input of structural and metabolic MRI techniques in understanding neuronal dysfunction in temporal lobe epilepsy

**F. Cendes**

*Department of Neurology, FCM, UNICAMP, Campinas, SP, Brazil*

---

It is still unclear why, when and how neuronal damage and dysfunction occur in patients with temporal lobe epilepsy (TLE). It is possible, for example, that not all types of seizures do cause harm, or yet, that some individuals are more resistant to seizure-induced damage than others. Genetic background, age and type of initial brain insult, and other environmental factors, most likely interact in a number of ways, making it difficult to determine what are the exact mechanisms of ongoing brain damage in TLE (Cendes, 2004). Furthermore, mechanisms that are responsible for, or influence, the development of an epileptic condition differ from those that actually precipitate acute epileptic seizures (Schwartzkroin, 1993). Presumably, the acute structural change produced in a region of cortical tissue is not in itself sufficient for causing chronic seizures. Another complication, is the fact that seizure-related damage may be expressed in a number of ways; and not necessarily represent neuronal loss or atrophy (Sutula, 2004; Nairismagi et al., 2004). For example, many patients with TLE who do not respond well to treatment have progressive memory loss and signs of diffuse cognitive impairment, as well as progressive increase of bilateral epileptiform discharges (Morrell, 1989). Cognitive and behavioural impairment occur even in patients without measurable brain atrophy by conventional magnetic resonance imaging (MRI). These observations suggest that focal epileptic discharges may lead to neuronal dysfunction remote from the seizure focus.

Recent structural and metabolic MRI techniques have been instrumental for the better understanding of mechanisms of neuronal damage and dysfunction in TLE.

## Structural MRI studies in patients with TLE associated with mesial temporal sclerosis

Retrospective studies have shown a significant relationship between a history of prolonged febrile seizures (FS) in early childhood and mesial temporal sclerosis (MTS), as determined by magnetic resonance imaging (MRI) or postoperative histopathology (Falconer, 1974; Abou-Khalil et al., 1993; Cendes et al., 1993; Kuks et al., 1993; Trenerry et al., 1993; Maher et al., 1995; Cendes and Andermann, 2002). However, population studies have shown different results (Camfield et al., 1994; Nelson and Ellenberg, 1976). The interpretation of these observations remains controversial (Maher and McLachlan, 1995; Shinnar, 1998; Sloviter and Pedley, 1998). One possibility is that the early FS damages the hippocampus and is therefore a cause of hippocampal sclerosis (Abou-Khalil et al., 1993; Hamati-Haddad and Abou-Khalil, 1998; VanLandingham et al., 1998). Another possibility is that the child has a prolonged FS because the hippocampus was previously damaged due to a prenatal or perinatal insult or to a genetic predisposition (Cendes et al., 1995; Berkovic et al., 1996; Davies et al., 1996; Fernandez et al., 1998; Sloviter and Pedley, 1998, Kobayashi et al., 2001; Baulac et al., 2004).

There is a strong correlation between MTS and the severity of the epilepsy in series of surgical patients. In addition, MTS identified by MRI has been associated with poor control of seizures by antiepileptic medication (Semah et al., 1998). However, the findings of MRI abnormalities in patients with good outcome or seizure remission, indicates that MTS is found not only in patients with medically refractory TLE (Franceschi et al., 1989; Kim et al., 1999; Briellmann et al., 2001; Kobayashi et al., 2001a; Kobayashi et al., 2001b; Kobayashi et al., 2002).

## Hippocampal volumetric measurements

Several cross-sectional MRI studies have shown an association between the severity of atrophy of the hippocampus, amygdala, and entorhinal cortex and the duration of epilepsy, seizure frequency, or lifetime seizure number (Tasch et al., 1999; Salmenpera et al., 2001; Theodore and Gaillard, 2002; Kalviainen and Salmenpera, 2002; Theodore et al., 2003). Cross-sectional MRI studies, however, have limitations for identifying the cause of atrophy: acute damage associated with the initial insult; underlying pathology; chronic progression of damage caused by the initial insult that may be independent of recurrent seizures; or direct consequence of seizures. Another problem is the inaccurate quantification of seizure frequency and seizure number. Longitudinal studies may overcome several of these limitations, and recent data have confirmed ongoing subtle volumetric changes in brain volume in partial epilepsies. In temporal lobe epilepsy, the progressive atrophy affects mainly the hippocampus ipsilateral to the seizure "focus", but also other structures (Briellmann et al., 2001; Liu et al., 2001; Liu et al., 2003a; Liu et al., 2002; Fuerst et al., 2003). However, even longitudinal studies must account for brain changes over time that may occur independently of epilepsy or ongoing seizures (Liu et al., 2003b).

Patients with MTLE have significant reduction of the volume of the cortical structures with close anatomical and functional connections to the hippocampus – that is, the entorhinal and perirhinal cortices (Bonilha *et al.*, 2003; Bernasconi *et al.*, 2001; Bernasconi *et al.*, 2003). Other structures, such as the parahippocampal and temporopolar cortices, seem to be less affected (Bonilha *et al.*, 2003).

Studies in familial mesial temporal lobe epilepsy (FMTLE) showed that MRI signs of MTS were present in affected individuals (Cendes *et al.*, 1998; Kobayashi *et al.*, 2001; Kobayashi *et al.*, 2003) and in asymptomatic family members (Kobayashi *et al.*, 2002). In fact, two of the asymptomatic individuals in whom we documented hippocampal atrophy (Kobayashi *et al.*, 2002) developed MTLE a few years after they had MRI (unpublished data), but the others did not. These findings support the view that hippocampal abnormalities are probably not the sole consequence of repeated seizures and, that genetically determined mechanisms might play an important role in the development of hippocampal damage, which may be hereditary, at least in the context of FMTLE (Kobayashi *et al.*, 2001; 2002; 2003).

The finding of hippocampal atrophy in asymptomatic individuals and patients with rare seizures in one end, and patients with refractory epilepsy in the other end of the spectrum of FMTLE, provides a unique opportunity to investigate the additional contribution of seizure frequency in memory deficits in patients with hippocampal atrophy. We performed MRI volumetric measurements and compared memory performances in patients with refractory *versus* benign FMTLE *versus* their asymptomatic first-degree relatives (Alessio *et al.*, 2004). We found that individuals with hippocampal atrophy had more severe memory deficits than those with normal hippocampi independently from clinical status (asymptomatic, benign or refractory epilepsy). Even those with hippocampal atrophy and good seizure control, seizure remission or asymptomatic had significantly worse memory function than patients without hippocampal atrophy but similar clinical presentation. However, the interaction of hippocampal atrophy and refractory seizures was related to worst memory performance.

## ■ Measurements of hippocampal signal

Studies with T2 signal quantification (relaxometry) showed a high sensitivity and specificity for hippocampal signal abnormalities in patients with TLE (Briellmann *et al.*, 2002; Van Paesschen *et al.*, 1997b). T2 signal abnormalities appears to correlate with gliosis and may not be directly related to the degree of neuronal loss (Van Paesschen *et al.*, 1997; Briellmann *et al.*, 2002).

We measured T1 and T2 signals in MRIs of 152 individuals (106 affected and 46 asymptomatics) from 36 unrelated families with FMTLE (Coan *et al.*, 2004). T2 signal changes were more frequent and more severe than T1 signal changes among affected and unaffected individuals; however, T1 signal changes appeared to discriminate better affected from unaffected individuals. This may indicate that significant T1 signal changes occur only in more advanced hippocampal pathology, which is consistent with our observation in patients with TLE undergoing pre-surgical investigation (Coan *et al.*, 2003). T2 signal abnormalities were not identified in all affected subjects with MTLE; in addition, they were present in 48% of unaffected individuals

(Coan et al., 2004). Furthermore, we observed that 55% of patients with normal hippocampal volumes had abnormal hippocampal signal (Coan et al., 2004). This altogether, may support the existence of less severe MTS or pre-existing abnormalities, that appear to be inherited in the context of these families (Kobayashi et al., 2001a, Kobayashi et al., 2002; Kobayashi et al., 2003), and is in agreement with findings of MRI texture analysis discussed below.

## ■ Hippocampal texture analysis

The texture of images refers to the appearance, structure and arrangement of the parts of an object within the image (Castellano et al., 2004). We may attribute the texture concept in a digital image to the distribution of grey-level values among the pixels of a given region of interest in the image. Texture analysis of MR images is a quantitative method that can be used to detect and quantify structural abnormalities in different tissues (Castellano et al., 2004). It makes possible to assess the degree of gray-tone modifications and the alterations of gray-tone spatial distribution in a given anatomical region of interest. This gray-tone variation is thought to correspond to underlying functional and anatomical changes (Bernasconi et al., 2001; Antel et al., 2003). In this setting, texture analysis may be sensitive to detect subtle changes in MRI and to extract more information than visual assessment.

In a group of 19 consecutive patients who underwent temporal lobectomy due to unilateral refractory MTLE, with histological confirmation of HS, texture analysis showed a significant difference of almost all texture parameters of hippocampi with histologically proven hippocampal sclerosis (HS) and hippocampi contralateral to the side of HS, compared to control group (Bonilha et al., 2003a). We have not observed however, differences between the hippocampi with HS and the contralateral hippocampi, even through the selection of the most discriminant features (Bonilha et al., 2003a). The observation of bilateral hippocampal abnormalities is concordant with the knowledge that hippocampal pathology results in asymmetrically bilateral texture alterations (Yu et al., 2001).

We have also found that texture analysis was significantly different between normal controls and subjects with FMTLE with a wide spectrum of clinical presentation and severity of hippocampal atrophy (Caselato et al., 2003). This difference was similar for both hippocampi as found in previous studies (Yu et al., 2001; Bonilha et al., 2003). Interestingly, this alteration was more pronounced in the non-affected subjects, relatives in first degree of the MTLE patients (Caselato et al., 2003). If confirmed, this could indicate, for example, that the abnormal texture reflects a tissue vulnerability determined by a genetic defect (in non-affected individuals) which could precede the development of the full blown hippocampal sclerosis; and the occurrence of clinical seizures. Once the MTS develops, albeit still abnormal compared to controls, there may be a modification of the hippocampal texture pattern. Therefore, this would explain the apparent discrepancy of more pronounced hippocampal texture abnormalities in non-affected individuals (who are at risk for developing TLE) as compared to the individuals with MRI signs of MTS belonging to families with FMTLE.

## Voxel based morphometry

Voxel based morphometry (VBM) is a recently described technique for evaluation of MRI morphometric differences between subjects or groups of subjects (Friston et al., 1995; Ashburner and Friston, 2000; Good et al., 2001). VBM is performed by the determination of the concentration of different brain tissues such as gray matter, white matter and cerebrospinal fluid (CSF). To estimate these concentrations, the VBM uses images previously corrected for inter-individual variability of brain shape and size according to a pre-defined stereotactic template (Collins et al., 1994). Subsequent to normalization, the scans from all the participants are in a common stereotactic space, allowing analysis among individuals and close correspondence to other neuroimaging studies. Next, the images undergo segmentation of tissue, which estimate the tissue concentration for each voxel (Good et al., 2001) preserving its quantity while ensuring a good spatial alignment between patients and controls. Finally, the images are convolved in order to minimize gyral inter-individual variability. This smoothing creates images that are more normally distributed and permits voxel-wise analysis. The resulting images are then compared using the convenient statistical test to search of differences between subjects or groups in the probability of each voxel being gray matter, or white matter or CSF.

Since partial epilepsies are disorders affecting the gray matter, VBM studies of partial epilepsies have focused on gray matter concentration (GMC). The primary goal of the use of VBM studies in partial epilepsies is to define areas within the brain that show different GMC in a group of patients with a similar form of partial epilepsies as compared to normal controls.

Recent studies showed that in patients with MTLE the reduction in GMC extends beyond the hippocampus ipsilateral to the seizure origin, involving cortical and subcortical structures connected to the hippocampus and parahippocampal region (Bernasconi et al., 2004; Bonilha et al., 2004).

## Proton magnetic resonance spectroscopy studies in TLE

Magnetic resonance spectroscopy (MRS) enables noninvasive measurements of certain compounds in living tissue. The noninvasive nature of MRS means that repeated measurements can be made, so that kinetic and longitudinal studies are possible in a single subject. In addition, one can study human tissues that are inaccessible except by invasive techniques. In the human brain, phosphate energy stores, intracellular pH, lactate concentration, and the neuronal marker N-Acetylaspartate (NAA) are examples of MRS-measurable variables that are important for both clinical and scientific purposes and cannot be studied easily by any other technique (Cendes et al., 2002).

Proton magnetic resonance spectroscopy (MRS) studies have shown focal reductions of N-Acetylaspartate (NAA) signal in patients with different forms of TLE, including those with normal MRI, as well as extra-temporal partial epilepsies. Both single-voxel and multivoxel $^1$H-MRS have high sensitivity for detecting low NAA indicative of neuronal dysfunction in focal epilepsies. Decreases in NAA correlate strongly with

EEG abnormalities and severity of cell loss, and may be a more sensitive measure than structural MRI. However, the NAA decrease is often more widespread than the epileptogenic focus. A major limitation of current proton MRS studies in epilepsy is the inability of covering the entire brain in a single acquisition, thus leading to major sampling bias. The area of maximal abnormality may reside further away, even when there is an abnormality inside of the volume of interest used for that particular exam. These observations, together with the fact of the often widespread NAA abnormality, need to be taken into account for the correct and adequate interpretation of proton MRS studies in the assessment of partial epilepsies (Cendes et al., 2002).

Proton MRS studies (Hugg et al., 1996; Cendes et al., 1997; Serles et al., 2001) have shown recovery of relative NAA either ipsilaterally or contralaterally after successful temporal lobe removal. This suggests that structural or functional changes associated with seizure activity may lead to depression of NAA in the ipsilateral or contralateral temporal lobe. These observations have potentially great significance for understanding the utility of imaging NAA in the presurgical lateralization of TLE. They suggest that reduction in NAA reflects not only the sequel of the initial injury to temporal lobe structures, but also an effect of the seizure activity itself (or other factors associated with the ongoing epileptic state). Still, what remains most interesting is the component of NAA decrease that is not directly related to neuronal loss.

Studies have also investigated the relationships between NAA and cognition in patients with epilepsy (Gadian et al., 1996; Incisa della Rocchetta et al., 1995; Martin et al., 1999; Sawrie et al., 2000; Sawrie et al., 2001). Incisa della (Rocchetta et al., 1995) found that patients with right TLE and a contralateral (i.e., left temporal) abnormality on $^1$H-MRS performed significantly worse on measures of episodic verbal memory than those patients with right onset but without a contralateral abnormality.

Studies using MRSI investigating whether TLE is a progressive disease have produced seemingly conflicting results. Vermathen et al. (2000) studied a group of patients with non-temporal neocortical epilepsy and showed that hippocampal NAA/Cr was not reduced, in contrast to patients with unilateral TLE. They argued that seizures did not cause secondary hippocampal damage. Garcia et al. (1997) found a negative correlation between NAA and seizure frequency in patients with both frontal and temporal epilepsy, although there was no correlation with duration of epilepsy. Tash et al. (1999) found that ipsilateral and contralateral NAA/Cr was negatively correlated with duration of temporal lobe epilepsy. Frequency of complex partial seizures was not correlated with MRS or MRI volumetric abnormalities. Patients with frequent generalized tonic-clonic seizures had lower NAA/Cr bilaterally and smaller hippocampal volumes ipsilaterally than patients with none or rare generalized tonic-clonic seizures (Tasch et al., 1999). This study suggests that temporal lobe epilepsy begins with an early injury, which occurs asymmetrically, and is followed by a gradual and progressive course of further neuronal loss and dysfunction. The etiology of the progression remains uncertain.

# Conclusion

Modern neuroimaging techniques, including high resolution structural MRI, proton magnetic resonance spectroscopy and other functional imaging modalities, have provided substantial new insights suggesting that the epileptogenic damage is both cause and consequence of repeated seizures. However, the causes of MTS and mechanisms of progression of damage are still unknown. Although there is a high incidence of complex FS among patients with MTS in retrospective studies, it is still not clear whether complex FS are an epiphenomenon or a causative factor. Recognition of the syndrome of FMTLE indicates a strong genetic role as one of the probable causes for the development of MTS.

# References

Abou-Khalil B, Andermann E, Andermann F, et al. Temporal lobe epilepsy after prolonged febrile convulsions: excellent outcome after surgical treatment. *Epilepsia* 1993; 34: 878-83.

Alessio A, Kobayashi E, Damasceno BP, et al. Evidence of memory impairment in asymptomatic individuals with hippocampal atrophy. *Epilepsy Behav* 2004; 5: 981-7.

Antel SB, Collins DL, Bernasconi N, et al. Automated detection of focal cortical dysplasia lesions using computational models of their MRI characteristics and texture analysis. *Neuroimage* 2003; 19: 1748-59.

Ashburner J, Friston KJ. Voxel-based morphometry – the methods. *Neuroimage* 2000; 11: 805-21.

Baulac S, Gourfinkel-An I, Nabbout R, et al. Fever, genes, and epilepsy. *Lancet Neurol* 2004; 3: 421-30.

Berkovic SF, Mcintosh A, Howell RA, et al. Familial temporal lobe epilepsy – a common disorder identified in twins. *Ann Neurol* 1996; 40: 227-35.

Bernasconi A, Antel SB, Collins DL, et al. Texture analysis and morphological processing of magnetic resonance imaging assist detection of focal cortical dysplasia in extra-temporal partial epilepsy. *Ann Neurol* 2001; 49: 770-5.

Bernasconi N, Bernasconi A, Caramanos Z, et al. Entorhinal cortex atrophy in epilepsy patients exhibiting normal hippocampal volumes. *Neurology* 2001; 56: 1335-9.

Bernasconi N, Bernasconi A, Caramanos Z et al. Mesial temporal damage in temporal lobe epilepsy: a volumetric MRI study of the hippocampus, amygdala and parahippocampal region. *Brain* 2003; 126: 462-9.

Bernasconi N, Duchesne S, Janke A, et al. Whole-brain voxel-based statistical analysis of gray matter and white matter in temporal lobe epilepsy. *Neuroimage* 2004; 23: 717-723.

Bonilha L, Kobayashi E, Castellano G, et al. Texture analysis of hippocampal sclerosis. *Epilepsia* 2003; 44: 1546-50.

Bonilha L, Kobayashi E, Rorden C, et al. Medial temporal lobe atrophy in patients with refractory temporal lobe epilepsy. *J Neurol Neurosurg Psychiatry* 2003; 74: 1627-30.

Bonilha L, Rorden C, Castellano G, et al. Voxel-based morphometry reveals gray matter network atrophy in refractory medial temporal lobe epilepsy. *Arch Neurol* 2004; 61: 1379-84.

Briellmann RS, Newton MR, Wellard RM, et al. Hippocampal sclerosis following brief generalized seizures in adulthood. *Neurology* 2001; 57: 315-7.

Briellmann RS, Kalnins RM, Berkovic SF, et al. Hippocampal pathology in refractory temporal lobe epilepsy: T2-weighted signal change reflects dentate gliosis. *Neurology* 2002; 58: 265-71.

Camfield P, Camfield C, Gordon K, et al. What types of epilepsy are preceded by febrile seizures? A population-based study of children. *Dev Med Child Neurol* 1994; 36: 887-92.

Caselato GR, Kobayashi E, Bonilha L, et al. Hippocampal texture analysis in patients with familial mesial temporal lobe epilepsy. *Arq Neuropsiquiatr* 2003; 61 (suppl 1): 83-7.

Castellano G, Bonilha L, Li LM, et al. Texture analysis of medical images. *Clin Radiol* 2004; 59: 1061-9.

Cendes F. Febrile seizures and mesial temporal sclerosis. *Curr Opin Neurol* 2004; 17: 161-4.

Cendes F, Andermann F, Dubeau F, et al. Early childhood prolonged febrile convulsions, atrophy and sclerosis of mesial structures and temporal lobe epilepsy: an MRI volumetric study. *Neurology* 1993; 43: 1083-7.

Cendes F, Cook MJ, Watson C, et al. Frequency and characteristics of dual pathology in patients with lesional epilepsy. *Neurology* 1995; 45: 2058-64.

Cendes F, Andermann F, Dubeau F, et al. Normalization of neuronal metabolic dysfunction after surgery for temporal lobe epilepsy. Evidence from proton MR spectroscopic imaging. *Neurology* 1997; 49: 1525-33.

Cendes F, Lopes-Cendes I, Andermann E, et al. Familial temporal lobe epilepsy: a clinically heterogeneous syndrome. *Neurology* 1998; 50: 554-7.

Cendes F, Andermann F. Do febrile seizures promote temporal lobe epilepsy? Retrospective studies. In: Baram TZ, Shinnar S, eds. *Febrile Seizures*. San Diego CA: Academic Press, 2002: 77-86.

Cendes F, Knowlton RC, Novotny E, et al. Magnetic Resonance Spectroscopy in Epilepsy: Clinical Issues. *Epilepsia* 2002; 43: 32-9.

Coan AC, Kobayashi E, Li LM, et al. Quantification of hippocampal signal intensity in patients with mesial temporal lobe epilepsy. *J Neuroimaging* 2003; 13: 228-33.

Coan AC, Kobayashi E, Lopes-Cendes I, et al. Abnormalities of hippocampal signal intensity in patients with familial mesial temporal lobe epilepsy. *Braz J Med Biol Res* 2004; 37: 827-32.

Collins DL, Neelin P, Peters TM, et al. Automatic 3D intersubject registration of MR volumetric data in standardized Talairach space. *J Comput Assist Tomogr* 1994; 18: 192-205.

Davies KG, Hermann BP, Dohan FC, et al. Relationship of hippocampal sclerosis to duration and age of onset of epilepsy, and childhood febrile seizures in temporal lobectomy patients. *Epilepsy Res* 1996; 24: 119-26.

Falconer MA. Mesial temporal (Ammon's horn) sclerosis as a common cause of epilepsy. Aetiology, treatment, and prevention. *Lancet* 1974; 2: 767-70.

Fernandez G, Effenberger O, Vinz B, et al. Hippocampal malformation as a cause of familial febrile convulsions and subsequent hippocampal sclerosis. *Neurology* 1998; 50: 909-17.

Franceschi M, Triulzi F, Ferini-Strambi L, et al. Focal cerebral lesions found by magnetic resonance imaging in cryptogenic nonrefractory temporal lobe epilepsy patients. *Epilepsia* 1989; 30: 540-6.

Friston KJ, Holmes AP, Worsley K, Poline JB, Frith CD, Frackowiak RSJ. Statistic parametric maps in functional imaging: A general linear approach. *Hum Brain Mapp* 1995; 2: 189-210.

Fuerst D, Shah J, Shah A, et al. Hippocampal sclerosis is a progressive disorder: a longitudinal volumetric MRI study. *Ann Neurol* 2003; 53: 413-6.

Gadian DG, Isaacs EB, Cross JH, et al. Lateralization of brain function in childhood revealed by magnetic resonance spectroscopy. *Neurology* 1996; 46: 974-7.

Garcia PA, Laxer KD, van der Grond J, et al. Correlation of seizure frequency with N-acetyl-aspartate levels determined by 1H magnetic resonance spectroscopic imaging. *Magn Reson Imaging* 1997; 15: 475-8.

Good CD, Johnsrude IS, Ashburner J, et al. A voxel-based morphometric study of ageing in 465 normal adult human brains. *Neuroimage* 2001; 14: 21-36.

Hamati-Haddad A, Abou-Khalil B. Epilepsy diagnosis and localization in patients with antecedent childhood febrile convulsions. *Neurology* 1998; 50: 917-22.

Hugg JW, Kuzniecky RI, Gilliam FG, et al. Normalization of contralateral metabolic function following temporal lobectomy demonstrated by H-1 magnetic resonance spectroscopic imaging. *Ann Neurol* 1996; 40: 236-9.

Incisa della Rocchetta A, Gadian DG, Connelly A, et al. Verbal memory impairment after right temporal lobe surgery: role of contralateral damage as revealed by 1H magnetic resonance spectroscopy and T2 relaxometry. *Neurology* 1995; 45: 797-802.

Jackson GD, Kim SE, Fitt GJ, et al. Hippocampal T(2) abnormalities correlate with antecedent events and help predict seizure intractability. *Dev Neurosci* 1999; 21: 200-6.

Jackson GD, Connelly A, Duncan JS, et al. Detection of hippocampal pathology in intractable partial epilepsy: increased sensitivity with quantitative magnetic resonance T2 relaxometry. *Neurology* 1993; 43: 1793-9.

Kalviainen R, Salmenpera T. Do recurrent seizures cause neuronal damage? A series of studies with MRI volumetry in adults with partial epilepsy. *Prog Brain Res* 2002; 135: 279-95.

Kim WJ, Park SC, Lee SJ, et al. The prognosis for control of seizures with medications in patients with MRI evidence for mesial temporal sclerosis. *Epilepsia* 1999; 40: 290-3.

Kobayashi E, Lopes-Cendes I, Guerreiro CA, et al. Seizure outcome and hippocampal atrophy in familial mesial temporal lobe epilepsy. *Neurology* 2001; 56: 166-72.

Kobayashi E, Guerreiro CA, Cendes F. Late onset temporal lobe epilepsy with MRI evidence of mesial temporal sclerosis following acute neurocysticercosis: case report. *Arq Neuropsiquiatr* 2001; 59: 255-8.

Kobayashi E, Li LM, Lopes-Cendes I, et al. Magnetic resonance imaging evidence of hippocampal sclerosis in asymptomatic, first-degree relatives of patients with familial mesial temporal lobe epilepsy. *Arch Neurol* 2002; 59: 1891-4.

Kobayashi E, D'Agostino MD, Lopes-Cendes I, et al. Hippocampal atrophy and T2-weighted signal changes in familial mesial temporal lobe epilepsy. *Neurology* 2003; 60: 405-9.

Kuks JB, Cook MJ, Fish DR, et al. Hippocampal sclerosis in epilepsy and childhood febrile seizures. *Lancet* 1993; 342: 1391-4.

Liu RS, Lemieux L, Bell GS, et al. A longitudinal quantitative MRI study of community-based patients with chronic epilepsy and newly diagnosed seizures: methodology and preliminary findings. *Neuroimage* 2001; 14: 231-43.

Liu RS, Lemieux L, Sander JW, et al. Seizure-associated hippocampal volume loss: a longitudinal magnetic resonance study of temporal lobe epilepsy. *Ann Neurol* 2002; 52: 861.

Liu RS, Lemieux L, Bell GS, et al. A longitudinal study of brain morphometrics using quantitative magnetic resonance imaging and difference image analysis. *Neuroimage* 2003; 20: 22-33.

Liu RS, Lemieux L, Bell GS, et al. Progressive neocortical damage in epilepsy. *Ann Neurol* 2003; 53: 312-324

Maher J, McLachlan RS. Febrile convulsions. Is seizure duration the most important predictor of temporal lobe epilepsy? *Brain* 1995; 118: 1521-8.

Martin RC, Sawrie S, Hugg J, et al. Cognitive correlates of $^1$H-MRSI-detected hippocampal abnormalities in temporal lobe epilepsy. *Neurology* 1999; 53: 2052-8.

Morrell F. Varieties of human secondary epileptogenesis. *J Clin Neurophysiol* 1989; 6: 227-75.

Nairismagi J, Grohn OH, Kettunen MI, et al. Progression of brain damage after status epilepticus and its association with epileptogenesis: a quantitative MRI study in a rat model of temporal lobe epilepsy. *Epilepsia* 2004; 45: 1024-34.

Nelson KB, Ellenberg JH. Predictors of epilepsy in children who have experienced febrile seizures. *N Engl J Med* 1976; 295: 1029-33.

Salmenpera T, Kalviainen R, Partanen K, et al. Hippocampal and amygdaloid damage in partial epilepsy: a cross-sectional MRI study of 241 patients. *Epilepsy Res* 2001; 46: 69-82.

Sawrie SM, Martin RC, Gilliam F, et al. Nonlinear trends in hippocampal metabolic function and verbal memory: evidence of cognitive reserve in temporal lobe epilepsy. *Epilepsy and Behavior* 2000; 1: 106-11.

Sawrie SM, Martin RC, Gilliam FG, et al. Visual confrontation naming and hippocampal function: A neural network study using quantitative (1)H magnetic resonance spectroscopy. *Brain* 2001; 123: 770-80.

Schwartzkroin PA. *Epilepsy: Models, mechanisms, and concepts.* Cambridge University Press, 1993.

Semah F, Picot MC, Adam C, et al. Is the underlying cause of epilepsy a major prognostic factor for recurrence? [see comments]. *Neurology* 1998; 51: 1256-62.

Serles W, Li LM, Antel SB, et al. Time course of postoperative recovery of N-acetyl-aspartate in temporal lobe epilepsy. *Epilepsia* 2001; 42: 190-7.

Shinnar S. Prolonged febrile seizures and mesial temporal sclerosis [editorial; comment]. *Ann Neurol* 1998; 43: 411-2.

Sloviter RS, Pedley TA. Subtle hippocampal malformation: importance in febrile seizures and development of epilepsy [editorial; comment]. *Neurology* 1998; 50: 846-9.

Sutula TP. Mechanisms of epilepsy progression: current theories and perspectives from neuroplasticity in adulthood and development. *Epilepsy Res* 2004; 60: 161-71.

Tasch E, Cendes F, Li LM et al. Neuroimaging evidence of progressive neuronal loss and dysfunction in temporal lobe epilepsy. *Ann Neurol* 1999; 45: 568-76.

Theodore WH, Gaillard WD. Neuroimaging and the progression of epilepsy. *Prog Brain Res* 2002; 135: 305-13.

Theodore WH, DeCarli C, Gaillard WD. Total cerebral volume is reduced in patients with localization-related epilepsy and a history of complex febrile seizures. *Arch Neurol* 2003; 60: 250-2.

Trenerry MR, Jack CR, Jr., Sharbrough FW, et al. Quantitative MRI hippocampal volumes: association with onset and duration of epilepsy, and febrile convulsions in temporal lobectomy patients. *Epilepsy Res* 1993; 15: 247-52.

VanLandingham KE, Heinz ER, Cavazos JE, et al. Magnetic resonance imaging evidence of hippocampal injury after prolonged focal febrile convulsions. *Ann Neurol* 1998; 43: 413-26.

Van Paesschen W, Connelly A, King MD, et al. The spectrum of hippocampal sclerosis: a quantitative magnetic resonance imaging study. *Ann Neurol* 1997; 41: 41-51.

Van Paesschen W, Revesz T, Duncan JS, et al. Quantitative neuropathology and quantitative magnetic resonance imaging of the hippocampus in temporal lobe epilepsy. *Ann Neurol* 1997; 42: 756-66.

Van Paesschen W, Duncan JS, Stevens JM, et al. Longitudinal quantitative hippocampal magnetic resonance imaging study of adults with newly diagnosed partial seizures: one-year follow-up results. *Epilepsia* 1998; 39: 633-9.

Vermathen P, Laxer KD, Matson GB, et al. Hippocampal structures: anteroposterior N-acetylaspartate differences in patients with epilepsy and control subjects as shown with proton MR spectroscopic imaging. *Radiology* 2000; 214 (2): 403-10.

Yu O, Mauss Y, Namer IJ, et al. Existence of contralateral abnormalities revealed by texture analysis in unilateral intractable hippocampal epilepsy. *Magn Reson Imaging* 2001; 19: 1305-10.

# Temporal lobe epilepsy and cognition in children: will fMRI be of some help for a better understanding of the mechanisms involved?

D.A. Weber[1], M.M. Berl[1], E.N. Moore[1], G.A. Gioia[1], E.K. Ritzl[2], N.B. Ratner[3], C. Vaidya[1,4], W. Davis Gaillard[1,2,3]

[1] Department of Neurosciences, Children's National Medical Center, George Washington University School of Medicine, Washington DC
[2] Clinical Epilepsy Section, NINDS, NIH, Bethesda
[3] Department of Hearing and Speech Sciences, University of Maryland, College Park
[4] Department of Psychology, Georgetown University, Washington DC, USA

---

This chapter will consider the effects of temporal lobe epilepsy on cognitive function in children as shown by functional neuroimaging methods. The focus will primarily be on language studies using functional magnetic resonance imaging (fMRI) as this is the most extensively studied cognitive domain. Other aspects of basic and higher cognitive function including executive function, emotional regulation, and memory can be studied using similar techniques, but they have not been employed in pediatric epilepsy populations. fMRI language investigations provide insight into factors affecting anomalous language lateralization commonly found in epilepsy populations and hold theoretical importance regarding understanding of organization and reorganization of higher cognitive processes. The majority of research to date has focused on adult populations – though the onset epilepsy is during childhood – but an increasing number of language studies are being performed in children. These studies demonstrate similar language networks in adults and children (Gaillard et al., 2000a; Gaillard et al., 2001b; Gaillard et al., 2002; Schlaggar et al., 2002; Ahmad et al., 2003; Gaillard et al., 2003a; Gaillard et al., 2003b; Brown et al., 2004). Although the primary focus will be on fMRI imaging techniques, a review of other pertinent data (intra-carotid amobarbital test (IAT or Wada procedure), electro-cortical stimulation (ECS)) will also be included. This paper will consider four different aspects of fMRI cognitive investigations in temporal lobe epilepsy (TLE):

- fMRI principles and validation by invasive modalities;
- Normal language patterns & language laterality;
- Language findings in epilepsy patient populations;
- And expanding areas of fMRI research.

Epilepsy is a prevalent neurological disorder found in approximately 1.5 percent of the population (Hauser, 1983). Upwards of 30 percent of individuals with epilepsy are at risk for exhibiting language impairment and processing difficulties (Adcock et al., 2003). There is evidence in cross sectional studies for progressive harmful effects in some localization related epilepsies, and temporal lobe epilepsy (TLE) in particular, including cognitive decline, progressive hippocampal atrophy, and reduced gray and white-matter volume (Cascino, 1991; Cook, 1992; Cendes, 1993; Marsh, 1997; Lawson, 2000; Hermann et al., 2002; Bernasconi, 2003; Liu, 2003; Theodore et al., 2003), and remote atrophy in temporal lobe projections such as fornix and thalamus (DeCarli, 1998; Natsume, 2003). There is also evidence for both regional and remote metabolic abnormalities identified with FDG-PET and MRS. In mesial temporal lobe epilepsy FDG-PET shows decreased glucose consumption in ipsilateral lateral temporal neocortex, thalamus and inferior frontal lobe, while MRS shows abnormalities in contralateral hippocampus (Theodore et al., 1988; DeCarli et al., 1995; Gaillard et al., 1995; Cendes et al., 1997b; Li et al., 2000).

The local and remote regional effects seen in TLE make plausible regional and remote effects on higher ordered cognitive functions mediated by these brain structures such as language, memory, and emotional regulation. Since epilepsy is primarily a pediatric disorder with ramifications that extend into adulthood, there are often harmful consequences for language, intellectual, and cognitive development during this sensitive window of development.

The nature of language impairments in children with TLE and adults with childhood onset epilepsy is well documented and detailed in accompanying chapters. There is continued debate to the extent to which language is able to successfully reorganize behaviorally in the right hemisphere in the setting of left temporal lobe epilepsy. Some investigators find evidence of incomplete restoration of language functions following transfer, while others find no such evidence of language skill impairment (Helmstaedter et al., 1994; Loring et al., 1999). While the resection of the left temporal lobe places patients at risk for further language impairments, improvement in VIQ following right temporal lobectomy in some adults points to a deleterious effect of epilepsy on language functions (Novelly et al., 1984; Baxendale, 2002). These studies alone are not able to answer questions related to the functional and structural reorganization of language. fMRI, in conjunction with neuropsychological assessment, is a versatile tool for noninvasive identification of areas of the brain implicated in language function and the disrupted language networks found in epilepsy populations.

# fMRI principles and validation by invasive modalities

## Principles of functional MRI

This section provides a brief review of fMRI principles, validity, and limitations to provide a background for the chapter; full reviews are available elsewhere (Cohen & Bookheimer, 1994; Moonen & Bandettini, 2000; Logothetis et al., 2001). fMRI primarily utilizes the blood oxygenation level-dependent (BOLD) technique that allows for indirect measurement of neuronal activity based on detecting associated signal changes induced by increases in blood volume, flow, and composition (through an increase in ratio of oxygenated to deoxygenated blood). Increases in dendritic synaptic activity are tightly linked to highly regulated local changes in blood flow. As a consequence, measurements are based on relative differences in signal between two conditions (experimental or target *versus* control or baseline). Areas involved in processing a task may not appear "activated" (meeting statistical criteria for difference in signal for target *versus* control task); areas "activated" may be associated with, but not critical to, the task. The temporal resolution, six seconds, precludes analysis of interaction between posterior and anterior language processing networks.

In order to identify common areas of activation with greater statistical power, group studies are traditionally employed (Gaillard et al., 2001a). These analyses typically involve modest study sample sizes (8-15) and data is analyzed in a common anatomic atlas. Random effects analysis allows the group finding to be extrapolated to broad populations. Group studies however, assume a homogenous population and assume that a uniform network exists for any given cognitive function. The multiple confounds found in patients populations suggest such approaches and results must be viewed with caution as they may be misleading (Gaillard, 2004a). The particular power of fMRI resides in individual subject analysis that, in turn, allows for the examination of the effect of developmental conditions and disease states in language processes.

Several methodological approaches distinguish child and patient based language studies. Isolating the area of interest on an individual basis depends upon the ability to detect change between experimental and control conditions. Patients must be able to perform the task, thus tasks may need to be adjusted for ability. The choice of an appropriate control for patients is also important and may require high contrast between conditions (Balsamo & Gaillard, 2002; Gaillard, 2004a). Refined methods with proper task selection may be used to parse out and target different aspects of language processing (Gaillard, 2004b).

## Validation of fMRI

It is known from previous intra-carotid amobarbital test studies, the standard for pre-operative assessment of language dominance, that localization related epilepsy is associated with a high incidence of inter-hemispheric reorganization of language (Rasmussen & Milner, 1977; Woods et al., 1988; Loring et al., 1999; Janszky et al., 2003b). These studies, involving substantial numbers of patients, find atypical language dominance in up to 33% of patients with left hemisphere epilepsy (approximately 20-25% of patients with left temporal lobe epilepsy), and 0-4% of patients with right hemisphere epilepsy. These studies also suggest that early brain lesions combined with atypical handedness are associated with greater likelihood of atypical language representation. Electro-cortical stimulation studies demonstrate intra-hemispheric reorganization of language in areas adjacent to Broca's (anterior and superior to Broca's) and Wernicke's (e.g. anterior, mid temporal); they also suggest intra-hemispheric reorganization may occur with onset of epilepsy later in childhood, after five or six years (Ojemann et al., 1989; Devinsky et al., 1993).

Epilepsy populations provided the opportunity to validate blood flow based functional mapping techniques, fMRI and $^{15}$O water PET. There is excellent, but not complete, agreement with invasive tests such as IAT (wada test) and ECS (electro-cortical stimulation). Repeated studies involving over 400 patients report high (over 90%) concordance rates between IAT and fMRI for determining language lateralization (Binder et al., 1996; Yetkin et al., 1998; Benson et al., 1999; Pujol et al., 1999; Lehericy et al., 2000; Carpentier et al., 2001; Gaillard et al., 2002; Rutten et al., 2002; Adcock et al., 2003; Fernandez et al., 2003; Woermann et al., 2003; Gaillard, 2004a). Investigations with fMRI, and trans-cranial doppler agree with patient based IAT findings for typical and atypical language dominance and agree with IAT predictions that atypical language would be found in 4-7% of right handed and 30% of left handed healthy volunteers (Rasmussen & Milner, 1977; Pujol et al., 1999; Springer et al., 1999; Knecht et al., 2000).

Overt disagreement between IAT and fMRI is rare, but may occur when the physiologic basis for the BOLD response is disrupted (Jayakar et al., 2002; Lehericy et al., 2002; Rother et al., 2002; Gaillard, 2004a). Important for this topic is the observation that a post-ictal state may affect functional imaging results (Jayakar et al., 2002). Partial disparity, reported in 10% of patient studies, occurs when one method is rated unilateral and the other bilateral. Part of the disparity seen revolves on defining "bilateral" language. Instances can be found where one or the other method (fMRI or IAT) was "correct" based on ECS or post operative outcome (Pardo & Fox, 1993; Jayakar et al., 2002; Lehericy et al., 2002; Gaillard et al., 2004; Kho et al., 2005). In these circumstances fMRI may be used in to provide complementary information to IAT regarding language lateralization (Ries et al., 2004; Kho et al., 2005). Finally, comparison between fMRI and ECS finds 90% sensitivity and 67% specificity, confirming a close link between disrupting brain function by ECS and eliciting function with fMRI (Bookheimer et al., 1997; Pouratian et al., 2002; Rutten et al., 2002).

fMRI confers important advantages over invasive methods. The entire brain may be imaged providing a means of localizing and identifying distributed brain networks both out of view to either IAT or ECS. Studying both normal and disease states adds to the limited information presently available regarding the organization of neuronal systems. Paradigms can probe several distinct aspects of language processing and can be repeated. fMRI allows for more extensive mapping of complex language function and examination of the relationship between disease progression and its impact on neural function and organization thus providing an effective means to enhance understanding of language and other cognitive functioning in temporal lobe epilepsy.

## Normal language patterns and language laterality

### Typical areas of activation and language tasks in children

Aspects of language commonly studied through fMRI include verbal fluency (semantic and phonologic), reading, story listening, sentence comprehension, and semantic/phonologic decision (Balsamo & Gaillard, 2002). When combined, these tasks identify the posterior "receptive" language regions found in left superior temporal sulcus implicated in language comprehension, and the anterior "expressive" areas found in the inferior frontal gyrus (IFG) implicated in word retrieval, planning, and grammatical processing (Geschwind & Galaburda, 1985; Gaillard, 2004a).

Verbal fluency tasks – semantic, phonologic, and verb generation from nouns – are among the most commonly reported language tasks used to identify frontal language areas in fMRI studies in adults and children (Harvey et al., 1999; Logan et al., 1999; Poldrack et al., 1999; Gaillard et al., 2000a; Keene et al., 2000; Holland et al., 2001; Gaillard et al., 2002; Liegeois et al., 2002; Schlaggar et al., 2002; Gaillard et al., 2003b; Brown et al., 2004; Wood et al., 2004). These tasks have been shown to reliably activate the dorsolateral prefrontal cortex and the ventrolateral cortex [inferior frontal gyrus (IFG)], but have variable temporal activation. Category decision tasks in children based on the Binder et al. paradigm (Binder et al., 1995; Binder et al., 1996) also show strongly lateralized activation in left fusiform, inferior temporal gyrus, in addition to IFG and MFG (Balsamo, 2003; Balsamo et al., 2003). Most verbal fluency and lexical decision tasks also show activation of supplementary motor cortex and anterior cingulate implicated in attention and motor planning (Gaillard et al., 2000a; Holland et al., 2001; Liegeois et al., 2002; Gaillard et al., 2003b; Wood et al., 2004).

Tasks that stress semantic comprehension are consistently associated with activation in the left middle temporal gyrus (MTG), and the left temporo-parietal area. Stories or a whole language approach results in identifying a more distributed network, and, although they are harder to monitor, the design is more robust for individual subject temporal activation. Children and adults show very similar patterns of activation and lateralization on listening comprehension tasks (Ulualp et al., 1998; Booth et al., 1999b; Booth et al., 2000; Balsamo et al., 2002; Ahmad et al., 2003). Reading single words with a decision identifies, in group maps, inferior temporal, middle temporal, and inferior frontal cortex (Shaywitz et al., 2002). Reading sentences and stories shows strong activation in fusiform, middle temporal gyrus, and varying degrees of mid frontal gyrus in children aged 5 to 12 years (Gaillard et al., 2001b; Gaillard et al., 2003b). Sentence reading is a strong identifier of the language cortex in the temporal region on an individual basis.

Patterns of activation seen in children are fundamentally similar to those found in adults. Minor differences are seen in degree of laterality in frontal cortex for fluency tasks in younger children (see below) and age and performance differences seen in association cortex (Gaillard et al., 2001b; Holland et al., 2001; Schlaggar et al., 2002; Ahmad et al., 2003; Gaillard et al., 2003b; Brown et al., 2004).

## Language lateralization in normal volunteers

Numerous studies have shown the impressive reorganization capacity and plasticity of the immature brain; however, differences in neurological outcomes between adults and children suggest the plasticity of the brain's functional capacity is limited. Unlike children, similar injuries to the left hemisphere in adults result in profound and persistent aphasia (Geschwind & Galaburda, 1985). Children experiencing injury to the left hemisphere early in life commonly develop normal language function, suggesting an equipotentiality for each hemisphere for language function. Conservative estimates of this window of neural plasticity extends through age five or six years (Muller & Courchesne, 2000; Balsamo et al., 2002; Janszky et al., 2003a; Gaillard et al., in press). Latitude of plasticity in part depends on when language laterality is established and consolidated. The age at which left hemisphere dominance for language is established remains debated.

fMRI may be used to identify the hemisphere of language dominance in healthy controls and in patients. Language lateralization is typically based on a region of interest (ROI) asymmetry index $[AI=(L-R)/(L+R]$. Although the threshold employed differs on methods (threshold used, voxel counts, mean t score) and laboratories, two standard deviations from the mean of the normative data AI, based on activated voxel counts, yields an effective asymmetry index threshold of 0.25 or 0.20 (Pujol et al., 1999; Springer et al., 1999; Gaillard et al., 2002; Gaillard, 2004a). Subregion analysis may be more informative than hemispheric ROIs (Binder et al., 1996; Hertz-Pannier et al., 1997; Gaillard et al., 2001b; Gaillard et al., 2002; Spreer et al., 2002; Gaillard et al., 2004). Language typically is a left hemispheric function, but laterality, and degree of laterality, of language is affected by age, handedness, and task complexity. Studies in children and adults report 10-30% of activation to occur in right hemisphere in typically left dominant individuals (Springer et al., 1999; Gaillard et al., 2000b; Holland et al., 2001; Ahmad et al., 2003; Gaillard et al., 2003c; Gaillard et al., 2003b).

Functional and anatomical asymmetries in the auditory association area and left planum temporale of neonates and infants suggest a hemisphere dominance for language is present from birth (Balsamo et al., 2002). Three month-old infants listening to stories, compared to reverse speech, activate left posterior superior temporal gyrus and left angular gyrus, similar to left-sided language areas in older children and adults activated by speech perception (Booth et al., 1999a; Booth et al., 2000; Gaillard et al., 2001b; Balsamo et al., 2002; Dehaene-Lambertz et al., 2002; Ahmad et al., 2003; Balsamo, 2003; Balsamo et al., 2003; Gaillard et al., 2003a). Several studies examining reading text and stories contrasted to appropriate controls find highly lateralized activation in children as young as five along the left superior temporal sulcus and in the mid temporal gyrus (Gaillard et al., 2001b; Gaillard et al., 2003a).

Some degree of activation in homologous regions in non-dominant cortex is seen for all tasks, and is threshold dependent (Gaillard et al., 2000b; Gaillard et al., 2001b; Gaillard et al., 2002; Ahmad et al., 2003; Gaillard et al., 2003b). Greater bilateral activation is also seen with increasing task difficulty (Just et al., 1996; Gaillard et al., 2001b). Conflicting evidence suggests language processing areas may be less consolidated and more bilateral in younger children, particularly in frontal regions (Gaillard et al., 2003b) The diffuse activation signal sometimes seen in children may reflect developmental maturation of synaptic connections (Gaillard et al., 2001a).

Although activation patterns for several different language processing tasks – verbal fluency, listening comprehension, reading – are fundamentally similar to adults and strongly left lateralized, several studies suggest that younger children, albeit left dominant, may exhibit greater bilateral activation due to recruitment in right homologous regions than seen in older children and adults. Most of these tasks target IFG and MFG. One such study examined frontal AI (voxel counts) in 8-12 year olds with verbal fluency (Gaillard et al., 2000a). Another study using a noun-verb generation fluency task also found lower AI (asymmetry index) based on mean ROI t score in younger children (Holland et al., 2001). Berl et al. found greater bilateral activation in frontal regions for younger children (4-6) for a category decision task, but not for other tasks that required language comprehension (Berl et al., in press). There is evidence from reading tasks that younger children may also recruit more right hemispheric areas to perform task than older children (Gaillard et al., 2003a). These findings may provide a possible explanation for the ability of younger children to recover from dominant hemisphere brain injury. There is one verbal fluency study performed that found language networks in adults and children are similarly lateralized and regionally restricted in the dorsolateral prefrontal cortex of the dominant hemisphere by age seven (Gaillard et al., 2003b). This study raises the concern that differing developmental findings may also reflect different imaging factors and performance issues pertaining to signal-noise determination. Elegant studies have looked at single word fluency and find age and performance related difference in children seven years though young adulthood; the overall network for processing these tasks is the same across ages, but some restricted regions in association cortex show age and performance effects. Laterality indices were not presented (Schlaggar et al., 2002; Brown et al., 2004).

It is widely assumed that the dominant hemisphere is responsible for all essential language functions; however varying degrees of or relative *versus* complete lateralization of language is possible. It is unclear whether increased activation of right regions represents a recruiting of additional processing for semantics or represents non-linguistic aspects of language processing (Gaillard et al., 2002).

## Handedness and language representation

Pujol and colleagues found left sided language lateralization in 96% of normal right-handed adult volunteers with 4% showing a bilateral activation pattern in a fMRI verbal fluency study targeting frontal language regions (50 right handed, 50 left handed). Left sided language lateralization was found in 76% of normal left-handed volunteers with 14% showing bilateral activation and 10% exhibiting right-hemisphere language dominance (Pujol et al., 1999). Left hemispheric language dominance is found in 94% of 100 right-handed healthy adults using a semantic decision task eliciting the bulk of activation in frontal areas (Springer et al., 1999). A follow up in 50 left handers found 8% right dominant, 14% bilateral, and 78% left dominant for language (Szaflarski et al., 2002). No published studies specifically examine receptive language laterality in temporal language processing areas. In four small series (n = 13-22 each) involving right handed healthy children 5-12 years old using listening, category decision and reading tasks over 86-95% of those showing activation had left dominance in temporal regions; 95% of 22 right handed adults demonstrated left temporal dominance for a reading task only (Gaillard et al., 2001b; Ahmad et al., 2003; Balsamo, 2003; Gaillard et al., 2003b).

# Language findings in epilepsy patient populations

## Lateralization and localization of language in epilepsy and other disease states

Several studies demonstrate atypical language organization in epilepsy populations. They show increased atypical language dominance, reveal the patterns of atypical language, and show the local and remote effects of epilepsy on language functions. The timing of intra- and inter-hemispheric transfer of language function appears most dependent upon age of insult with limited capacity for re-organization into late childhood and early adolescence.

Seventeen to 33 percent of adults with childhood onset localization related epilepsy exhibit atypical language representation identified by fMRI (Table I) (Springer et al., 1999; Adcock et al., 2003; Woermann et al., 2003; Gaillard, 2004a; Thivard et al., 2005). There are fewer reports, with smaller patient numbers, regarding atypical language in right hemisphere focus epilepsy populations; these studies report 0-11% atypical language dominance (Table I). Many of these reports do not detail MRI findings or nature of early brain insult, thus it is difficult to distinguish between affect of epilepsy or its remote cause on language networks.

## Patterns of atypical language activation and language dominance

Several patterns of activation can be identified that represent atypical language dominance (Table II). All activation for atypical language dominance is seen in homologous regions in the right hemisphere. Only rarely is activation seen outside the distributed language network (Berl et al., 2004; Gaillard, 2004a). Right sided dominant activation in frontal and temporal regions occurs in one fifth of patients. The other patterns represent different aspects of bilateral language:

– Bilateral activation of both frontal and temporal regions;
– Bifrontal activation with unilateral temporal activation or the converse, bitemporal with unilateral frontal activation;
– Crossed dominance (diaschisis of activation) between the temporal and frontal regions (Baciu et al., 2003; Gaillard et al., 2004; Ries et al., 2004; Thivard et al., 2005);
– and rarely, a task dependent pattern, where one task is right, another task, left dominant with the degree of activation reflecting the paradigm employed (e.g. reading comprehension versus, auditory comprehension) (Berl et al., 2004; Gaillard, 2004a).

Table I. fMRI studies documenting atypical language.

| FMRI Study | Task | Number Patients | TLE | Atypical Language All | Atypical Language L focus | Atypical Language R focus |
|---|---|---|---|---|---|---|
| Springer | SD | 50 (23L) | 93% | 22% | | |
| Woermann | VF | 100 (82L) | 76% | 29% | 30% | 22% |
| Adcock | VF | 19 (12L) | All | | 33% | |
| Thivard | VF/Listen | 36 (18L) | All | 19% | 28% | 11% |
| Gaillard | RRN | 50 (30L) | 86% | 14% | 23% | 0% |

SD = single word semantic decision; VF = verbal fluency; Listen=Listening to stories; RRN = reading response naming (what is a long yellow fruit?). R = right; L = left.

Table II. Patterns of atypical language organization (n = 33).
Atypical location representing an immature or variant network is rare (3%).

| Pattern | Sub-Pattern | Percent | Percent |
|---|---|---|---|
| Right Dominant: Frontal & Temporal | | | 18% |
| Bilateral: Bilateral Frontal & Unilateral Temporal | | | 39% |
| | Right Temporal | 15% | |
| | Left Temporal | 24% | |
| Bilateral: Bilateral Temporal & Unilateral Frontal | | | 9% |
| Bilateral: Bilateral Frontal & Bilateral Temporal | | | 9% |
| Bilateral: Crossed Dominance, Frontal & Temporal | | | 15% |
| Bilateral: Task Dependent | | | 9% |

Table III. MRI, seizure focus, and atypical language, combined NIH & CNMC experience

| Atypical Language in Left Hemisphere Partial Epilepsy (n = 88) | | | |
|---|---|---|---|
| MRI | Number (n = 90) | Atypical Language (n = 27) | Percent Atypical Language (30%) |
| Normal | 30 | 9 | 31% |
| MTS | 26 | 6 | 23% |
| Dysplasia | 8 | 1 | 13% |
| Tumor | 14 | 2** | 14% |
| Stroke | 5* | 5 | 100% |
| Vascular Malformation | 2 | 0 | 0% |
| Inflammation | 2 | 1 | 50% |

* 1 child MTS and dysplasia, 1 child MTS.
** 1 child STG resection age 2.

Bilateral activation is a continuum. It is unknown whether the bilateral activation seen is necessary or sufficient to sustain language, and is likely to differ across patients (Gaillard et al., 2002; Gaillard, 2004a). These observations highlight the different lateralizing roles of frontal and temporal processing areas for language.

## Local, remote and non-specific effects of epilepsy on language organization

Several studies note increased right activation in epilepsy patients. Few have examined specific regional effects. Thivard et al. (2005) examined different tasks targeted at frontal networks (verbal fluency vs rest) and temporal networks (listening vs reverse speech) in 17 healthy controls, 18 patients with LTLE (17 childhood onset), and 18 patients with RTLE (12 childhood onset); 31 had mesial temporal sclerosis, and five had dysplasia. They found, as a group, reduced AI in temporal regions for LTLE and a trend for reduced AI in frontal regions. For those patients with atypical language (5 left, 2 right) there was a greater reduction in temporal than frontal regions that the authors interpreted as a greater local effect of TLE on language functions, but did not consider the more bilateral nature of the verbal fluency task. Regional AIs for TLE with normal language and healthy controls were not different. Patients with atypical language dominance had better cognitive measures suggesting a deleterious cognitive effect on those unable to transfer language to the left.

A recent study from our group found both focal and widespread effects on hemispheric and regional distribution of language processing, suggesting compensatory mechanisms (Gaillard et al., 2003c). This study involved 50 patients (30 left, 20 right; 24 children, 26 adults, predominantly TLE; 21 normal MRI, 19 MTS, 10 small low grade tumor, focal dysplasia, or vascular malformation) compared to 33 healthy volunteers (12 children). A covert reading response paradigm (what is a long yellow fruit) targeted to activate left temporal, LIFG and LMG allowed investigation of receptive and expressive processing. No differences were found between adults and children. 23% of RTLE had atypical language dominance and none of RTLE patients. Patients with left focus, but who retained left language, had a lower AI compared to controls for all three regions suggesting a effect on temporal and frontal networks (*Figure 1*). Patients with left focus but atypical language had lowered AI by definition, but all AIs were similarly reduced. The right focus/left language group had AI similar to normal controls for IFG, but unexpectedly lower AIs than healthy controls in temporal and MFG ROIs and thus comparable to left focus/left language group for these regions. Patients activated more voxels than healthy controls. Several observations may be drawn from this data. A left focus has both a local and a remote effect on transferring language function to right hemisphere in temporal and frontal regions – an effect also seen to a lesser degree even though language is preserved as left dominant. The right focus/left language temporal lobe findings suggest an effect on local and contralateral temporal networks. The reduced AI in MFG for both left and right focus may suggest a non-specific affect on working memory. The reduced IFG AI in the left focus/left language group likely represents a remote effect on ipsilateral frontal language functions. The overall increase in voxels suggests that greater recruitment and resources are required to preserve performance for epilepsy patients in general.

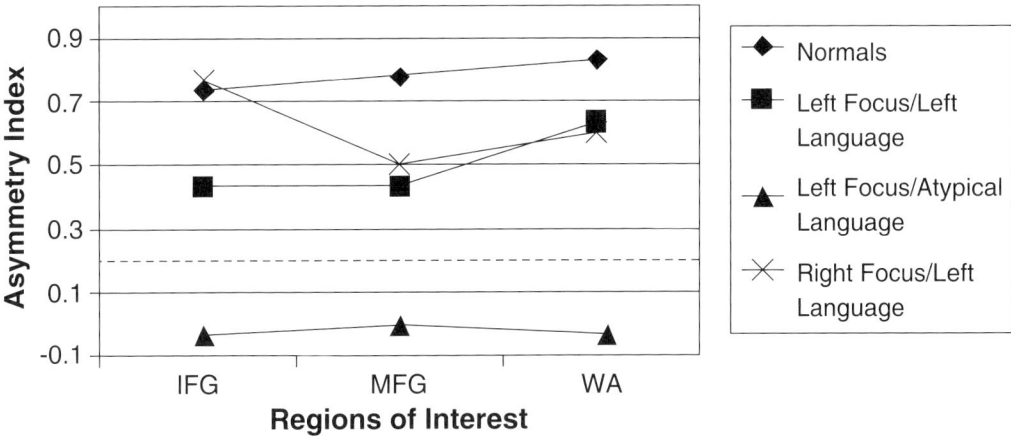

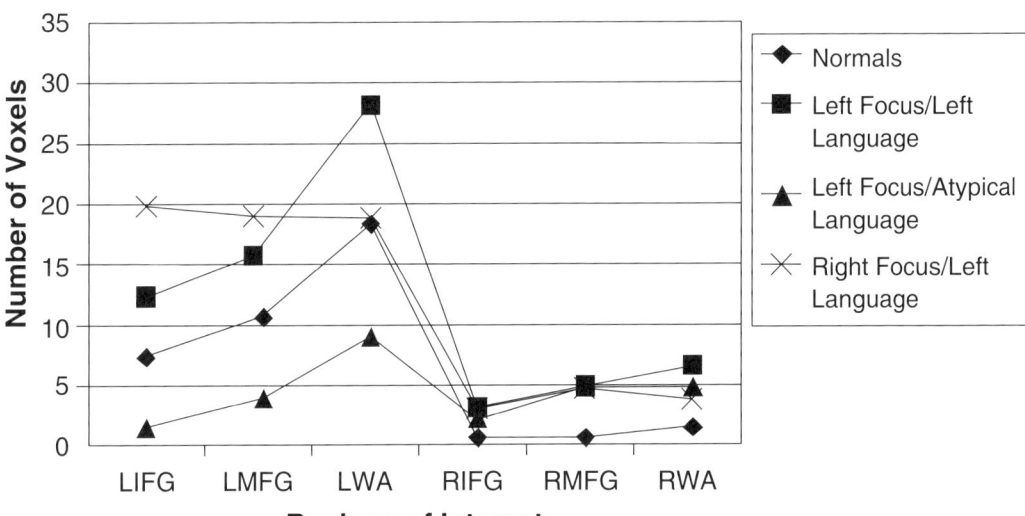

**Figure 1. Asymmetry indices (AI) and voxel counts in three brain regions implicated in language processing.**
Data from four groups is shown: Normal controls are diamonds, right hemisphere focus/left language epilepsy patients are crosses, left hemisphere focus/left language epilepsy patients are squares, and, left hemisphere focus/atypical language epilepsy patients are triangles. Regions of interest include Right (R) and Left (L) Inferior Frontal Gyrus (IFG), Mid Frontal Gyrus (MFG), Wernicke's Area (WA) (left mid/superior temporal gyrus/inferior parietal lobe). Dashed line for AI is 0.2 and represents threshold for typical (> 0.2) and atypical (< 0.2) language dominance. The threshold 0.2 is based on 2SD normal volunteer regional data for pooled language tasks.

The results may represent a medication effect, neuro-cognitive differences, or an effect of epilepsy. These findings are not attributable to motion. There is no strong correlation with cognitive and behavioral measures, though as a group the patients had lower VIQ than patients.

Further evidence for compensatory mechanisms is found in another study comparing semantic and phonemic tasks in RTLE and LTLE. Billingsley et al. found adolescent and adult patients with left temporal lobe epilepsy exhibited more left dorsolateral prefrontal activity than controls for their semantic task (single word semantic decision), but not their phonologic task, and showed an increased signal change in the right middle temporal areas as well. Patients with right temporal lobe epilepsy had poorer performance on measures of linguistic skills compared with controls (Billingsley et al., 2001). A verbal memory encoding task showed less left hippocampal activation for LTLE patients but greater left dorsolateral pre-frontal activation, thus providing additional supporting evidence for compensatory cognitive strategies in TLE (Dupont et al., 2000).

Intra-hemispheric re-organization is harder to establish. Data from our lab does not find significant change in the maxima locus of activation (location, magnitude, and extent) for a reading response naming task in temporal or frontal regions for localization related epilepsy (n = 15, predominantly temporal lobe, child and adult) compared to healthy child and adult controls (n = 38, 16 children). Activation, when it occurred in the right hemisphere, was in homologous regions.

## Effect of epilepsy *vs* remote symptomatic cause on language organization

Exploring mechanisms of different disease processes provides insight into intra – inter hemispheric language reorganization and shifts in strategies pursued to preserve language function. There are several factors that appear related to atypical language. Patients with atypical language have a higher incidence of atypical handedness and younger age of seizure onset that those with typical language (Gaillard, 2004a). In this setting atypical handedness may represent early brain injury. Correlation cannot be found with AI or voxel counts with age of seizure onset or duration of epilepsy (Gaillard et al., 2003c). Yet closer examination of our series 133 patients (58 < 16 years) identified 36 patients with atypical language, 33 of whom had a history of early seizure onset, atypical handedness, history of developmental lesion (dysplasia, low grade tumor), mesial temporal sclerosis/or brain insult all attributable before age six years. Two other fMRI studies in adults find earlier age of seizure onset (Springer et al., 1999; Woermann et al., 2003) and early history of predisposing factors (Woermann et al., 2003) in patients with bilateral or right language. This data supports the view that early brain insults, injury, and seizure onset are important factors for inter-hemispheric language reorganization.

Examination of our series of 149 (56 < 16 years old) patients with fMRI tasks finds an effect of lesion type with likelihood of language reorganization *(Table III)*. All our patients with early left hemisphere stroke had atypical language organization. One third of patients with neocortical epilepsy had atypical language, and one fifth of patients with mesial temporal sclerosis. The evidence for dysplasia and tumors is more problematic. We found 14% of tumors associated with language re-organization, one who had undergone resection of left STG at age two, and only one patient with dysplasia.

One other investigation describes a low incidence of language reorganization in children with focal developmental dysplasia and low grade tumors (Labate et al., 2004). In contrast, a study of 14 children with dysplasia found a high likelihood of atypical language: One intra-hemispheric, four right dominant, and nine bilateral. There was no correlation with degree of reorganization and severity of microscopic pathological changes. This study only looked at patients with dysplasia in expected left language areas (Smith et al., 2004). Three important observations can be made: *first*, dysplasia can sustain language function (Janszky et al., 2003b; Keene et al., 2004; Smith et al., 2004); *second*, rarely is activation displaced to the margins of the lesion; *third*, it appears that the location and extent of dysplasia is more important than pathology. It would be useful to compare dysplasia with and without seizures to examine role of epilepsy in the process.

Mesial temporal sclerosis may play a role in the unexpectedly high reports (10%) of atypical language in RTLE (Woermann et al., 2003; Thivard et al., 2005) (2/17 or 12% in our experience). This observation suggests remote effects of RTLE on left temporal language networks, discussed above, which may be mitigated by right temporal lobectomy (Novelly et al., 1984; Gaillard et al., 2003c), or reflect the bilateral nature of the disease observed with MR spectroscopy (Cendes et al., 1997a). The higher incidence of re-organization in patients with neocortical epilepsy, often non-lesional, as seen in our series and others (Woermann et al., 2003), also suggests a specific effect of epilepsy.

A study of ten children with developmental lesions examined the effect of lesion location on verbal fluency activation (Liegeois et al., 2004). Four out of five children with temporal lobe lesions removed from Wernicke's area (mesial temporal sclerosis, arachnoid cysts, mesial encephalomalacia) had right dominant activation. Only one in five children with lesions in Broca's area had atypical language. The one child with atypical language and a frontal lesion had a large dysplastic lesion encompassing frontal lobe whereas the other frontal lesions (dysplasia, vascular) were limited in extent. All the temporal patients had TLE, lending further support to remote epilepsy effects. The study included a task design that only probed at areas involved in frontal activation (verbal fluency) and as such inferences regarding other areas cannot be made.

Evidence for factors modulating language re-organization may be found in patients with congenital stroke. Children with left middle cerebral artery strokes have reorganization of language to homologous temporal cortex ascertained with a listening task (Booth et al., 1999b; Booth et al., 2000). Elegant studies in adults with peri-natal ischemia confirm reorganization is constrained to homologous regions in the right hemisphere (Staudt et al., 2002). Inter-hemispheric reorganization of frontal networks identified with a verbal fluency task was proportional to the extent of frontal peri-ventricular white matter injury, whereas temporal areas identified with listening to stories, remained left hemisphere dominant (Staudt et al., 2001). Disruption of white matter tracts is likely relevant in this circumstance as cortical mechanisms are for other settings (Catani et al., 2005).

Two case studies provide additional insight into the timing and capacity of language re-organization. The first concerns an eight year old with a left frontal brain tumor who developed bilateral frontal activation with a shift to right biased activation, assessed with a verbal fluency task, during the year following diagnosis. The child's twin sibling remained left dominant for the task. Although the twin exhibited an increase in right hemisphere activation, this transfer of language function did not result in full recovery of language (Anderson et al., 2002). The second case is a child with Rasmussen's encephalitis with onset after age five year six months years who experienced progressive aphasia and ultimately underwent a dominant hemispherectomy at age nine. Preoperative verbal fluency performed at age six years eight months (VIQ 118) demonstrated left frontal activation, fMRI post-op at age ten years six months (VIQ 64, limited verbal recovery) showed right frontal activation for verbal fluency tasks (Hertz-Pannier, 2002). In cases with Rasmussen's encephalitis it is difficult to distinguish co-morbid disease processes and epilepsy.

Most fMRI studies have examined age of onset of seizures, and duration of epilepsy. Studies have not attempted to examine seizure severity as measured by seizure counts. Investigations have not examined the effect of inter-ictal discharges and epileptogenesis on brain function. Yet event related interictal spike fMRI allows for mapping of interictal spikes. These methods not only identify BOLD effect on spike location but also on their propagated effect providing a window to examine remote perturbation on cerebral function (Krakow et al., 1999; Krakow et al., 2001; Aghakhani et al., 2004). A final cautionary note should be made regarding the effect altered coupling of blood flow and metabolism seen in TLE may have on the BOLD response and our ability to map language in affected temporal or other regions (Gaillard et al., 1995; Jayakar et al., 2002).

Cerebral plasticity and the capacity of the non-dominant right hemisphere to sustain language functions varies according to the complexity of functions requiring compensation, the extent of dominant hemisphere lesion, and the age of onset of functional/structural damage (Muller & Courchesne, 2000). The functional imaging data suggests several factors that influence language reorganization. Both epilepsy and remote symptomatic cause play a role in language reorganization. Early brain insult or seizure onset appears to be the most important. The nature of remote symptomatic cause also plays an important influence on reorganization. The high incidence of atypical language dominance in non-lesional neocortical epilepsy suggests a direct effect of seizures or the underlying epileptogenic process. It is unclear whether the right activation represents a persistent immature pattern, or whether language may shift to the right. In those patients with complete "transfer" or dominance, right regions sustain function. In other settings, and with later injury, the right may assume some, but not all language function, giving rise to the notion of a critical period for the right hemisphere to sustain function. In this view normal maturation is the persistence of language in the left and loss of independent language processing in the right. The role on intra-hemispheric reorganization presumed to occur with later injury or seizure onset, and limited to margins of language processing areas, has not yet been studied rigorously. With functional imaging the evidence suggests the distributed network for language has some latitude for compensation; activation outside this network and language areas is rare and constrains the extent and degree of language reorganization.

## Expanding areas of fMRI epilepsy research

The other cognitive domain of specific relevance to temporal lobe epilepsy is memory. No temporal lobe based fMRI memory studies have been performed in children. Studies in adults demonstrate the ability to activate mesial temporal structures (Stern et al., 1996; Brewer et al., 1998), and provide application to epilepsy populations. As with language, different aspects of memory can be probed in patients such as implicit, explicit memory, and memory encoding and retrieval (Bellgowan et al., 1998; Detre et al., 1998; Dupont et al., 2000; Dupont et al., 2001; Golby et al., 2001; Jokeit et al., 2001; Golby et al., 2002; Janszky et al., 2004; Rabin et al., 2004). On an individual basis, and unlike language, each paradigm employed has had only fair agreement with IAT. Although fMRI memory cannot predict overall memory outcomes, individual paradigms do predict post-operative performance for the specific fMRI task (Janszky et al., 2004; Rabin et al., 2004).

These studies are beginning to address the challenging issues of functional adequacy and functional reserve for memory. Further studies are also examining compensatory mechanism for memory processing as seen in language (Dupont et al., 2000).

Employing fMRI to study other aspects of cognitive function including executive function, emotional regulation, and memory will provide greater insight into the organization of higher order cognitive structures.

## Conclusions

fMRI provides a comprehensive view of language processing with anatomic and functional specificity that allows insight into plasticity for reorganization found in epilepsy populations. Reorganization of language is confined to the widely distributed network known to support language and to homologous regions in the right, typically nondominant, hemisphere. Furthermore, inter-hemispheric reorganization is more likely to occur with either remote brain insult or epilepsy onset before age six years. There is a diminishing capacity to sustain functional capacity with reorganization of language to the right following injury after age six.

Destructive processes such as stroke and inflammation are more likely to drive reorganization. Developmental processes such as tumors and dysplasia are less likely to lead to inter-hemispheric reorganization. When re-organization of language is seen in patients with dysplasia, the location and extent of lesion appears more important than severity of microscopic pathology.

Non-lesional neocortical epilepsy is associated with inter-hemispheric reorganization in one third of patients arguing for a direct effect of epilepsy itself on affecting the organization of language networks. There is further evidence that epilepsy, its remote cause, or its treatment, has remote and non-specific affects on language processing, manifest in altered regional weighting of activity and reflecting compensatory brain mechanisms. It is not known, however, why one form or epilepsy is more likely to be associated with atypical language than another.

fMRI's use is not limited to identification of language processing areas. Future applications will be applied to memory, emotional regulation (anxiety, depression), working memory, visual spatial processing, and attention. These studies are likely to reveal the specific, remote, and non-specific effects of epilepsy on brain function, similar to effects seen with language processing.

**Supported by NINDS RO1 NS44280; Mental Retardation and Developmental Disabilities Center Grant NICHD P30HD40677, General Clinical Research Center Grant MO1RR020359, and the Clinical Epilepsy Section, NINDS, NIH.**

# References

Adcock JE, Wise RG, Oxbury JM, Oxbury SM, Matthews PM. Quantitative fMRI assessment of the differences in lateralization of language-related brain activation in patients with temporal lobe epilepsy. *Neuroimage* 2003; 18 (2): 423-38.

Aghakhani Y, Bagshaw AP, Benar CG, Hawco C, Andermann F, Dubeau F, et al. fMRI activation during spike and wave discharges in idiopathic generalized epilepsy. *Brain* 2004; 127 (5): 1127-44.

Ahmad Z, Balsamo LM, Sachs BC, Xu B, Gaillard WD. Auditory comprehension of language in young children: Neural networks identified with fMRI. *Neurology* 2003; 60 (10): 1598-605.

Anderson DP, Harvey S, Sailing MM, Anderson V, Jacobs R, Abbott DF, et al. Differential functional magnetic resonance imagine language activation in twins discordant for a left frontal tumor. *Journal of Child Neurology* 2002; 17 (10): 766-9.

Baciu MV, Watson JM, McDermott KB, Wetzel RD, Attarian H, Moran CJ, et al. Functional MRI reveals an interhemispheric dissociation of frontal and temporal language regions in a patient with focal epilepsy. *Epilepsy Behav* 2003; 4 (6): 776-80.

Balsamo L. Neural representation and function of language in children with new onset partial epilepsy. *Psychology* 2003; Dissertation American University: 127.

Balsamo LM, Gaillard WD. The utility of functional magnetic resonance imaging in epilepsy and language. *Curr Neurol Neurosci Rep* 2002; 2 (2): 142-9.

Balsamo LM, Xu B, Sachs B, Gaillard WD. Language networks underlying auditory based category decision in children identified with fMRI. *Annals of Neurology* 2003; 54 (suppl 7): S105.

Balsamo LM, Xu B, Grandin CB, Petrella JR, Braniecki SH, Elliott TK, et al. A functional magnetic resonance imaging study of left hemisphere language dominance in children. *Arch Neurol* 2002; 59 (7): 1168-74.

Baxendale S. The role of functional MRI in the presurgical investigation of temporal lobe epilepsy patients: a clinical perspective and review. *J Clin Exp Neuropsychol* 2002; 24 (5): 664-76.

Bellgowan PS, Binder JR, Swanson SJ, Hammeke TA, Springer JA, Frost JA, et al. Side of seizure focus predicts left medial temporal lobe activation during verbal encoding. *Neurology* 1998; 51 (2): 479-84.

Benson RR, FitzGerald DB, LeSeuer LL, Kennedy DN, Kwong KK, Buchbinder BR, et al. Language dominance determined by whole brain functional MRI in patients with brain lesions. *Neurology* 1999; 52: 798-809.

Berl M, Balsamo B, Xu B, Moore EN, Weinstein SL, Conry JA, et al. Seizure focus affects regional language networks assessed by fMRI. In: ed. in press. Neurology.

Berl MM, Moore EN, Xu B, Pearl PL, Conry JA, Weinstein SL, et al. Atypical language dominance and patterns of reorganization in epilepsy as assessed by a panel of fMRI tasks. *Epilepsia* 2004; 45 (suppl 7): 306.

Bernasconi N, Bernasconi A, Caramanos Z, Antel SB, Andermann F, Arnold DL. Mesial temporal damage in temporal lobe epilepsy: a volumetic MRI study of the hippocampus, amygdala and parahippocampal region. *Brain* 2003; 126: 465-69.

Billingsley RL, McAndrews MP, Crawley AP, Mikulis DJ. Functional MRI of phonological and semantic processing in temporal lobe epilepsy. *Brain* 2001; 124: 1218-27.

Binder J, Rao S, Hammeke T, Frost JA, Bandettini P, Jesmanowicz A, et al. Lateralized human brain language systems demonstrated by task subtraction functional magnetic resonance imaging. *Arch Neurology* 1995; 52: 593-601.

Binder JR, Swanson SJ, Hammeke TA, Morris GL, Mueller WM, Fischer M, et al. Determination of language dominance using functional MRI: A comparison with the Wada test. *Neurology* 1996; 46: 978-84.

Bookheimer SY, Dapretto M, Black K, Cohen MS. FMRI of language patients with aggressive brain tumors. *Soc Neurosci Abs* 1997; 23.

Booth JR, Macwhinney B, Thulborn KR, Sacco K, Voyvodic J, Feldman HM. Functional organization of activation patterns in children: whole brain fMRI imaging during three different cognitive tasks. *Prog Neuropsychopharmacol Biol Psychiatry* 1999a; 23 (4): 669-82.

Booth JR, Feldman HM, Macwhinney B, Thulborn KR, Sacco K, Voyvodic J. Functional activation patterns in adults, children, and pediatric patients with brain lesions. *Prog Neuropsychopharm Biol Psych* 1999b; 23: 669-82.

Booth JR, MacWhinney B, Thulborn KR, Sacco K, Voyvodic JT, Feldman HM. Developmental and lesion effects in brain activation during sentence comprehension and mental rotation. *Dev Neuropsychol* 2000; 18 (2): 139-69.

Brewer JB, Zhao Z, Desmond JE, Glover GH, Gabrieli JDE. Making memories: Brain activity that predicts how well visual experience will be remembered. *Science* 1998; 281: 1185-7.

Brown TT, Lugar HM, Coalson RS, Miezin FM, Petersen S, Schlaggar BL. Developmental changes in human cerebral functional organization for word generation. *Cereb Cortex* 2004; electronic publication, Aug 5.

Carpentier A, Pugh KR, Westerveld M, Studholme C, Skrinjar O, Thompson JL, et al. Functional MRI of Language Processing: dependence on input modality and temporal lobe epilepsy. *Epilepsia* 2001; 42 (10): 1241-54.

Cascino GD, Jack CR Jr, Parisi JE, et al. Magnetic resonance imaging-based volume studies in temporal lobe epilepsy: pathological correlations. *Ann Neurol* 1991; 30: 31-6.

Catani M, Jones DK, Ffytche DH. Perisylvian language networks of the human brain. *Annals of Neurology* 2005; 57 (1): 8-16.

Cendes F, Andermann F, Dubeau F. Normalization of neuronal metabolic dysfunction after surgery for temporal lobe epilepsy. Evidence from proton MR spectroscopic imaging. *Neurology* 1997a; 49: 1525-33.

Cendes F, Caramanos Z, Andermann F, Dubeau F, Arnold DL. Proton magnetic resonance spectroscopic imaging and magnetic resonance imaging volumetry in the lateralization of temporal lobe epilepsy: a series of 100 patients. *Ann Neurol* 1997b; 42 (5): 737-46.

Cendes F, Andermann F, Gloor P, et al. MRI volumetric measurement of amygdala and hippocampus in temporal lobe epilepsy. *Neurology* 1993; 43: 719-25.

Cohen MS, Bookheimer SY. Localization of brain function using magnetic resonance imaging. *Trends Neurosci* 1994; 17 (7): 268-77.

Cook MJ, Fish DR, Shorvon SD, Staughan K, Stevens JM. Hippocampal volumetric and morphometric studies in frontal and temporal lobe epilepsy. *Brain* 1992; 155 (Pt 4): 1001-15.

DeCarli C, McIntosh AR, Blaxton TA. Use of positron emission tomography for the evaluation of epilepsy. *Neuroimaging Clin N Am* 1995; 5: 623-45.

DeCarli C, Hatta J, Fazilat S, Gaillard WD, Theodore WH. Extratemporal atrophy in patients with complex partial seizures of left temporal origin. *Ann Neurol* 1998; 43 (1): 41-5.

Dehaene-Lambertz G, Dehaene S, Hertz-Pannier L. Functional neuroimaging of speech perception in infants. *Science* 2002; 298: 2013-5.

Detre JA, Maccotta L, King D, Alsop DC, D'Esposito M, Zarahn E, et al. Functional MRI lateralization of memory in temporal lobe epilepsy. *Neurology* 1998; 50: 926-32.

Devinsky O, Perrine K, Llinas R, Luciano DJ, Dogali M. Anterior temporal lobe language areas in patients with early onset temporal lobe epilepsy. *Ann of Neurol* 1993; 34: 727-32.

Dupont S, Samson Y, Van de Moortele PF, Samson S, Poline JB, Adam C, et al. Delayed verbal memory retrieval: a functional MRI study in epileptic patients with structural lesions of the left medial temporal lobe. *Neuroimage* 2001; 14 (5): 995-1003.

Dupont S, Van de Moortele PF, Samson S, Hasboun D, Poline JB, Adam C, et al. Episodic memory in left temporal lobe epilepsy: a functional MRI study. *Brain* 2000; 123 (Pt 8): 1722-32.

Fernandez G, Specht K, Weis S, Tendolkar I, Reuber M, Fell J, et al. Intrasubject reproducibility of presurgical language lateralization and mapping using fMRI. *Neurology* 2003; 60 (6): 969-75.

Gaillard WD. Functional MR imaging of language, memory, and sensorimotor cortex. *Neuroimaging Clin N Am* 2004a; 14 (3): 471-85.

Gaillard WD, Grandin CB, Xu B. Developmental aspects of pediatric fMRI: considerations for image acquisition, analysis, and interpretation. *Neuroimage* 2001a; 13 (2): 239-49.

Gaillard WD, Balsamo LM, Ibrahim Z, Sachs BC, Xu B. fMRI identifies regional specialization of neural networks for reading in young children. *Neurology* 2003a; 60 (1): 94-100.

Gaillard WD, Moore EN, Weber DA, Ritzl EK, Berl MM. fMRI of normal and pathological language development. *Second residential Course on Developmental Cognitive Neuro-Sciences*. Paris: John Libbey Eurotext (in press).

Gaillard WD, Hertz-Pannier L, Mott SH, Barnett AS, LeBihan D, Theodore W. Functional anatomy of cognitve development: fMRI of verbal fluency in clhidren and adults. *Neurology* 2000a; 54: 108-5.

Gaillard WD, Hertz-Pannier L, Mott SH, Barnett AS, LeBihan D, Theodore WH. Functional anatomy of cognitive development: fMRI of verbal fluency in children and adults. *Neurology* 2000b; 54 (1): 180-5.

Gaillard WD, Fazilat S, White S, Malow B, Sato S, Reeves P, et al. Interictal metabolism and blood flow are uncoupled in temporal lobe cortex of patients with complex partial epilepsy. *Neurology* 1995; 45 (10): 1841-7.

Gaillard WD, Pugliese M, Grandin CB, Braniecki SH, Kondapaneni P, Hunter K, et al. Cortical localization of reading in normal children: an fMRI language study. *Neurology* 2001b; 57 (1): 47-54.

Gaillard WD, Sachs BC, Whitnah JR, Ahmad Z, Balsamo LM, Petrella JR, et al. Developmental aspects of language processing: fMRI of verbal fluency in children and adults. *Hum Brain Mapp* 2003b; 18 (3): 176-85.

Gaillard WD, Berl MM, Sachs B, Balsamo L, Xu B, Grandin CB, et al. Reduced degree of language dominance in left hemisphere localization related epilepsy assessed by a fMRI reading comprehension task. *Epilepsia* 2003c; 44 (9): 88.

Gaillard WD, Balsamo L, Xu B, McKinney C, Papero PH, Weinstein S, et al. fMRI language task panel improves determination of language dominance. *Neurology* 2004; 63 (8): 1403-8.

Gaillard WD, Balsamo L, Xu B, Grandin CB, Braniecki SH, Papero PH, et al. Language dominance in partial epilepsy patients identified with an fMRI reading task. *Neurology* 2002; 59 (2): 256-65.

Geschwind N, Galaburda AM. Cerebral lateralization. Biological mechanisms, associations, and pathology: A hypothesis and a program for research. *Arch Neurol* 1985; 42: 428-59.

Golby AJ, Poldrack RA, Illes J, Chen D, Desmond JE, Gabrieli JD. Memory lateralization in medial temporal lobe epilepsy assessed by functional MRI. *Epilepsia* 2002; 43 (8): 855-63.

Golby AJ, Poldrack RA, Brewer JB, Spencer D, Desmond JE, Aron AP, et al. Material-specific lateralization in the medial temporal lobe and prefrontal cortex during memory encoding. *Brain* 2001; 124 (Pt 9): 1841-54.

Harvey AS, Anderson D, Jackson G. Functional MRI lateralization of expressive language in children with partial epilepsy and left hemisphere lesions. *Epilepsia* 1999; 40: 183.

Hauser WA, Annegers JF, Anderson VE. Epidemiology and the genetics of epilepsy. *Res Publ Assoc Res Nerv Ment Dis* 1983; 61: 267-94.

Helmstaedter C, Kurthen M, Linke DB, Elger CE. Right hemisphere restitution of language and memory functions in right hemisphere language-dominant patients with left temporal lobe epilepsy. *Brain* 1994; 117 (Pt 4): 729-37.

Hermann BP, Seidenberg M, Bell B. The neurodevelopmental impact of childhood onset temporal lobe epilepsy on brain structure and function and the risk of progressive cognitive effects. *Prog Brain Res* 2002; 135: 429-38.

Hertz-Pannier L, Gaillard WD, Mott S, Cuenod CA, Bookheimer S, Weinstein S, et al. Assessment of Language Hemispheric Dominance in Children with Epilepsy using Functional MRI. *Neurology* 1997; 48: 1003-12.

Holland SK, Plante E, Weber Byars A, Strawsburg RH, Schmithorst VJ, Ball WS. Normal fMRI brain activation patterns in children performing a verb generation task. *Neuroimage* 2001; 14: 837-43.

Janszky J, Jokeit H, Heinemann D, Schulz R, Woermann FG, Ebner A. Epileptic activity influences the speech organization in medial temporal lobe epilepsy. *Brain* 2003a; 126 (Pt 9): 2043-51.

Janszky J, Jokeit H, Konstantina K, Mertens M, Ebner A, Pohlmann-Edan B, et al. Functional MRI predicts memory performance after right mesiotemporal epilepsy surgery. *Epilepsia* 2004; 46 (2): 244-50.

Janszky J, Ebner A, Kruse B, Mertens M, Jokeit H, Seitz RJ, et al. Functional organization of the brain with malformations of cortical development. *Ann Neurol* 2003b; 53 (6): 759-67.

Jayakar P, Bernal B, Santiago Medina L, Altman N. False lateralization of language cortex on functional MRI after a cluster of focal seizures. *Neurology* 2002; 58 (3): 490-92.

Jokeit H, Okujava M, Woermann FG. Memory fMRI lateralizes temporal lobe epilepsy. *Neurology* 2001; 57 (10): 1786-93.

Just MA, Carpenter PA, Keller TA, Eddy WF, Thulborn KR. Brain activity modulated by sentence comprehension. *Science* 1996; 274: 114-6.

Keene DL, Logan WJ, McAndrews MP. A comparison of three functional MRI language paradigms in children. *Epilepsia* 2000; 41: 193.

Keene DL, Olds J, Logan WJ. Functional MRI study of verbal fluency in a patient with subcortical laminar heterotopia. *Can J Neurol Sci* 2004; 31 (2): 261-4.

Kho KH, Leijten FS, Rutten GJ, Vermeulen J, Van Rijen P, Ramsey NF. Discrepant findings for Wada test and functional magnetic resonance imaging with regard to language function: use of electrocortical stimulation mapping to confirm results. *J Neurosurg* 2005; 102 (1): 169-73.

Knecht S, Deppee D, Drager L, Bobe H, Lohmann H, Ringelstein EB, et al. Language Lateralization in healthy right-handers. *Brain* 2000; 123: 74-81.

Krakow K, Messina D, Lemieux L, Duncan JS, Fish DR. Functional MRI activation of individual interictal epileptiform spikes. *Neuroimage* 2001; 13 (3): 502-5.

Krakow K, Woermann FG, Symms MR, Allen PJ, Lemieux L, Barker GJ, et al. EEG-triggered functional MRI of interictal epileptiform activity in patients with partial seizures. *Brain* 1999; 122: 1679-88.

Labate A, Briellmann R, Waites AB, Harvey AS, Jackson G. Temporal lobe developmental tumors: an fMRI study for language lateralization. *Epilepsia* 2004; 41: 1456-62.

Lawson JA, Vogrin S, Bleasel AF, Cook MJ, Bye AM. Cerebral and cerebellar volume reduction in children with intractable epilepsy. *Epilepsia* 2000; 41: 1456-62.

Lehericy S, Cohen L, Bazin B, Samson S, Giacomini E, Rougetet R, et al. Functional MR evaluation of temporal and frontal language dominance compared with the Wada test. *Neurology* 2000; 54 (8): 1625-33.

Lehericy S, Biondi A, Sourour N, Vlaicu M, Tezenas du Montcel S, Cohen L, et al. Arteriovenous brain malformations: Is functional MR imaging reliable for studying language reorganization in patients? Initial observations. *Radiology* 2002; 223 (3): 672-82.

Li LM, Cendes F, Andermann F, Dubeau F, Arnold DL. Spatial extent of neuronal metabolic dysfunction measured by proton MR spectroscopic imaging in patients with localization-related epilepsy. *Epilepsia* 2000; 41 (6): 666-74.

Liegeois F, Connelly A, Salmond CH, Gadian DG, Vargha-Khadem F, Baldeweg T. A direct test for lateralization of language activation using fMRI: comparison with invasive assessments in children with epilepsy. *Neuroimage* 2002; 17 (4): 1861-7.

Liegeois F, Connelly A, Cross JH, Boyd SG, Gadian DG, Vargha-Khadem F, et al. Language reorganization in children with early-onset lesions of the left hemisphere: an fMRI study. *Brain* 2004; 127 (Pt 6): 1229-36.

Liu RS, Lemieux, L, Bell GS, et al. Progressive neocortical damage in epilepsy. *Ann Neurol* 2003; 53: 312-24.

Logan WJ, Smith MI, McAndrews MP. Lateralization of language in chidren with functional MRI compared to intracarotid amobarbital procedures. *Epilepsia* 1999; 40: 44.

Logothetis NK, Pauls J, Augath M, Trinath T, Oeltermann A. Neurophysiological investigation of the basis of the fMRI signal. *Nature* 2001; 412: 150-7.

Loring DW, Strauss E, Hermann BP, Perrine K, Trenerry MR, Barr WB, et al. Effects of anomalous language representation on neuropsychological performance in temporal lobe epilepsy. *Neurology* 1999; 53 (2): 260-77.

Marsh L, Morrell MJ, Shear PK, et al. Cortical and hippocampal volume deficits in temporal lobe epilepsy. *Epilepsia* 1997; 38: 576-87.

Moonen CTW, Bandettini PA. *Functional MRI*. Heidelberg, Springer, 2000.

Muller RA, Courchesne E. *The duplicity of plasticity: A conceptual approach to the study of early lesion and developmental disorders*. New York, Cambridge UP, 2000.

Natsume J, Bernasconi N, Andermann F, Bernasconi A. MRI volumetry of the thalamus in temporal, extratemporal, and idiopathic generalized epilepsy. *Neurology* 2003; 60: 1296-300.

Novelly RA, Augustine EA, Mattson RH, Glasser GH, Williamson PD, Spencer DD, et al. Selective memory improvement and impairment in temporal lobectomy for epilepsy. *Annals of Neurology* 1984; 15: 64-7.

Ojemann G, Ojemann J, Lettich E, Berger M. Cortical language localization in left, dominant hemisphere. An electrical stimulation mapping investigation in 117 patients. *J Neurosurg* 1989; 71 (3): 316-26.

Pardo JV, Fox PT. Preoperative assessment of the cerebral hemispheric dominance for language with CBF PET. *Hum Brain Mapp* 1993; 1: 57-68.

Poldrack RA, Wagner AD, Prull MW, Desmond JE, Glover GH, Gabrieli JD. Functional specialization for semantic and phonological processing in the left inferior prefrontal cortex. *Neuroimage* 1999; 97: 21-23.

Pouratian N, Bookheimer SY, Rex DE, Martin NA, Toga AW. Utility of preoperative functional magnetic resonance imagine for identifying language cortices in patients with vascular malformations. *J Neursurg* 2002; 97: 21-32.

Pujol J, Deus J, Losilla J, Capdevila A. Cerebral lateralization of language in normal left-handed people studied by functional MRI. *Neurology* 1999; 52 (5): 1038-43.

Rabin ML, Narayan VM, Kimberg DY, Casasanto DJ, Glosser G, Tracy JI, et al. Functional MRI predicts post-surgical memory following temporal lobectomy. *Brain* 2004; 127: 2286-98.

Rasmussen T, Milner B. The role of early left-sided brain injury in determining lateralization of cerebral speech functions. *Annals of New York Academy of Science* 1977; 229: 335-69.

Ries M, Boop FA, Griebel ML, Zou P, Phillips NS, Johnson SC, et al. Functional MRI and Wada determination of language lateralization: A case of crossed dominance. *Epilepsia* 2004; 45 (1): 85-9.

Rother J, Knab R, Hamzei F, Fiehler J, Reichenbach JR, Buchel C, et al. Negative dip in BOLD fMRI is caused by blood flow – oxygen consumption uncoupling in humans. *Neuroimage* 2002; 15 (1): 98-102.

Rutten GJ, Ramsey NF. Reproducibility of fMRI-determined language lateralization in individual subjects. *Brain Lang* 2002; 296: 1476-79.

Schlaggar BL, Brown TT, Lugar HM, Visscher KM, Miezin FM, Petersen SE. Functional neuroanatomical differences between adults and school-age children in the processing of single words. *Science* 2002; 296 (5572): 1476-9.

Shaywitz BA, Shaywitz SE, Pugh KR, Mencl WE, Fulbright RK, Skudlarski P, et al. Disruption of posterior brain systems for reading in children with developmental dyslexia. *Biol Psychiatry* 2002; 52 (2): 101-10.

Smith ML, Bernal B, Duchowny M, Dunoyer C, Jayakar P, Altman NR. Severity of focal cortical dysplasia and functional organization of the brain. *Epilepsia* 2004; 45: 357.

Spreer J, Arnold S, Quiske A, Wohlfarth R, Ziyeh S, Altenmuller D, et al. Determination of hemisphere dominance for language: comparison of frontal and temporal fMRI activation with intracarotid amytal testing. *Neuroradiology* 2002; 44 (6): 467-74.

Springer JA, Binder JR, Hammeke TA, Swanson SJ, Frost JA, Bellgowan PS, et al. Language dominance in neurologically normal and epilepsy subjects: a functional MRI study. *Brain* 1999; 122 (Pt 11): 2033-46.

Staudt M, Grodd W, Niemann G, Wildgruber D, Erb M, Krageloh-Mann I. Early left periventricular brain lesions induce right hemispheric organization of speech. *Neurology* 2001; 57: 122-25.

Staudt M, Lidzba K, Wolfgang G, Wildgruber D, Michael E, Krageloh-Mann I. Right-hemispheric organization of language following early left-sided brain lesions: Functional MRI topography. *NeuroImage* 2002; 16: 954-67.

Stern CE, Corkin S, González RG, Guimaraes AR, Baker JA, Jennings PJ, et al. The hippocampal formation participates in novel picture encoding: Evidence from functional magnetic resonance imaging. *Proc Natl Acad Sci USA* 1996; 93: 8660-5.

Szaflarski JP, Binder JR, Possing ET, McKiernan KA, Ward BD, Hammeke TA. Language lateralization in left-handed and ambidextrous people: fMRI data. *Neurology* 2002; 59 (2): 238-44.

Theodore WH, Fishbein D, Dubinsky R. Patterns of cerebral glucose metabolism in patients with partial seizures. *Neurology* 1988; 38: 1201-6.

Theodore WH, DeCarli C, Gaillard WD. Total cerebral volume is reduced in patients with localization-related epilepsy and a history of complex febrile seizures. *Arch Neurol* 2003; 60: 250-2.

Thivard L, Hombrouck J, Montcel T, Delmaire C, Cohen L, Samson S, et al. Productive and perceptive language reorganization in temporal lobe epilepsy. *Neuroimage* 2005; 24: 841-51.

Ulualp SO, Biswal BB, Yetkin FZ, Kidder TM. Functional Magnetic Resonance Imaging of Auditory Cortex in Children. *Laryngoscope* 1998; 108: 1782-6.

Woermann FG, Jokeit H, Luerding R, Freitag H, Schulz R, Guertler S, et al. Language lateralization by Wada test and fMRI in 100 patients with epilepsy. *Neurology* 2003; 61 (5): 699-701.

Wood AG, Harvey AS, Wellard RM, Abbott DF, Anderson V, Kean M, et al. Language cortex activation in normal children. *Neurology* 2004; 63 (6): 1035-44.

Woods RP, Dodrill CB, Ojemann GA. Brain injury, handedness, and speech lateralization in a series of amobarbital studies. *Ann Neurol* 1988; 23: 510-8.

Yetkin FZ, Swanson S, Fischer M, Akansel G, Morris G, Mueller W, et al. Functional MR of frontal lobe activation: comparison with Wada language results. *Am J Neuroradiol* 1998; 19: 1095-8.

# Temporal lobe epilepsy and cognitive dysfunction: what do we learn from PET studies in children?

E. Asano, H.T. Chugani

*Departments of Pediatrics, Neurology and Radiology, and the PET Center, Children's Hospital of Michigan, Wayne State University, Detroit, Michigan, USA*

---

Positron emission tomography (PET) is a noninvasive functional imaging tool which can measure regional uptake and affinity of ligands or metabolic substrates in brain. PET has been utilized clinically to localize epileptogenic foci, to evaluate the integrity of brain regions outside the epileptic focus and to predict postoperative cognitive dysfunction in patients with intractable focal epilepsy being evaluated for surgical resection. The most widely available PET tracer for presurgical evaluation of both adults and children with intractable focal epilepsy is 2-deoxy-2-[$^{18}$F]fluoro-D-glucose (FDG). Other PET tracers include [$^{11}$C]flumazenil (FMZ) which binds to GABA$_A$ receptors (Muzik et al., 2000; Juhasz et al., 2001b; Asano et al., 2002), and alpha-[$^{11}$C]methyl-L-tryptophan (AMT) which measures tryptophan metabolism (Chugani et al., 1998; Asano et al., 2001a; Juhasz et al., 2003). Other PET tracers with the potential for detecting epileptic brain regions include: ligands for opioid receptors (Frost et al., 1988), histamine H1 receptors (Iinuma et al., 1993), monoamine oxidase type B enzyme (Kumlien et al., 1995), N-methyl-D-aspartate receptors (Kumlien et al., 1999), peripheral-type benzodiazepine receptors (Sauvageau et al., 2002), and serotonin 1A receptors (Toczek et al., 2003).

Cognitive aspects in patients with epilepsy have been investigated mainly using FDG PET, whereas other PET tracers have been used to provide a better localization of epileptogenic cortex. In this review, we will summarize the findings of previous PET studies which investigated cognitive aspects of adults with temporal lobe epilepsy (TLE) as well as children with various epilepsy syndromes, and discuss the clinical implications of these findings for children with TLE.

## ■ Role of FDG PET in presurgical evaluation for adults with intractable TLE

TLE is one of the most common forms of epilepsy and is often medically intractable (Semah et al., 1998). Hippocampal sclerosis is the most common pathologic finding in adults with mesial temporal lobe epilepsy (M TLE), and temporal lobectomy is effective for the control of medically refractory seizures in these patients (Wiebe et al., 2001). One of the major roles of FDG PET in epilepsy surgery for adults and children with TLE is to detect dysfunctional cortical regions showing interictal hypometabolism that generally correspond to the location of epileptic foci (Theodore et al., 1986; Henry et al., 1993a). It is generally accepted that interictal FDG PET is very sensitive in demonstrating unilaterally decreased temporal lobe glucose metabolism in 80-90% of adults with M TLE (Theodore et al., 1986; Gaillard et al., 1995; Henry et al., 1993a; Knowlton et al., 1997). A previous study which compared FDG PET and intracranial EEG recordings in TLE showed an overall high sensitivity of FDG PET for detecting the epileptogenic temporal lobe as defined by ictal intracranial EEG (Henry et al., 1993c). In fact, FDG PET is able to correctly lateralize and localize the temporal epileptic focus in the majority of cases, and its sensitivity surpasses that of MRI, including hippocampal volumetry and proton magnetic resonance spectroscopy, in unilateral TLE (Gaillard et al., 1995; Knowlton et al., 1997). The presence of interictal glucose hypometabolism confined to a temporal lobe, in general, can predict a favorable postsurgical seizure outcome (Theodore et al., 1992; Koutroumanidis et al., 1998; van Bogaert et al., 2000; Theodore et al., 2001). Conversely, the presence of interictal glucose hypometabolism involving the bilateral temporal lobes is associated with poorer surgical outcome presumably due to the presence of independent bilateral epileptogenic foci (Koutroumanidis et al., 2000; Choi et al., 2003). Due to its high lateralizing and localizing value in TLE, FDG PET imaging has contributed to a significant reduction in the number of TLE patients who require extensive intracranial EEG monitoring.

Cognitive aspects of TLE have been well studied in the adult population. Adults with unilateral TLE of long duration occasionally show widespread neocortical hypometabolism on the side of the epileptic focus (e.g. lateral temporal, insular, parietal, frontal cortex) as well as thalamic hypometabolism, even though temporal lobe resection is sufficient to obtain seizure-free outcome (Henry et al., 1993b; Ryvlin et al., 1998; Chassoux et al., 2004, Benedek et al., 2004). These findings suggest that not all hypometabolic brain regions are epileptic, but that such extratemporal neocortical hypometabolism may be associated with cognitive dysfunction in adults with longstanding TLE. A previous FDG PET study showed that severity (defined by asymmetry index) of glucose hypometabolism in the left lateral temporal lobe and left thalamus was correlated to impairment of verbal IQ (Rausch et al., 1994). Another FDG PET study showed that severe glucose hypometabolism (defined as > 10% asymmetry) of the prefrontal region was associated with a history of secondary generalized tonic clonic seizures and a significant reduction of verbal and performance IQ (Jokeit et al., 1997). Association between glucose metabolism and cognitive function was also demonstrated in a postsurgical follow-up study of adults with left TLE (Griffith et al., 2000), which noted a postoperative verbal memory decline in 33% of adults when the hypometabolic left temporal lobe showed at least 10% asymmetry on glucose metabolism, and in 89% of adults when the hypometabolic left temporal lobe showed less than 10% asymmetry on glucose metabolism. This finding suggests that FDG PET may be useful to predict a postoperative cognitive dysfunction in adults with TLE.

## ■ Children with TLE are different from adults with TLE

Major distinctions between adults and children with TLE include the underlying etiology for seizures. Hippocampal sclerosis is less common in children with medically refractory TLE compared to brain malformation and low-grade brain tumor (*Figure 1A*; Wyllie et al., 1998; Mohamed et al., 2001). Approximately 80% of children who underwent a temporal lobectomy for uncontrolled seizures due to hippocampal sclerosis had mild cortical dysplasia in the lateral temporal neocortex (*Figure 1B*; Mohamed et al., 2001). On the other hand, a large portion of children with new-onset TLE have cryptogenetic etiology (Harvey et al., 1997; Gaillard et al., 2002; Sztriha et al., 2002). Such etiologic differences may complicate any experimental protocol designed to assess cognitive aspects of a series of children with TLE.

It should also be noted that children are capable of reorganizing cognitive functions to a greater degree compared to adults because of developmental brain plasticity. Considerable brain plasticity also occurs in adults but, in general, this is less robust than that seen in children. For example, recovery from language deficits due to a massive neuronal destruction involving the entire left hemisphere can be expected in children, if the right hemisphere is intact and capable of reorganizing language functions (Boatman et al., 1999; Kossoff et al., 2002). Therefore, cognitive function of children with TLE may also highly depend on the integrity of the presumed healthy hemisphere including the temporal lobe.

## ■ Pathophysiology of glucose hypometabolism in focal epilepsy

Although FDG PET has been widely used as one of the essential diagnostic tools for patients with intractable focal epilepsy including TLE, the pathophysiology of interictal glucose hypometabolism has not been completely understood (Koepp and Woermann 2005). Interictal glucose hypometabolism at least partially reflects volume loss in the affected temporal lobe structures such as a sclerotic hippocampus or atrophic temporal neocortex (Knowlton et al., 2001). Yet, the severity of interictal hypometabolism in patients with TLE may not be simply dependent on neuronal loss (Henry et al., 1994; Theodore et al., 2001), but may be correlated to duration of epilepsy (Gaillard et al., 2002; Chassoux et al., 2004; Benedek et al., 2004), effects of diaschisis (Tatsch et al., 2003), or ictal discharge generation and spread pathways (Chassoux et al., 2004). Interictal spike frequency during FDG PET scanning may also influence PET findings. It has been known that a small subset of PET studies result in a focal glucose hypermetabolism in the presumed epileptic temporal lobe, which is associated with active interictal spike-wave activity on EEG during PET scanning (Chugani

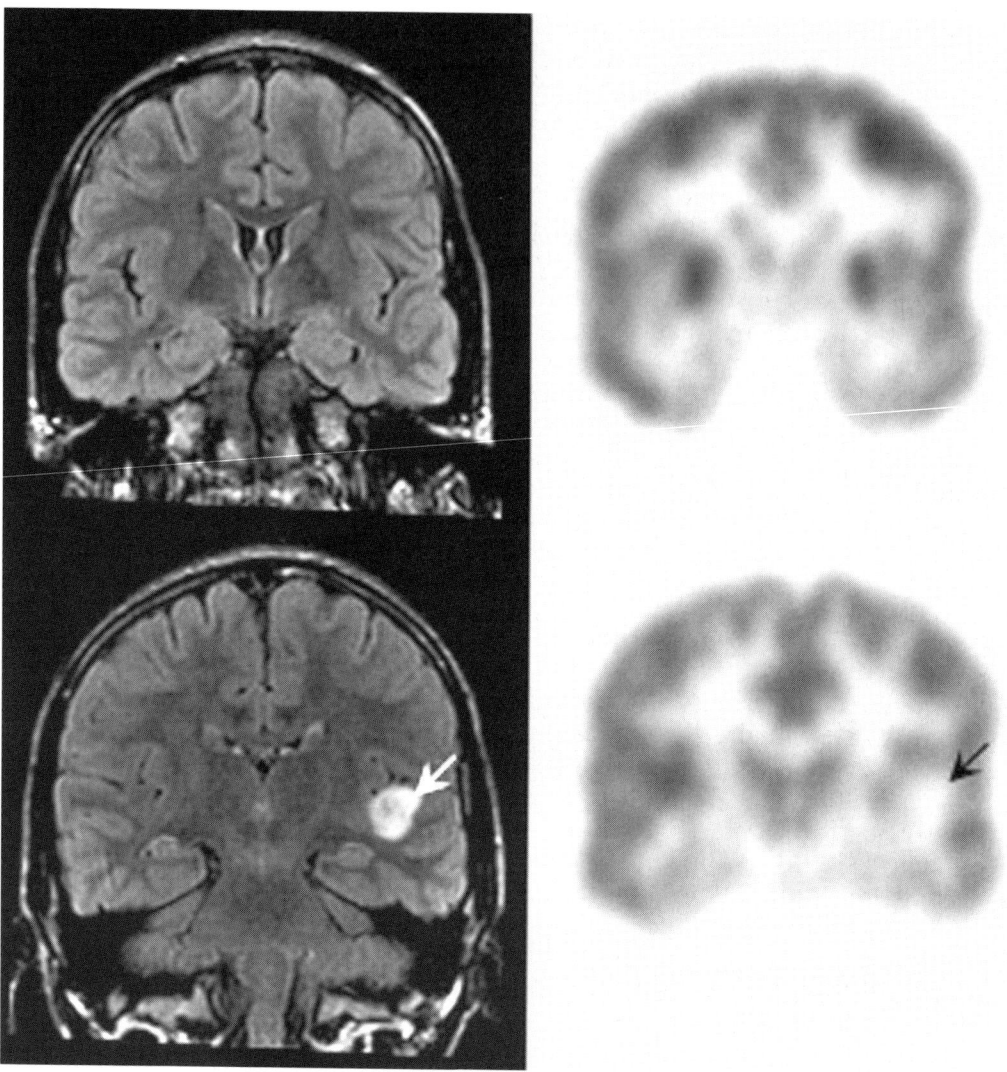

**Figure 1A. Etiologic variation in children with temporal lobe epilepsy.**
Fluid-attenuated inversion recovery (FLAIR) MRI and FDG PET images in a 15-year-old boy with intractable temporal lobe epilepsy. MRI shows a well-defined hyperintense lesion in the left superior temporal gyrus (arrow). PET shows severe glucose hypometabolism confined to the lesion as well as the surrounding cortex (arrow). Surgical resection of the lesion and the surrounding superior temporal gyrus resulted in a seizure-free outcome without postoperative deficits. A diagnosis of dysembryoplastic neuroepithelial tumor was made on pathology.

*et al.*, 1993). A previous study showed that the asymmetry of interictal spike frequency between the presumed epileptic and healthy temporal lobes was negatively correlated with the asymmetry of interictal glucose metabolism on FDG PET (Hong *et al.*, 2002). These findings may suggest that interictal glucose hypometabolism in the epileptic

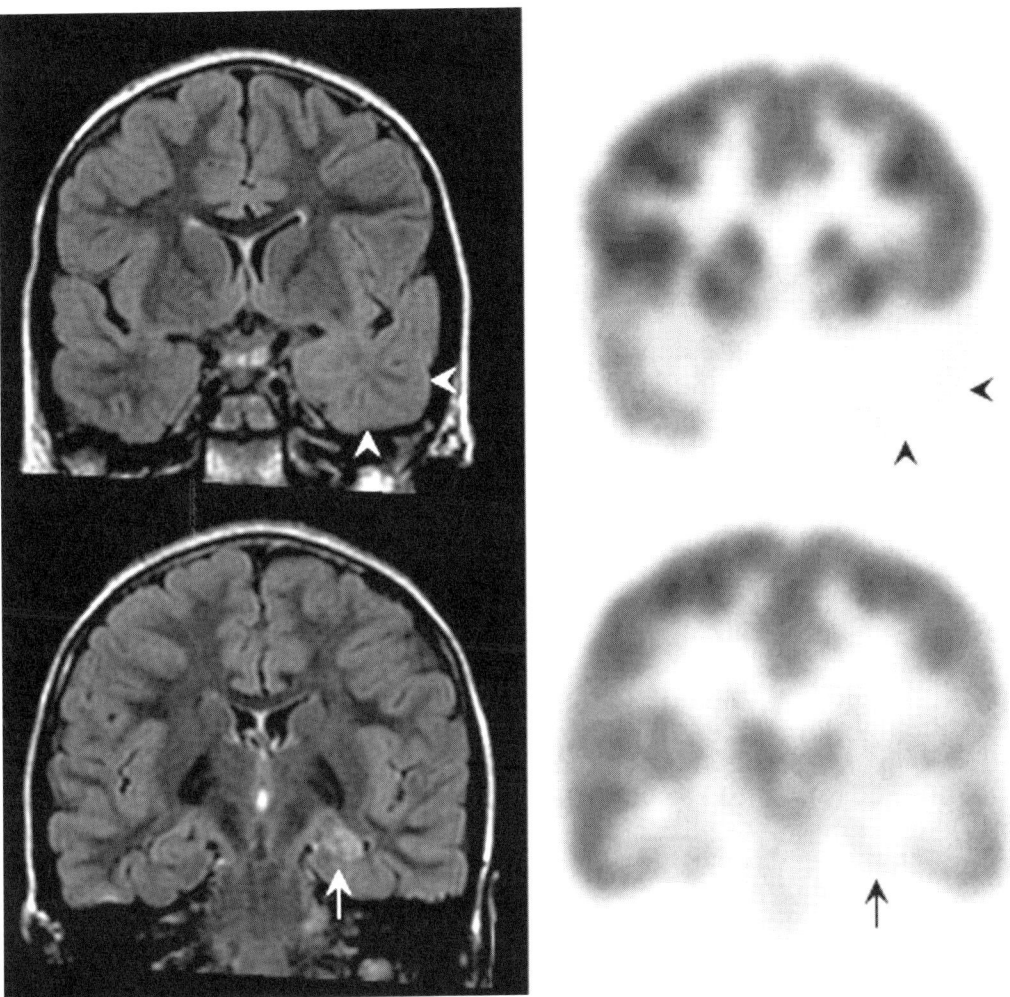

**Figure 1B. Etiologic variation in children with temporal lobe epilepsy.**
FLAIR MRI and FDG PET images in a 9-year-old girl with diagnosis of intractable temporal lobe epilepsy associated with dual pathology and attention deficit hyperactivity disorder. MRI shows evidence of hippocampal sclerosis in the left side (arrow) and cortical dysplasia in the left temporal neocortex (arrowheads). PET shows severe glucose hypometabolism in the left hippocampus as well as temporal neocortex corresponding to the structural lesion on MRI. PET also shows mild glucose hypometabolism in the left thalamus and temporal neocortex outside the structural lesion on MRI. The patient is currently scheduled for epilepsy surgery.

temporal region might be transiently masked or even reversed by increased energy consumption by an active epileptogenic focus. Therefore, EEG monitoring is recommended during FDG tracer uptake period for appropriate interpretation of falsely lateralized PET findings (Chugani et al., 1993).

## ■ PET studies in children with various epilepsy syndromes

Very few PET studies have focused on cognitive aspects in a series of children with pure TLE. Instead, several previous PET studies demonstrated an association between specific abnormal PET patterns including temporal lobe abnormalities and specific behavioral phenotypes in children with various epilepsy syndromes. We will now discuss the implications of these findings for children with TLE.

### Tuberous sclerosis complex

Tuberous sclerosis complex (TSC) is an autosomal dominant inherited disorder, now known to result from mutations in at least two different genes, TSC1 (Fryer et al., 1987; van Slegtenhorst et al., 1997) and TSC2 (Kandt et al., 1992). In the brain, cortical lesions in TSC include not only tubers (Huttenlocher and Heydemann 1984), but also microscopic abnormalities such as microdysgenesis, heterotopic grey matter, and lamination defects (Machado-Salas 1984, Asano et al., 2000). Deeper brain lesions, such as subependymal nodules and subependymal giant cell astrocytomas, are also prominent (Asano et al., 2003). Neurological sequelae of these brain lesions include epilepsy, mental retardation and autism in some cases. Our previous PET study of 26 children with TSC (Asano et al., 2001b) showed that the autistic group had decreased glucose metabolism in the lateral temporal gyri bilaterally (Figure 2), increased glucose metabolism in the deep cerebellar nuclei bilaterally, and increased AMT tracer uptake in the caudate nuclei bilaterally, compared to a mentally-retarded non-autistic group with TSC. In addition, glucose hypometabolism in the bilateral temporal gyri was significantly associated with communication disturbances. Glucose hypermetabolism in the deep cerebellar nuclei and increased AMT uptake in the caudate nuclei were both related to stereotypical behaviors and impaired social interaction, as well as communication disturbances in children with TSC. Our findings are consistent with a number of other reported observations in the TSC population. For example, an association has been demonstrated between structural and electrographic temporal abnormalities and autistic phenotype in children with TSC (Bolton and Griffiths 1997, Bolton et al., 2002; Curatolo et al., 2004; Seri et al., 1999). An association between the presence of cerebellar tubers and autistic phenotype in children with TSC has also been reported (Weber et al., 2000). Furthermore, a potential role of the caudate nucleus in some autistic features such as stereotypical behaviors has been implied in previous studies using MR imaging and spectroscopy (Kates et al., 1998; Levitt et al., 2003).

### Sturge-Weber syndrome

Sturge-Weber syndrome is a neurocutaneous disorder characterized by leptomeningeal angiomatosis, glaucoma, and ipsilateral facial capillary hemangioma (port-wine stain) in the distribution of the trigeminal nerve (Arzimanoglou and Aicardi 1992). In approximately 85% of cases with Sturge-Weber syndrome, the leptomeningeal angioma is unilateral, typically in the posterior head region (Boltshauser et al., 1976). The lack of normal cortical veins, together with the angioma, may lead to stasis and thrombosis, resulting in hypoxia and chronic ischemia and leading to progressive clinical symptoms (Comi, 2003). Neurologic complications often include epilepsy,

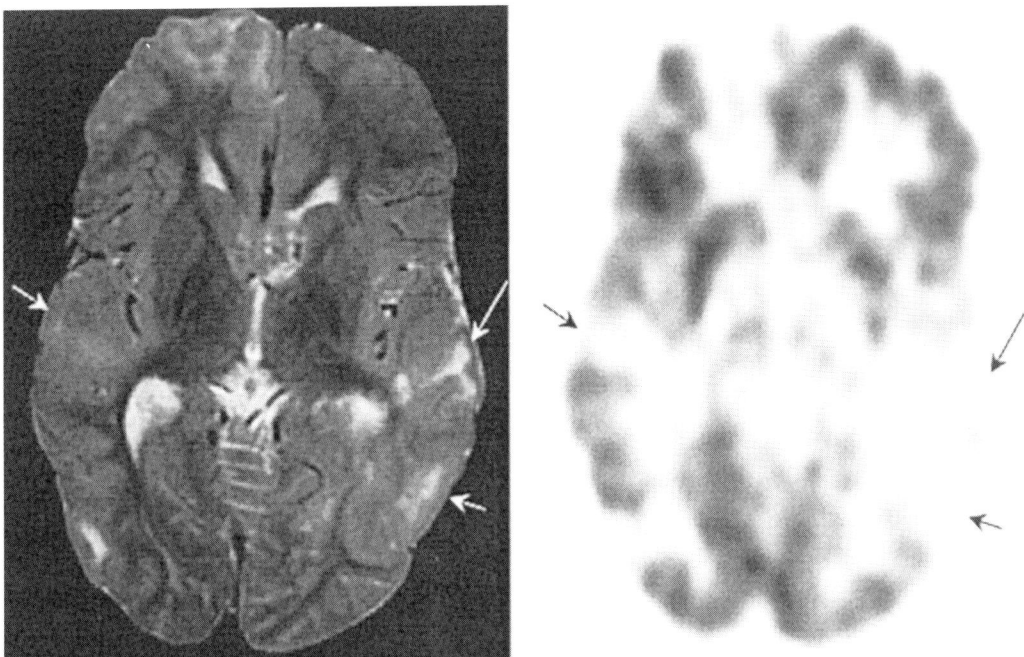

**Figure 2. MRI and FDG PET images in a 6-year-old boy with diagnosis of tuberous sclerosis, intractable epilepsy and autism.**
(A) T2-wighted MR image shows multiple cortical tubers in the left and right temporal, the right frontal and the right occipital lobes. (B) FDG PET image shows severe hypometabolism corresponding to the cortical tubers (arrows) as well as mild hypometabolism bilaterally in the non-tuberous temporal regions.

progressive mental retardation, contralateral hemiparesis, hemiplegia, and hemianopsia (Arzimanoglou and Aicardi, 1992). Focal epilepsy affects approximately 80% of patients with SWS, and seizures begin during infancy in many cases (Kossoff et al., 2002). Using FDG PET, we previously studied 13 children with unilateral cerebral involvement of Sturge-Weber syndrome and determined the clinical significance of mildly hypometabolic cortical areas (defined as 10-20% decrease compared to the contralateral homotopic regions) and severely hypometabolic areas (> 20% decrease) (Lee et al., 2001). In short, the severity of epilepsy and cognitive impairment was related to the size of not severely but mildly hypometabolic cortical regions. At first glance, these findings may appear paradoxical. However, these data are consistent with the classic theory that nociferous cortex is more detrimental to the brain than the *absence* of the same brain region (Penfield, 1952). These findings might have clinical implications in children with TLE; surgical removal of the epileptic temporal lobe which is giving rise to frequent seizures and showing abundant interictal epileptiform discharges might result in a better cognitive outcome compared to such a nociferous and dysfunctional temporal lobe which is left in place. Early demise of the affected cortex or hemisphere (either spontaneously or with surgical resection) may allow the contralateral hemisphere to reorganize more effectively, leading to better cognitive outcome (Arzimanoglou et al., 2000; Lee et al., 2001).

## Landau-Kleffner syndrome

Landau-Kleffner syndrome is a pediatric epilepsy syndrome characterized by acquired aphasia following normal acquisition of language skills and epileptic discharges, more prominent in the temporal regions on interictal EEG (Commission on Classification and Terminology of the International League Against Epilepsy, 1989). In some, the clinical syndrome is associated with Electrical Status Epilepticus during slow sleep but again with a temporal prominance. Patients with Landau-Kleffner syndrome may or may not have a history of clinical seizures. A previous PET study of 17 children with Landau-Kleffner syndrome demonstrated that bilateral glucose hypometabolism in the temporal regions is the most common finding (da Silva et al., 1997), but a small subset of patients had focal glucose hypermetabolism involving a unilateral temporal lobe showing frequent interictal spike activity. Association between interictal bitemporal glucose hypometabolism and language impairment is consistent with the observation that the severity of bitemporal glucose hypometabolism was correlated to the severity of communication skills in children with TSC (Asano et al., 2001b). It remains uncertain whether focal glucose hypermetabolism as well as hypometabolism on interictal FDG PET is a transient finding due to frequent interictal epileptiform activity or a persistent finding related to the underlying etiology. Surgical intervention, such as multiple subpial transections, for patients with Landau-Kleffner syndrome is currently controversial, since the majority of cases are associated with multifocal independent interictal spike activity. Resective surgery in children with Landau-Kleffner syndrome might be warranted in selected cases showing concordance between focal abnormalities on electrographic, functional and structural investigations.

## Aggressive behavior in children with focal epilepsy

Interictal aggressive behavior is one of the most challenging manifestations in children with focal epilepsy, since it can be a major contributor to poor social adaptation (Herman, 1982). Aggression was found to be associated with early-onset TLE (Herzberg and Fenwick, 1988), suggesting that either seizures or underlying etiologies may affect the developing brain and facilitate aggressive behavior. Certain antiepileptic drugs may also induce aggressive behavior, even if they improve seizure control (Alper et al., 2002). Our pilot FDG PET study of seven children with focal epilepsy (including three children with TLE) showed an association between interictal aggressive behavior and bilateral prefrontal and temporal neocortical brain glucose hypometabolism, with relative preservation of metabolism in medial temporal lobe structures (Figure 3; Juhasz et al., 2001a). This study also demonstrated a negative correlation between the severity of aggression and glucose metabolism of the left temporal neocortex as well as bilateral medial prefrontal cortex. A previous volumetric MRI study showed that the left frontal lobe was smaller in aggressive children with epilepsy compared to this region in non-aggressive children (Woermann et al., 2000). Based on the above findings, we speculate that a widespread dysfunction of neocortical regions, which normally exert an inhibitory effect on aggressive impulse from the limbic structures such as amygdala, may be responsible for interictal aggression. In other words, medial temporal lobe structures, which show relatively preserved metabolic activity, may be "disinhibited". This pattern of glucose metabolism is to be

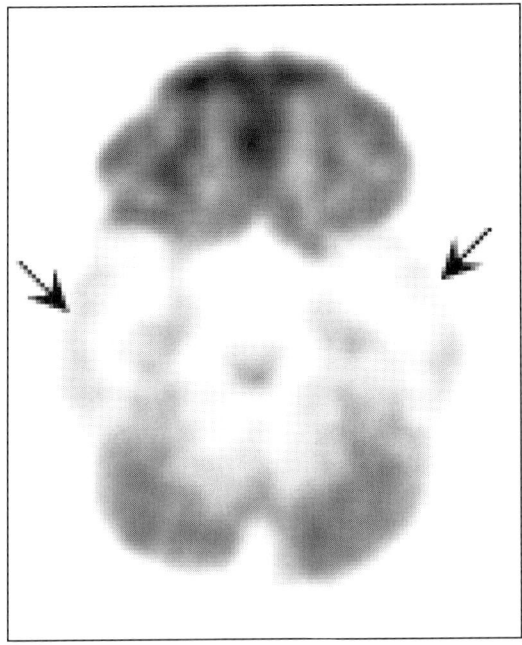

**Figure 3. FDG PET image in an 11-year-old girl with intractable tonic seizures, developmental delays and interictal aggressive behaviors.**
PET shows glucose hypometabolism involving the bilateral temporal lobes sparing the medial structures.

distinguished from that showing hypometabolism in *both* lateral and medial temporal lobe structures, which is a pattern associated with autistic or pervasive phenotype (Chugani *et al.*, 1996; DeLong and Heinz, 1997).

## Effects of medications on PET imaging

The majority of antiepileptic drugs have been reported to induce global reduction (10-30%) of glucose metabolism on FDG PET in adults (Gaillard *et al.*, 1996; Spanaki *et al.*, 1999). A previous FMZ PET study showed a decrease in $GABA_A$-receptor binding involving widespread cortical regions and cerebellum in children taking vigabatrin (Juhasz *et al.*, 2001c). It should be noted that general anesthesia using propofol during FDG uptake period may alter focal PET findings (Juengling *et al.*, 2002). In this study of 30 children with severe myoclonic epilepsy, statistically significant hypometabolic areas were found in the medial parieto-occipital cortex bilaterally, including the lingual gyrus, cuneus, posterior cingulate and middle occipital gyrus in all sedated children. In our institute, if necessary, children receive intravenous sedative agents not during an FDG tracer uptake period but during a subsequent scanning period. With this approach, sedation will not affect the pattern or rate of glucose metabolism. The potential effects of antiepileptic drugs as well as sedation on PET imaging should be taken into consideration in a study of cognitive aspects in children with focal epilepsy.

## ■ Concluding remarks

It is likely that a number of factors such as underlying etiology, interictal epileptiform activity, severity of seizures and medications contribute to FDG PET imaging patterns (Koepp and Woermann, 2005). We have learned that there are several PET imaging patterns more or less specific to certain clinical phenotypes in children with focal epilepsy. Bitemporal hypometabolism may be associated with impairment of language skills (da Silva et al., 1997; Asano et al., 2001b). Bitemporal hypometabolism involving the limbic structures such as amygdala and hippocampus may be associated with autistic features including impairment of social interaction (Chugani et al., 1996; DeLong and Heinz, 1997). Children with glucose hypometabolism in bilateral homotopic temporal lobes are least likely to achieve normal development postoperatively, even if surgical resection of the epileptogenic zone results in seizure-free outcome (Chugani et al., 1996; Szabo et al., 1999). Bitemporal hypometabolism sparing the medial structures may be associated with interictal aggression (Juhasz et al., 2001a).

One of the most important fundamental questions in the application of PET for the study of cognitive aspects in children with focal epilepsy is to clarify the effect of interictal epileptiform activity during FDG PET tracer uptake period. The cutoff threshold of interictal spike frequency for inducing focal glucose *hypermetabolism* is not known in patients with focal epilepsy, and much work needs to be done to clarify this issue. Finally, it is also important to establish a standardized model using FDG PET to predict cognitive function in children with focal epilepsy.

## References

Alper KR, Barry JJ, Balabanov AJ. Treatment of psychosis, aggression, and irritability in patients with epilepsy. *Epilepsy Behav* 2002; 3: 13-8.

Arzimanoglou A, Aicardi J. The epilepsy of Sturge-Weber syndrome: clinical features and treatment in 23 patients. *Acta Neurol Scand* 1992; 140 (suppl): 18-22.

Arzimanoglou A, Andermann F, Aicardi J, Sainte-Rose C, Beaulieu MA, Villemure JC, et al. Sturge-Weber syndrome: indications and results of surgery in 20 patients. *Neurology* 2000; 55: 1472-9.

Asano E, Chugani DC, Muzik O, Shen C, Juhász C, Janisse J, et al. Multimodality imaging for improved detection of epileptogenic foci in tuberous sclerosis complex. *Neurology* 2000; 54: 1976-84.

Asano E, Chugani DC, Juhasz C, Muzik O, Chugani HT. Surgical treatment of West syndrome. *Brain Dev* 2001a; 23: 668-76.

Asano E, Chugani DC, Muzik O, Behen M, Janisse J, Rothermel R, et al. Autism in tuberous sclerosis complex is related to both cortical and subcortical dysfunction. *Neurology* 2001b; 57: 1269-77.

Asano E, Juhász C, Chugani DC, Muzik O, Chugani HT. Positron Emission Tomography Localization for Epilepsy Surgery. In: Reisin RC et al., ed. *Advances in Clinical Neurophysiology*. Elsevier Science B. V., 2002: 351-8.

Asano E, Chugani DC, Chugani HT. Positron Emission Tomography. In: Curatolo P, ed. *Tuberous Sclerosis Complex*. Cambridge: Mac Keith Press, 2003: 124-35.

Benedek K, Juhasz C, Muzik O, Chugani DC, Chugani HT. Metabolic changes of subcortical structures in intractable focal epilepsy. *Epilepsia* 2004; 45: 1100-5.

Boatman D, Freeman J, Vining E, Pulsifer M, Miglioretti D, Minahan R, et al. Language recovery after left hemispherectomy in children with late-onset seizures. *Ann Neurol* 1999; 46: 579-86.

Bolton PF, Griffiths PD. Association of tuberous sclerosis of temporal lobes with autism and atypical autism. *Lancet* 1997; 349: 392-5.

Bolton PF, Park RJ, Higgins JN, Griffiths PD, Pickles A. Neuro-epileptic determinants of autism spectrum disorders in tuberous sclerosis complex. *Brain* 2002; 125: 1247-55.

Boltshauser E, Wilson J, Hoare RD. Sturge-Weber syndrome with bilateral intracranial calcification. *J Neurol Neurosurg Psychiatry* 1976; 39: 429-35.

Chassoux F, Semah F, Bouilleret V, Landre E, Devaux B, Turak B, et al. Metabolic changes and electro-clinical patterns in mesio-temporal lobe epilepsy: a correlative study. *Brain* 2004; 127: 164-174.

Choi JY, Kim SJ, Hong SB, Seo DW, Hong SC, Kim BT, Kim SE. Extratemporal hypometabolism on FDG PET in temporal lobe epilepsy as a predictor of seizure outcome after temporal lobectomy. *Eur J Nucl Med Mol Imaging* 2003; 30: 581-7.

Chugani DC, Chugani HT, Muzik O, Shah JR, Shah AK, Canady A, et al. Imaging epileptogenic tubers in children with tuberous sclerosis complex using alpha-[11C]methyl-L-tryptophan positron emission tomography. *Ann Neurol* 1998; 44: 858-66.

Chugani HT, Shewmon DA, Khanna S, Phelps ME. Interictal and postictal focal hypermetabolism on positron emission tomography. *Pediatr Neurol* 1993; 9: 10-5.

Chugani HT, Da Silva E, Chugani DC. Infantile spasms: III. Prognostic implications of bitemporal hypometabolism on positron emission tomography. *Ann Neurol* 1996; 39: 643-9.

Comi AM. Pathophysiology of Sturge-Weber syndrome. *J Child Neurol* 2003; 18: 509-16.

Commission on Classification and Terminology of the International League Against Epilepsy. Proposal for revised classification of epilepsies and epileptic syndromes. *Epilepsia* 1989; 30: 389-99.

Curatolo P, Porfirio MC, Manzi B, Seri S. Autism in tuberous sclerosis. *Eur J Paediatr Neurol* 2004; 8: 327-32.

da Silva EA, Chugani DC, Muzik O, Chugani HT. Landau-Kleffner syndrome: metabolic abnormalities in temporal lobe are a common feature. *J Child Neurol* 1997; 12: 489-95.

DeLong GR, Heinz ER. The clinical syndrome of early-life bilateral hippocampal sclerosis. *Ann Neurol* 1997; 42: 11-7.

Frost JJ, Mayberg HS, Fisher RS, Douglass KH, Dannals RF, Links JM, et al. Mu-opiate receptors measured by positron emission tomography are increased in temporal lobe epilepsy. *Ann Neurol* 1988; 23: 231-7.

Fryer AE, Chalmers A, Connor JM, Fraser I, Povey S, Yates AD, et al. Evidence that the gene for tuberous sclerosis is on chromosome 9. *Lancet* 1987; 1: 659-61.

Gaillard WD, Bhatia S, Bookheimer SY, Fazilat S, Sato S, Theodore WH. FDG-PET and volumetric MRI in the evaluation of patients with partial epilepsy. *Neurology* 1995; 45: 123-6.

Gaillard WD, Zeffiro T, Fazilat S, DeCarli C, Theodore WH. Effect of valproate on cerebral metabolism and blood flow: an 18F-2-deoxyglucose and 15O water positron emission tomography study. *Epilepsia* 1996; 37: 515-1.

Gaillard WD, Kopylev L, Weinstein S, Conry J, Pearl PL, Spanaki MV, et al. Low incidence of abnormal (18)FDG-PET in children with new-onset partial epilepsy: a prospective study. *Neurology* 2002; 58: 717-22.

Griffith HR, Perlman SB, Woodard AR, Rutecki PA, Jones JC, Ramirez LF, et al. Preoperative FDG-PET temporal lobe hypometabolism and verbal memory after temporal lobectomy. *Neurology* 2000; 54: 1161-5.

Harvey AS, Berkovic SF, Wrennall JA, Hopkins IJ. Temporal lobe epilepsy in childhood: clinical, EEG, and neuroimaging findings and syndrome classification in a cohort with new-onset seizures. *Neurology* 1997; 49: 960-8.

Henry TR, Chugani HT, Abou-Khalil BW, et al. Positron emission tomography. In: Engel J Jr, ed. *Surgical treatment of the epilepsies*, 2nd ed., New York: Raven Press, 1993a: 211-43.

Henry TR, Frey KA, Sackellares JC, Gilman S, Koeppe RA, Brunberg JA, et al. In vivo cerebral metabolism and central benzodiazepine-receptor binding in temporal lobe epilepsy. *Neurology* 1993b; 43: 1998-2006.

Henry TR, Mazziotta JC, Engel J Jr. Interictal metabolic anatomy of mesial temporal lobe epilepsy. *Arch Neurol* 1993c; 50: 582-9.

Henry TR, Babb TL, Engel J Jr, Mazziotta JC, Phelps ME, Crandall PH. Hippocampal neuronal loss and regional hypometabolism in temporal lobe epilepsy. *Ann Neurol* 1994; 36: 925-7.

Hermann BP. Neuropsychological functioning and psychopathology in children with epilepsy. *Epilepsia* 1982; 23: 545-54.

Herzberg JL, Fenwick PB. The aetiology of aggression in temporal-lobe epilepsy. *Br J Psychiatry* 1988; 153: 50-5.

Hong SB, Han HJ, Roh SY, Seo DW, Kim SE, Kim MH. Hypometabolism and interictal spikes during positron emission tomography scanning in temporal lobe epilepsy. *Eur Neurol* 2002; 48: 65-70.

Huttenlocher PR, Heydemann PT. Fine structure of cortical tubers in tuberous sclerosis: a Golgi study. *Ann Neurol* 1984; 16: 595-602.

Iinuma K, Yokoyama H, Otsuki T, Yanai K, Watanabe T, Ido T, Itoh M. Histamine H1 receptors in complex partial seizures. *Lancet* 1993; 341: 238.

Jokeit H, Seitz RJ, Markowitsch HJ, Neumann N, Witte OW, Ebner A. Prefrontal asymmetric interictal glucose hypometabolism and cognitive impairment in patients with temporal lobe epilepsy. *Brain* 1997; 120: 2283-94.

Juengling FD, Kassubek J, Martens-Le Bouar H, Reinhardt MJ, Krause T, et al. Cerebral regional hypometabolism caused by propofol-induced sedation in children with severe myoclonic epilepsy: a study using fluorodeoxyglucose positron emission tomography and statistical parametric mapping. *Neurosci Lett* 2002; 335: 79-82.

Juhasz C, Behen ME, Muzik O, Chugani DC, Chugani HT. Bilateral medial prefrontal and temporal neocortical hypometabolism in children with epilepsy and aggression. *Epilepsia* 2001a; 42: 991-1001.

Juhasz C, Chugani DC, Muzik O, Shah A, Shah J, Watson C, Chugani HT. Relationship of flumazenil and glucose PET abnormalities to neocortical epilepsy surgery outcome. *Neurology* 2001b; 56: 1650-8.

Juhasz C, Muzik O, Chugani DC, Shen C, Janisse J, Chugani HT. Prolonged vigabatrin treatment modifies developmental changes of GABA(A)-receptor binding in young children with epilepsy. *Epilepsia* 2001c; 42: 1320-6.

Juhasz C, Chugani DC, Muzik O, Shah A, Asano E, Mangner TJ, et al. Alpha-methyl-L-tryptophan PET detects epileptogenic cortex in children with intractable epilepsy. *Neurology* 2003; 60: 960-8.

Kandt RS, Haines JL, Smith M, Northrup H, Gardner RJ, Short MP, et al. Linkage of an important gene locus for tuberous sclerosis to a chromosome 16 marker for polycystic kidney disease. *Nat Genet* 1992; 2: 37-41.

Kates WR, Mostofsky SH, Zimmerman AW, Mazzocco MM, Landa R, Warsofsky IS, et al. Neuroanatomical and neurocognitive differences in a pair of monozygous twins discordant for strictly defined autism. *Ann Neurol* 1998; 43: 782-91.

Knowlton RC, Laxer KD, Ende G, Hawkins RA, Wong ST, Matson GB, et al. Presurgical multimodality neuroimaging in electroencephalographic lateralized temporal lobe epilepsy. *Ann Neurol* 1997; 42: 829-37.

Knowlton RC, Laxer KD, Klein G, Sawrie S, Ende G, Hawkins RA, et al. In vivo hippocampal glucose metabolism in mesial temporal lobe epilepsy. *Neurology* 2001; 57: 1184-90.

Koepp MJ, Woermann FG. Imaging structure and function in refractory focal epilepsy. *Lancet Neurol* 2005; 4: 42-53.

Kossoff EH, Buck C, Freeman JM. Outcomes of 32 hemispherectomies for Sturge-Weber syndrome worldwide. *Neurology* 2002; 59: 1735-8.

Koutroumanidis M, Binnie CD, Elwes RD, Polkey CE, Seed P, Alarcon G, et al. Interictal regional slow activity in temporal lobe epilepsy correlates with lateral temporal hypometabolism as imaged with 18FDG PET: neurophysiological and metabolic implications. *J Neurol Neurosurg Psychiatry* 1998; 65: 170-6.

Koutroumanidis M, Hennessy MJ, Seed PT, Elwes RD, Jarosz J, Morris RG, et al. Significance of interictal bilateral temporal hypometabolism in temporal lobe epilepsy. *Neurology* 2000; 54: 1811-21.

Kumlien E, Bergstrom M, Lilja A, Andersson J, Szekeres V, Westerberg CE, et al. Positron emission tomography with [11C]deuterium-deprenyl in temporal lobe epilepsy. *Epilepsia* 1995; 36: 712-21.

Kumlien E, Hartvig P, Valind S, Oye I, Tedroff J, Langstrom B. NMDA-receptor activity visualized with (S)-[N-methyl-11C]ketamine and positron emission tomography in patients with medial temporal lobe epilepsy. *Epilepsia* 1999; 40: 30-7.

Lee JS, Asano E, Muzik O, Chugani DC, Juhasz C, Pfund Z, et al. Sturge-Weber syndrome: correlation between clinical course and FDG PET findings. *Neurology* 2001; 57: 189-95.

Levitt JG, O'Neill J, Blanton RE, Smalley S, Fadale D, McCracken JT, et al. Proton magnetic resonance spectroscopic imaging of the brain in childhood autism. *Biol Psychiatry* 2003; 54: 1355-66.

Machado-Salas JP. Abnormal dendritic patterns and aberrant spine development in Bourneville's disease--a Golgi survey. *Clin Neuropathol* 1984; 3: 52-8.

Mohamed A, Wyllie E, Ruggieri P, Kotagal P, Babb T, Hilbig A, et al. Temporal lobe epilepsy due to hippocampal sclerosis in pediatric candidates for epilepsy surgery. *Neurology* 2001; 56: 1643-9.

Muzik O, da Silva EA, Juhász C, Chugani DC, Shah J, Nagy F, et al. Intracranial EEG *versus* flumazenil and glucose PET in children with extratemporal lobe epilepsy. *Neurology* 2000; 54: 171-9.

Penfield W. Ablation of abnormal cortex in cerebral palsy. *J Neurol Neurosurg Psychiatry* 1952; 15: 73-8.

Rausch R, Henry TR, Ary CM, Engel J Jr, Mazziotta J. Asymmetric interictal glucose hypometabolism and cognitive performance in epileptic patients. *Arch Neurol* 1994; 51: 139-44.

Ryvlin P, Bouvard S, Le Bars D, De Lamerie G, Gregoire MC, Kahane P, et al. Clinical utility of flumazenil-PET *versus* [18F]fluorodeoxyglucose-PET and MRI in refractory partial epilepsy. A prospective study in 100 patients. *Brain* 1998; 121: 2067-81.

Sauvageau A, Desjardins P, Lozeva V, Rose C, Hazell AS, Bouthillier A, Butterwort RF. Increased expression of "peripheral-type" benzodiazepine receptors in human temporal lobe epilepsy: implications for PET imaging of hippocampal sclerosis. *Metab Brain Dis* 2002; 17: 3-11.

Semah F, Picot MC, Adam C, Broglin D, Arzimanoglou A, Bazin B, et al. Is the underlying cause of epilepsy a major prognostic factor for recurrence? *Neurology* 1998; 51: 1256-62.

Seri S, Cerquiglini A, Pisani F, Curatolo P. Autism in tuberous sclerosis: evoked potential evidence for a deficit in auditory sensory processing. *Clin Neurophysiol* 1999; 110: 1825-30.

Spanaki MV, Siegel H, Kopylev L, Fazilat S, Dean A, Liow K, et al. The effect of vigabatrin (gamma-vinyl GABA) on cerebral blood flow and metabolism. *Neurology* 1999; 53: 1518-22.

Szabo CA, Wyllie E, Dolske M, Stanford LD, Kotagal P, Comair YG. Epilepsy surgery in children with pervasive developmental disorder. *Pediatr Neurol* 1999; 20: 349-53.

Sztriha L, Gururaj AK, Bener A, Nork M. Temporal lobe epilepsy in children: etiology in a cohort with new-onset seizures. *Epilepsia* 2002; 43: 75-80.

Tatsch K, Koch W, Linke R, Poepperl G, Peters N, Holtmannspoetter M, Dichgans M. Cortical hypometabolism and crossed cerebellar diaschisis suggest subcortically induced disconnection in CADASIL: an 18F-FDG PET study. *J Nucl Med* 2003; 44: 862-9.

Theodore WH, Dorwart R, Holmes M, Porter RJ, DiChiro G. Neuroimaging in refractory partial seizures: comparison of PET, CT, and MRI. *Neurology* 1986; 36: 750-9.

Theodore WH, Sato S, Kufta C, Balish MB, Bromfield EB, Leiderman DB. Temporal lobectomy for uncontrolled seizures: the role of positron emission tomography. *Ann Neurol* 1992; 32: 789-94.

Theodore WH, Sato S, Kufta CV, Gaillard WD, Kelley K. FDG-positron emission tomography and invasive EEG: seizure focus detection and surgical outcome. *Epilepsia* 1997; 38: 81-6.

Theodore WH, Gaillard WD, De Carli C, Bhatia S, Hatta J. Hippocampal volume and glucose metabolism in temporal lobe epileptic foci. *Epilepsia* 2001; 42: 130-2.

Toczek MT, Carson RE, Lang L, Ma Y, Spanaki MV, Der MG, et al. PET imaging of 5-HT1A receptor binding in patients with temporal lobe epilepsy. *Neurology* 2003; 60: 749-56.

Van Bogaert P, Massager N, Tugendhaft P, Wikler D, Damhaut P, Levivier M, et al. Statistical parametric mapping of regional glucose metabolism in mesial temporal lobe epilepsy. *Neuroimage* 2000; 12: 129-38.

van Slegtenhorst M, de Hoogt R, Hermans C, Nellist M, Janssen B, Verhoef S, et al. Identification of the tuberous sclerosis gene TSC1 on chromosome 9q34. *Science* 1997; 277: 805-8.

Weber AM, Egelhoff JC, McKellop JM, Franz DN. Autism and the cerebellum: evidence from tuberous sclerosis. *J Autism Dev Disord* 2000; 30: 511-7.

Woermann FG, van Elst LT, Koepp MJ, Free SL, Thompson PJ, Trimble MR, Duncan JS. Reduction of frontal neocortical grey matter associated with affective aggression in patients with temporal lobe epilepsy: an objective voxel by voxel analysis of automatically segmented MRI. *J Neurol Neurosurg Psychiatry* 2000; 68: 162-9.

Wyllie E, Comair YG, Kotagal P, Bulacio J, Bingaman W, Ruggieri P. Seizure outcome after epilepsy surgery in children and adolescents. *Ann Neurol* 1998; 44: 740-8.

Wiebe S, Blume WT, Girvin JP, Eliasziw M. Effectiveness and Efficiency of Surgery for Temporal Lobe Epilepsy Study Group. A randomized, controlled trial of surgery for temporal-lobe epilepsy. *N Engl J Med* 2001; 345: 311-8.

# What future for neuroimaging techniques in evaluating cognition in children

**P. Ryvlin[1], A. Montavont[1], A. Arzimanoglou[2]**

[1] Department of Functional Neurology and Epileptology, Hospices Civils de Lyon and Université Claude-Bernard Lyon 1, Lyon, France
[2] Epilepsy Unit, Child Neurology and Metabolic Diseases Dpt., University Hospital Robert-Debré (AP-HP), Paris, France

---

Neuroimaging techniques, which have been used to investigate cognitive functions in patients with epilepsy primarily include PET studies of glucose metabolism, using [$^{18}$F]Fluorodesoxyglucose (FDG), as well as morphological and functional MRI.

Most FDG-PET studies were performed in adult patients, showing correlation between temporal or prefrontal hypometabolism and altered memory performance or decreased IQ (Salanova et al., 1992, 2001; Raush et al., 1994; Jokeit et al., 1997; Griffith et al., 2000; Hong et al., 2000). Some studies were also performed in specific childhood epileptic conditions, such as tuberous sclerosis complex (TSC) and idiopathic epileptic spasms, Sturge-Weber and Laudau Kleffner syndromes, as well as continuous spike and waves discharges during sleep (CSWS), again showing correlation between various types of FDG-PET abnormalities and neuropsychological deficits (Maquet et al., 1995; Chugani et al., 1996; da Silva et al., 1997; Lee et al., 2001; Asano et al., 2001; De Tiège et al., 2004; and see Asano and Chugani in this volume for review). Only a few children with TLE were investigated with the aim to correlate cerebral metabolic dysfunction with behavioural disorders (Juhasz et al., 2001).

Functional MRI (fMRI) has been extensively used in adults and children with epilepsy to study the reorganisation of language neural networks (Springer et al., 1999; Billingsley et al., 2001; Gaillard et al., 2002; Hertz-Pannier et al., 2002; Liegeois et al., 2002; Adcock et al., 2003; Baciu et al., 2003; Janszky et al., 2003; Woermann et al., 2003; Ries et al., 2004; Smith et al., 2004; Thivard et al., 2005, and see Weber et al. in this volume for review). Memory functions were also assessed with fMRI in a number of epilepsy studies, but not speci in children with TLE (Bellgowan et al., 1998; Detre et al., 1998; Dupont et al., 2000, 2001; Jokeit et al., 2001; Golby et al., 2002; Janszky et al., 2004; Rabin et al., 2004).

Similarly, a number of series have correlated the degree of hippocampal atrophy or of decreased N-acetyl-aspartate with cognitive dysfunction, using volumetric MRI and MR spectroscopy (MRS), respectively (Lencz et al., 1992; Incisa della Rocchetta et al., 1995; Gadian et al., 1996; Kilpatric et al., 1997; Abrahams et al., 1999; Martin et al., 1999a, 1999b; Namer et al., 1999; Pauli et al., 2000; Sawrie et al., 2000, 2001a, 2001b; Kikuchi et al., 2001; Wendel et al., 2001; Alessio et al., 2004a, 2004b; Hanoglu et al., 2004). However, these series provided only limited data in children with TLE. Conversely, a correlation was observed in children with epilepsy, between the presence of bi-temporal MRI abnormalities and autistic disorders, in particular in TSC patients (Bolton and Griffiths, 1997; DeLong and Heinz, 1997; Bolton et al., 2002; Curatolo et al., 2004).

Overall, FDG-PET, standard MRI and fMRI protocols, as well as MRS, still offer many opportunities to investigate cognitive disturbances in children with TLE. However, this review will focus on other relevant neuroimaging tools which could provide new insights in the pathophysiology of such disturbances, including more recent PET tracers, as well as developmental and training based MRI and fMRI investigations.

## ■ Recent and future PET tracers

Several PET tracers hold promise for the study of cognitive functions, some of which were previously studied in epilepsy with the aim to identify the seizure onset zone, such as [$^{11}$C]flumazenil, while other remain in development. One major limitation of PET studies in children must be stressed, however, ie the lack of age matched control data, for obvious ethical reasons. Accordingly, the use of radio-isotope investigation for the sole purpose of clinical research, as well as the repetition of PET studies in the same individual, should not be encouraged in children with epilepsy. It remains that some PET studies might be justified from a clinical point of view, in the context of a pre-surgical evaluation, offering the possibility to correlate the data to various neuropsychological endpoints.

### [$^{11}$C]flumazenil-PET (FMZ-PET) studies of benzodiazepine (BZD) receptors

FMZ-PET entered the field of epilepsy in the late eighties as a potential marker of GABAergic dysfunction, given that FMZ specifically binds to the BZD allosteric site at the GABAA receptor complex (Savic et al., 1988) However, it was rapidly considered as a mere marker of neuronal density (Henry et al., 1993; Sette et al., 1993; Heiss et al., 2000). As a matter of fact, decreased [$^{11}$C]-FMZ binding was consistently observed in the atrophic hippocampus in temporal lobe epilepsy (TLE) (Savic et al., 1993; Koepp et al., 1996; Debets et al., 1997; Ryvlin et al., 1998), and was found to correlate with autoradiographic measurements of [3H]-FMZ binding performed on surgically removed tissue (Koepp et al., 1998). Correlations were also reported between in vitro [3H]-FMZ binding and neuronal cell count in human epileptogenic hippocampi (Burdette et al., 1995). However, these correlations were not replicated when in vivo PET measurement of [$^{11}$C]-FMZ distribution volume was directly compared to the histologically assessed neuronal loss (Koepp et al., 1997), suggesting that part of the FMZ-PET abnormalities observed in epileptic patients might reflect functional changes of BZD receptors. Such functional changes were also suggested by various observations indicating the possibility of seizure-induced down regulation of BZD receptors (Savic et al., 1996, 1998; Ryvlin et al., 1998, 1999; Koepp et al., 2000). More recently, we demonstrated that significant short term changes of [$^{11}$C]-FMZ binding could be detected at one week interval in the epileptogenic hippocampus of patients with epilepsy, as well as in the temporal pole of control subjects (Bouvard et al., 2005).

The fact that [$^{11}$C]-FMZ PET can indirectly disclose short term regulation of the GABAA receptor complex, raise the possibility of investigating some aspects of cognition with this tracer. Indeed, the GABAergic system has been recognised to play a major role in generating and modulating several oscillatory rhythms (Buzsaki, 2001; Klausberger et al., 2003; Traub et al., 2003; Hajos et al., 2004; Lagier et al., 2004), including the gamma band oscillations which are thought to subserve part of the inter-regional binding processes underlying many cognitive functions (Tallon-Baudry et al., 1997; Tallon-Baudry and Bertrand, 1999; Singer, 1999; Engel and Singer, 2001; Engel et al., 2001; Lachaux et al., 2000, 2005; Jung et al., 2005). Protocols aiming at testing the relation between [$^{11}$C]-FMZ binding and cognitive dysfunction in TLE should take into account the associated MRI abnormalities, since the latter represent an important confounding factor. Ideally, the resulting data should be compared to the fMRI BOLD response and related gamma oscillations recorded by intracerebral EEG or magnetoencephalography, in response to the cognitive task under consideration. However, it is not unlikely that data derived from these various sources of information will correlate with each other in a way preventing the delineation of any causal relationship. The above general comments apply to all further PET tracers.

## Investigating the serotoninergic system

A number of PET tracers targeting the serotoninergic system have been recently used in patients with epilepsy. [$^{11}$C]α-methyl-L-tryptophan (AMT) was first evaluated as a potential marker of serotonin (5-HT) synthesis (Chugani and Chugani, 2000). However, the focal increased AMT uptake observed in the epileptogenic zone of some patients with TSC, cortical dysplasias, or cryptogenic partial epilepsy, rather appear to reflect an abnormal regulation of the kynurenin metabolic pathway than an increased 5-HT synthesis (Chugani et al., 1998; Fedi et al., 2001, 2003; Juhasz et al., 2003; Natsume et al., 2003). A correlation was found in TSC patients between the presence of bilateral increased AMT uptake in the caudate and autistic features (Asano et al., 2001).

Other groups have investigated the 5-HT1A receptor subtype, using either [$^{11}$C]WAY100635, [$^{18}$F]FCWAY, or the [$^{18}$F]MPPF (Toczek et al., 2003; Merlet et al., 2004a, 2004b; Savic et al., 2004; Giovacchini et al., 2005). All three molecules are selective antagonists of 5-HT1A receptors, with marked binding over limbic brain regions and within the brainstem raphe nuclei which contain most of the serotoninergic neurones. A marked decreased binding of these tracers has been consistently observed in the epileptogenic temporal lobe of adult TLE patients, in particular over the mesial temporal structures where it appears more pronounced than the associated glucose hypometabolism (Toczek et al., 2003; Merlet et al., 2004a, 2004b; Savic et al., 2004; Giovacchini et al., 2005). This abnormality was also found to correlate with the degree of associated mood disorders, as measured by the Beck Depression Inventory II (BDI-2). It could also possibly correlate with specific cognitive dysfunction, according to the potential role of 5-HT in learning and memory. However, the latter seems to be mainly conveyed by the 5-HT6 receptor subtype (Russel and Dias, 2002; Lindner et al., 2003; Wooley et al., 2004; King et al., 2004), providing strong incentive to develop a specific tracer for this molecular target.

## Desperately looking for NMDA receptors

The quest for an appropriate PET tracer of NMDA receptors has been active for over two decades, without any success until recently. Indeed, the group of Hammersmith in London has developed a specific antagonist, the [$^{11}$C]CNS5161, which might enable a robust quantification of these receptors. If validated, this PET tracer will certainly open new avenues of research in the field of cognition and epilepsy.

## Futuristic PET tracers for the brain

Many molecular targets other than neurotransmission might also prove informative in that field. Recent trends in PET research include the design of radiolabelled oligonucleotides or nucleic acid aptamers (Tavitian et al., 1998; Cerchia et al., 2002), as well as markers of apoptosis (Hofstra et al., 2000). The former type of PET tracer could conceivably enable the visualisation of mRNAs, but a number of important methodological issues hamper their practical application to in vivo brain imaging. Non invasive investigation of neuronal apoptosis could participate to a better understanding of cognitive disorders, but the available tracer, Annexin-V, has only been validated for peripheral cardio-vascular imaging (Hofstra et al., 2000; Narula et al., 2001; Kietselaer et al., 2004; Keen et al., 2005).

## ■ Emerging MRI and fMRI techniques

The major limitations of PET studies in children pave the way for a more dynamic and fruitful research in MR imaging. Several methodological advances participate to these progress, including the development of new sequences, contrast agents which might label some of the molecular targets previously discussed for PET studies, and increased field strength up to 7 teslas or more. Brain MRI and fMRI at 7 teslas already proved possible in human, and more sensitive than with lower field strength (Yacoub et al., 2001a, 2001b). However, whether a 7 teslas magnetic field is perfectly safe for children with epilepsy remains an open question. Another open avenue of MRI research derives from the extraordinary progress accomplished during the last four years in the study of brain development, both from a morphological and functional point of view.

## Morphological development of the brain

MRI volumetric studies across age have demonstrated asynchronous and non linear changes in the regional volume of gray and white matters, rather than an homogeneous increase until young adulthood followed by a linear decrease with aging as previously anticipated from the overall brain size changes (Paus, 2005). It was first shown that the white matter tracts of the internal capsule and left arcuate fasciculus increased in size between the age of 4 and 17 years old (Paus et al., 1999). The group of Sowell and collaborators have extensively studied this issue and provided the largest series of MRI measurements across life span (Sowell et al., 2001a, 2001b, 2002, 2003, 2004). They investigated 176 normal subjects, aged 7 to 87 years old (Sowell et al., 2003). White matter proved to increase in size until the age of 40. Conversely, the gray matter volume appeared to diminish from early childhood, at a rate which varies between brain regions, as confirmed by other investigators (Gogtay et al., 2004). The reduction in gray matter volume first predominated over the sensorimotor cortex, and more broadly along the superior frontal sulcus. Conversely, the left posterior temporal region followed a dramatically different evolution, with an increased in gray matter volume until the age of 30. This regional gradient only partly parallels that observed in synaptic maturation where the transition from synaptogenesis to synaptic pruning first occur in sensorimotor cortex, followed by temporal and parietal associative areas, to end up in the prefrontal cortex (Casey et al., 2005). In fact, intra-cortical myelination, rather than synaptic changes, is the most prominent contributor to the apparent decrease in gray matter volume observed during childhood and adolescence (Paus, 2005). One has to remember that axons and dendrites represent more than half of the total cortical volume. Myelination of these intra-cortical fibers will modify the MRI signal towards that of the white matter, resulting in more pronounced partial volume effect, and an overall reduction of gray matter MR signal density. Intra-cortical myelination also represents one of the major aspects of brain maturation, which continue throughout adolescence in several brain regions involved in emotional and cognitive control.

The age related physiological changes of brain volumes and maturation might be modulated by environmental factors. Several studies have reported correlation between the size of a specific brain region and the subjects' performance in various related tasks, though no conclusion could be drawn regarding the direction of such structure-function relationship (Paus, 2005). More intriguing however, is the observation of an intra-individual increased gray matter density of the lateral occipital cortex after three months of daily juggling (Draganski et al., 2004).

These research truly offer novel opportunities for physicians involved in the investigation and care of children with TLE at risk for developing cognitive dysfunction. We now envision the possibility to monitor the brain maturation of individual children with TLE, provided appropriate field strength and optimised sequences to specifically tackle the intra-cortical myelination process, and to compare this dynamic brain development over time to that of age and sex matched controls. This method might enable an earlier detection of focal brain dysfunction, as compared with other standard investigations, and more robust correlations with neuropsychological findings.

## Functional development of the brain

Dramatic changes in the pattern of fMRI activation are also observed as a function of *age* and *training*. For instance, in a task of interference suppression, children aged 8 to 12, predominantly activated the left dorso-lateral frontal cortex as well as the left anterior insula, whereas adults activated a comparable network in the right hemisphere (Bunge, 2002). In addition, the degree of activation correlated with performance in both groups, though children performed at a lower level on average. These results suggest that the brain regions recruited during specific cognitive tasks will change during brain maturation (Casey et al., 2005). As a rule, regions whose brain activity correlates with task performance become more focal or fine-tuned, whereas regions not correlated with performance decrease in activity with age (Casey et al., 2005).

Short term training of a few weeks duration, also proved to modify the pattern of fMRI activation in response to the same task. Specifically, working memory training resulted in an increased activation in the left dorso-lateral frontal cortex, and the superior parietal lobule, bilaterally (Olesen et al., 2004).

As for morphological MRI, the observation of an age and activity-dependent plasticity of the BOLD response should promote longitudinal fMRI studies in children with TLE, in particular during adolescence where major hemispheric shift of activation seems to occur.

## Social cognition, biological motion and the theory of mind

Advances in the understanding of the neural substrates of biological motion and social cognition have resulted in important progress in autism, where a bilateral dysfunction of the superior temporal region has been identified (Zilbovicius et al., 2000). Indeed, the superior temporal sulcus (STS) was found to play a major role in decoding socially salient visual cues in normal individuals, though the temporal pole and the paracingulate gyrus were also found to be involved in specific paradigms (Gallagher et al., 2000; Allison et al., 2002; Gallagher and Frith, 2003; Gallese et al., 2004). Whether an epilepsy-related alteration in social cognition contributes to the overall psycho-intellectual burden of TLE is an important question which has not yet been fully addressed. The pioneering work of Laurent and collaborators reported in this book indicates that this might well be the case. Investigating this issue with fMRI should be the next step.

## ■ Concluding remarks

The rapidly evolving field of neuroimaging offer multiple emerging opportunities to investigate the complex issue of cognitive dysfunction in children with TLE. While PET might still provide valuable information, using either old, recent, or very new tracers, MRI and fMRI clearly carry the greatest challenges for the next five years, thanks to the possibility to perform longitudinal controlled studies. The dynamic dimension of cognitive evaluation, which remains an essential part of any valid neuropsychological assessment, must now enter the imaging arena.

# References

Abrahams S, Morris RG, Polkey CE, Jarosz JM, Cox TC, Graves M, Pickering A. Hippocampal involvement in spatial and working memory: a structural MRI analysis of patients with unilateral mesial temporal lobe sclerosis. *Brain Cogn* 1999; 41: 39-65.

Adcock JE, Wise RG, Oxbury JM, Oxbury SM, Matthews PM. Quantitative fMRI assessment of the differences in lateralization of language-related brain activation in patients with temporal lobe epilepsy. *Neuroimage* 2003; 18(2): 423-38.

Alessio A, Damasceno BP, Camargo CH, Kobayashi E, Guerreiro CA, Cendes F. Differences in memory performance and other clinical characteristics in patients with mesial temporal lobe epilepsy with and without hippocampal atrophy. *Epilepsy Behav* 2004; 5: 22-7.

Alessio A, Kobayashi E, Damasceno BP, Lopes-Cendes I, Cendes F. Evidence of memory impairment in asymptomatic individuals with hippocampal atrophy. *Epilepsy Behav* 2004; 5: 981-7.

Allison T, Puce A, McCarthy G. Social perception from visual cues: role of the STS region. *Trends Cogn Sci* 2000; 4: 267-78.

Asano E, Chugani DC, Muzik O, Behen M, Janisse J, Rothermel R, Mangner TJ, Chakraborty PK, Chugani HT. Autism in tuberous sclerosis complex is related to both cortical and subcortical dysfunction. *Neurology* 2001; 57: 1269-77.

Baciu MV, Watson JM, McDermott KB, Wetzel RD, Attarian H, Moran CJ, *et al*. Functional MRI reveals an interhemispheric dissociation of frontal and temporal language regions in a patient with focal epilepsy. *Epilepsy Behav* 2003; 4(6): 776-80.

Bellgowan PS, Binder JR, Swanson SJ, Hammeke TA, Springer JA, Frost JA, *et al*. Side of seizure focus predicts left medial temporal lobe activation during verbal encoding. *Neurology* 1998; 51(2): 479-84.

Billingsley RL, McAndrews MP, Crawley AP, Mikulis DJ. Functional MRI of phonological and semantic processing in temporal lobe epilepsy. *Brain* 2001; 124(Pt 6): 1218-27.

Bolton PF, Griffiths PD. Association of tuberous sclerosis of temporal lobes with autism and atypical autism. *Lancet* 1997; 349: 392-5.

Bolton PF, Park RJ, Higgins JN, Griffiths PD, Pickles A. Neuro-epileptic determinants of autism spectrum disorders in tuberous sclerosis complex. *Brain* 2002; 125: 1247-55.

Bouvard S, Costes N, Bonnefoi F, Lavenne F, Mauguière F, Delforge J, Ryvlin P. Seizure Related Short-Term Plasticity of Benzodiazepine Receptors in Partial Epilepsy: A [$^{11}$C]Flumazenil-PET study. *Brain* 2005; 128: 1330-43.

Burdette DE, Sakurai SY, Henry TR, *et al*. Temporal lobe central benzodiazepine binding in unilateral mesial temporal lobe epilepsy. *Neurology* 1995; 45: 934-41.

Bunge SA. Immature frontal lobe contributions to cognitive control in children: Evidence from fMRI. *Neuron* 2002; 33: 301-11.

Buzsaki G. Hippocampal GABAergic interneurons: a physiological perspective. *Neurochem Res* 2001; 26: 899-905.

Casey BJ, Tottenham N, Liston C, Durston S. Imaging the developing brain: what have we learned about cognitive development? *Trends Cogn Sci* 2005; 9: 104-10.

Cerchia L, Hamm J, Libri D, Tavitian B, de Franciscis V. Nucleic acid aptamers in cancer medicine. *FEBS Lett* 2002; 528: 12-6.

Chugani DC, Chugani HT. PET: mapping of serotonin synthesis. *Adv Neurol* 2000; 83: 165-71.

Chugani HT, Da Silva E, Chugani DC. Infantile spasms: III. Prognostic implications of bitemporal hypometabolism on positron emission tomography. *Ann Neurol* 1996; 39: 643-9.

Chugani DC, Chugani HT, Muzik O, *et al*. Imaging epileptogenic tubers in children with tuberous sclerosis complex using alpha-[$^{11}$C]methyl-L-tryptophan PET. *Ann Neurol* 1998; 44: 858-66.

Curatolo P, Porfirio MC, Manzi B, Seri S. Autism in tuberous sclerosis. *Eur J Paediatr Neurol* 2004; 8: 327-32.

Da Silva EA, Chugani DC, Muzik O, Chugani HT. Landau-Kleffner syndrome: metabolic abnormalities in temporal lobe are a common feature. *J Child Neurol* 1997; 12: 489-95.

DeLong GR, Heinz ER. The clinical syndrome of early-life bilateral hippocampal sclerosis. *Ann Neurol* 1997; 12: 11-7.

De Tiege X, Goldman S, Laureys S, Verheulpen D, Chiron C, Wetzburger C, Paquier P, Chaigne D, Poznanski N, Jambaque I, Hirsch E, Dulac O, Van Bogaert P. Regional cerebral glucose metabolism in epilepsies with continuous spikes and waves during sleep. *Neurology* 2004; 63: 853-7.

Debets RM, Sadzot B, Van Isselt JW, et al. Is [11C]Flumazenil PET superior to 18FDG PET and 123I-iomazenil SPECT in presurgical evaluation of temporal lobe epilepsy? *J Neurol Neurosurg Psychiatr* 1997; 62: 141-50.

Detre JA, Maccotta L, King D, Alsop DC, D'Esposito M, Zarahn E, et al. Functional MRI lateralization of memory in temporal lobe epilepsy. *Neurology* 1998; 50: 926-32.

Draganski B, Gaser C, Busch V, Schuierer G, Bogdahn U, May A. Neuroplasticity: changes in grey matter induced by training. *Nature* 2004; 427: 311-2.

Dupont S, Van de Moortele PF, Samson S, Hasboun D, Poline JB, Adam C, et al. Episodic memory in left temporal lobe epilepsy: a functional MRI study. *Brain* 2000; 123: 1722-32.

Dupont S, Samson Y, Van de Moortele PF, Samson S, Poline JB, Adam C, et al. Delayed verbal memory retrieval: a functional MRI study in epileptic patients with structural lesions of the left medial temporal lobe. *Neuroimage* 2001; 14: 995-1003.

Engel AK, Fries P, Singer W. Dynamic predictions: oscillations and synchrony in top-down processing. *Nat Rev Neurosci* 2001; 2: 704-16.

Engel AK, Singer W. Temporal binding and the neural correlates of sensory awareness. *Trends Cogn Sci* 2001; 5: 16-25.

Fedi M, Reutens DC, Andermann F, et al. Alpha-[11C]Methyl-L-tryptophan PET identifies the epileptogenic tuber and correlates with interictal spike frequency. *Epilepsy Res* 2003; 52: 203-13.

Fedi M, Reutens DC, Okazawa H, et al. Localizing value of alpha-methyl-L-tryptophan PET in intractable epilepsy of neocortical origin. *Neurology* 2001; 57: 1629-36.

Gadian DG, Isaacs EB, Cross JH, et al. Lateralization of brain function in childhood revealed by magnetic resonance spectroscopy. *Neurology* 1996; 46: 974-7.

Gaillard WD, Balsamo L, Xu B, Grandin CB, Braniecki SH, Papero PH, et al. Language dominance in partial epilepsy patients identified with an fMRI reading task. *Neurology* 2002; 59: 256-65.

Gallagher HL, Frith CD. Functional imaging of "theory of mind". *Trends Cogn Sci* 2003; 7: 77-83.

Gallagher HL, Happe F, Brunswick N, Fletcher PC, Frith U, Frith CD. Reading the mind in cartoons and stories: an fMRI study of theory of mind' in verbal and nonverbal tasks. *Neuropsychologia* 2000; 38: 11-21.

Gallese V, Keysers C, Rizzolatti G. A unifying view of the basis of social cognition. *Trends Cogn Sci* 2004; 8: 396-403.

Giovacchini G, Toczek MT, Bonwetsch R, Bagic A, Lang L, Fraser C, Reeves-Tyer P, Herscovitch P, Eckelman WC, Carson RE, Theodore WH. 5-HT1A receptors are reduced in temporal lobe epilepsy after partial-volume correction. *J Nucl Med* 2005; 46: 1128-35.

Gogtay N, Giedd JN, Lusk L, Hayashi KM, Greenstein D, Vaituzis AC, Nugent TF 3rd, Herman DH, Clasen LS, Toga AW, Rapoport JL, Thompson PM. Dynamic mapping of human cortical development during childhood through early adulthood. *Proc Natl Acad Sci USA* 2004; 101: 8174-9.

Golby AJ, Poldrack RA, Illes J, Chen D, Desmond JE, Gabrieli JD. Memory lateralization in medial temporal lobe epilepsy assessed by functional MRI. *Epilepsia* 2002; 43: 85563.

Griffith HR, Perlman SB, Woodard AR, et al. Preoperative FDG-PET temporal lobe hypometabolism and verbal memory after temporal lobectomy. *Neurology* 2000; 54: 1161-5.

Hajos N, Palhalmi J, Mann EO, Nemeth B, Paulsen O, Freund TF. Spike timing of distinct types of GABAergic interneuron during hippocampal gamma oscillations *in vitro*. *J Neurosci* 2004; 24: 9127-37.

Hanoglu L, Ozkara C, Keskinkilic C, Altin U, Uzan M, Tuzgen S, Dincer A, Ozyurt E. Correlation between 1H MRS and memory before and after surgery in mesial temporal lobe epilepsy with hippocampal sclerosis. *Epilepsia* 2004; 45: 632-40.

Heiss WD, Kracht L, Grond M, et al., Early [(11)C]Flumazenil/H(2)O positron emission tomography predicts irreversible ischemic cortical damage in stroke patients receiving acute thrombolytic therapy. *Stroke* 2000; 31: 366-9.

Henry TR, Frey KA, Sackellares JC, et al. In vivo cerebral metabolism and central benzodiazepine receptor binding in temporal lobe epilepsy. *Neurology* 1993; 43: 1998-2006.

Hertz-Pannier L, Gaillard WD, Mott S, Cuenod CA, Bookheimer S, Weinstein S, et al. Assessment of Language Hemispheric Dominance in Children with Epilepsy using Functional MRI. *Neurology* 1997; 48: 1003-12.

Hofstra L, Liem IH, Dumont EA, Boersma HH, van Heerde WL, Doevendans PA, De Muinck E, Wellens HJ, Kemerink GJ, Reutelingsperger CP, Heidendal GA. Visualisation of cell death in vivo in patients with acute myocardial infarction. *Lancet* 2000; 356: 209-12.

Hong SB, Roh SY, Kim SE, Seo DW. Correlation of temporal lobe glucose metabolism with the Wada memory test. *Epilepsia* 2000; 41: 1554-9.

Incisa della Rocchetta A, Gadian DG, Connelly A, Polkey CE, Jackson GD, Watkins KE, Johnson CL, Mishkin M, Vargha-Khadem F. Verbal memory impairment after right temporal lobe surgery: role of contralateral damage as revealed by 1H magnetic resonance spectroscopy and T2 relaxometry. *Neurology* 1995; 45: 797-802.

Janszky J, Ebner A, Kruse B, Mertens M, Jokeit H, Seitz RJ, et al. Functional organization of the brain with malformations of cortical development. *Ann Neurol* 2003; 53: 759-67.

Janszky J, Jokeit H, Konstantina K, Mertens M, Ebner A, Pohlmann-Edan B, et al. Functional MRI predicts memory performance after right mesiotemporal epilepsy surgery. *Epilepsia* 2004; 46: 244-50.

Jokeit H, Seitz RJ, Markowitsch HJ, Neumann N, Witte OW, Ebner A. Prefrontal asymmetric interictal glucose hypometabolism and cognitive impairment in patients with temporal lobe epilepsy. *Brain* 1997; 120: 2283-94.

Jokeit H, Okujava M, Woermann FG. Memory fMRI lateralizes temporal lobe epilepsy. *Neurology* 2001; 57: 1786-93.

Juhasz C, Behen ME, Muzik O, Chugani DC, Chugani HT. Bilateral medial prefrontal and temporal neocortical hypometabolism in children with epilepsy and aggression. *Epilepsia* 2001; 42: 991-1001.

Juhasz C, Chugani DC, Muzik O, Shah A, Asano E, Mangner TJ, Chakraborty PK, Sood S, Chugani HT. Alpha-methyl-L-tryptophan PET detects epileptogenic cortex in children with intractable epilepsy. *Neurology* 2003; 60: 960-8.

Jung J, Hudry J, Ryvlin P, Royet JP, Bertrand O, Lachaux JP. Functional Significance of Olfactory-induced Oscillations in the Human Amygdala. *Cereb Cortex* 2005 (In press).

Keen HG, Dekker BA, Disley L, Hastings D, Lyons S, Reader AJ, Ottewell P, Watson A, Zweit J. Imaging apoptosis *in vivo* using 124I-annexin V and PET. *Nucl Med Biol* 2005; 32: 395-402.

Kietselaer BL, Reutelingsperger CP, Heidendal GA, Daemen MJ, Mess WH, Hofstra L, Narula J. Noninvasive detection of plaque instability with use of radiolabeled annexin A5 in patients with carotid-artery atherosclerosis. *N Engl J Med* 2004; 350: 1472-3.

Kikuchi S, Kubota F, Hattori S, Oya N, Mikuni M. A study of the relationship between metabolism using 1H-MRS and function using several neuropsychological tests in temporal lobe epilepsy. *Seizure* 2001; 10: 188-93.

Kilpatrick C, Murrie V, Cook M, Andrewes D, Desmond P, Hopper J. Degree of left hippocampal atrophy correlates with severity of neuropsychological deficits. *Seizure* 1997; 6: 213-8.

King MV, Sleight AJ, Woolley ML, Topham IA, Marsden CA, Fone KC. 5-HT6 receptor antagonists reverse delay-dependent deficits in novel object discrimination by enhancing consolidation - an effect sensitive to NMDA receptor antagonism. *Neuropharmacology* 2004; 47: 195-204.

Klausberger T, Magill PJ, Marton LF, Roberts JD, Cobden PM, Buzsaki G, Somogyi P. Brain-state- and cell-type-specific firing of hippocampal interneurons in vivo. Nature 2003; 421: 844-8.

Koepp MJ, Richardson MP, Brooks DJ, et al. Cerebral benzodiazepine receptors in hippocampal sclerosis: An objective in vivo analysis. Brain 1996; 119: 1677-87.

Koepp MJ, Richardson MP, Labbé C, et al. $^{11}$C-flumazenil PET, volumetric MRI, and quantitative pathology in mesial temporal lobe epilepsy. Neurology 1997; 49: 764-73.

Koepp MJ, Kieran SP, Hand BS, et al. In vivo [$^{11}$C]flumazenil-PET correlates with ex vivo [$^3$H]flumazenil autoradiography in hippocampal sclerosis. Ann Neurol 1998; 43: 618-26.

Koepp MJ, Hammers A, Labbé C, et al. $^{11}$C-flumazenil PET in patients with refractory temporal lobe epilepsy and normal MRI. Neurology 2000; 54: 332-9.

Lachaux JP, Rodriguez E, Martinerie J, Adam C, Hasboun D, Varela FJ. A quantitative study of gamma-band activity in human intracranial recordings triggered by visual stimuli. Eur J Neurosci 2000; 12: 2608-22.

Lachaux JP, George N, Tallon-Baudry C, Martinerie J, Hugueville L, Minotti L, Kahane P, Renault B. The many faces of the gamma band response to complex visual stimuli. Neuroimage 2005; 25: 491-501.

Lagier S, Carleton A, Lledo PM. Interplay between local GABAergic interneurons and relay neurons generates gamma oscillations in the rat olfactory bulb. J Neurosci 2004; 24: 4382-92.

Lee JS, Asano E, Muzik O, Chugani DC, Juhasz C, Pfund Z, Philip S, Behen M, Chugani HT. Sturge-Weber syndrome: correlation between clinical course and FDG PET findings. Neurology 2001; 57: 189-95.

Lee JS, Asano E, Muzik O, Chugani DC, Juhasz C, Pfund Z, Philip S, Behen M, Chugani HT. Sturge-Weber syndrome: correlation between clinical course and FDG PET findings. Neurology 2001; 57: 189-95.

Lencz T, McCarthy G, Bronen RA, Scott TM, Inserni JA, Sass KJ, Novelly RA, Kim JH, Spencer DD. Quantitative magnetic resonance imaging in temporal lobe epilepsy: relationship to neuropathology and neuropsychological function. Ann Neurol 1992; 31: 629-37.

Liegeois F, Connelly A, Salmond CH, Gadian DG, Vargha-Khadem F, Baldeweg T. A direct test for lateralization of language activation using fMRI: comparison with invasive assessments in children with epilepsy. Neuroimage 2002; 17: 1861-7.

Lindner MD, Hodges DB Jr, Hogan JB, Orie AF, Corsa JA, Barten DM, Polson C, Robertson BJ, Guss VL, Gillman KW, Starrett JE Jr, Gribkoff VK. An assessment of the effects of serotonin 6 (5-HT6) receptor antagonists in rodent models of learning. J Pharmacol Exp Ther 2003; 307: 682-91.

Maquet P, Hirsch E, Metz-Lutz MN, Motte J, Dive D, Marescaux C, Franck G. Regional cerebral glucose metabolism in children with deterioration of one or more cognitive functions and continuous spike-and-wave discharges during sleep. Brain 1995; 118: 1497-520.

Martin RC, Hugg JW, Roth DL, Bilir E, Gilliam FG, Faught E, Kuzniecky RI. MRI extrahippocampal volumes and visual memory: correlations independent of MRI hippocampal volumes in temporal lobe epilepsy patients. J Int Neuropsychol Soc 1999; 5: 540-8.

Martin RC, Sawrie S, Hugg J, Gilliam F, Faught E, Kuzniecky R. Cognitive correlates of 1H MRSI-detected hippocampal abnormalities in temporal lobe epilepsy. Neurology 1999; 53: 2052-8.

Merlet I, Ostrowsky K, Costes N, Ryvlin P, Isnard J, Faillenot I, Lavenne F, Dufournel D, Le Bars D, Mauguiere F. 5-HT1A receptor binding and intracerebral activity in temporal lobe epilepsy: an [$^{18}$F]MPPF-PET study. Brain 2004a; 127: 900-13.

Merlet I, Ryvlin P, Costes N, Dufournel D, Isnard J, Faillenot I, Ostrowsky K, Lavenne F, Le Bars D, Mauguiere F. Statistical parametric mapping of 5-HT1A receptor binding in temporal lobe epilepsy with hippocampal ictal onset on intracranial EEG. Neuroimage 2004b; 22: 886-96.

Namer IJ, Bolo NR, Sellal F, Nguyen VH, Nedelec JF, Hirsch E, Marescaux C. Combined measurements of hippocampal N-acetyl-aspartate and T2 relaxation time in the evaluation of mesial temporal lobe epilepsy: correlation with clinical severity and memory performances. Epilepsia 1999; 40: 1424-32.

Narula J, Acio ER, Narula N, Samuels LE, Fyfe B, Wood D, Fitzpatrick JM, Raghunath PN, Tomaszewski JE, Kelly C, Steinmetz N, Green A, Tait JF, Leppo J, Blankenberg FG, Jain D, Strauss HW. Annexin-V imaging for noninvasive detection of cardiac allograft rejection. Nat Med 2001; 7: 1347-52.

Natsume J, Kumakura Y, Bernasconi N, Soucy JP, Nakai A, Rosa P, Fedi M, Dubeau F, Andermann F, Lisbona R, Bernasconi A, Diksic M.. Alpha-[$^{11}$C] methyl-L-tryptophan and glucose metabolism in patients with temporal lobe epilepsy. *Neurology* 2003; 60, 756-61.

Olesen PJ, Westerberg H, Klingberg T. Increased prefrontal and parietal activity after training of working memory. *Nat Neurosci* 2004; 7: 75-9.

Pauli E, Eberhardt KW, Schafer I, Tomandl B, Huk WJ, Stefan H. Chemical shift imaging spectroscopy and memory function in temporal lobe epilepsy. *Epilepsia* 2000; 41: 282-9.

Paus et al. Structural maturation of neural pathways in children and adolescents: *in vivo* study. *Science* 1999; 283: 1908-11.

Paus T. Mapping brain maturation and cognitive development during adolescence. *Trends Cogn Sci* 2005; 9: 60-8.

Rabin ML, Narayan VM, Kimberg DY, Casasanto DJ, Glosser G, Tracy JI, et al. Functional MRI predicts post-surgical memory following temporal lobectomy. *Brain* 2004; 127: 2286-98.

Rausch R, Henry TR, Ary CM, Engel J Jr, Mazziotta J. Asymmetric interictal glucose hypometabolism and cognitive performance in epileptic patients. *Arch Neurol* 1994; 51: 139-44.

Ries M, Boop FA, Griebel ML, Zou P, Phillips NS, Johnson SC, et al. Functional MRI and Wada determination of language lateralization: A case of crossed dominance. *Epilepsia* 2004; 45: 85-9.

Russell MG, Dias R. Memories are made of this (perhaps): a review of serotonin 5-HT(6) receptor ligands and their biological functions. *Curr Top Med Chem* 2002; 2: 643-54.

Ryvlin P, Bouvard S, Le Bars D, et al. Clinical utility of Flumazenil-PET versus $^{18}$F-fluorodesoxyglucose-PET and MRI in refractory partial epilepsy: a prospective study in 100 patients. *Brain* 1998; 121: 2067-81.

Ryvlin P, Bouvard S, Le Bars D, Mauguière F. False lateralization of 11C-flumazenil PET in temporal lobe epilepsy with no hippocampal atrophy. *Neurology* 1999; 53: 1882-5.

Salanova V, Morris HH 3rd, Rehm P, Wyllie E, Dinner DS, Luders H, Gilmore-Pollak W. Comparison of the intracarotid amobarbital procedure and interictal cerebral 18-fluorodeoxyglucose positron emission tomography scans in refractory temporal lobe epilepsy. *Epilepsia* 1992; 33: 635-8.

Salanova V, Markand O, Worth R. Focal functional deficits in temporal lobe epilepsy on PET scans and the intracarotid amobarbital procedure: comparison of patients with unitemporal epilepsy with those requiring intracranial recordings. *Epilepsia* 2001; 42: 198-203.

Savic I, Roland P, Sedvall G, et al. In vivo demonstration of reduced benzodiazepine receptor binding in human epileptic foci. *Lancet* 1988; 8616: 863-6.

Savic I, Ingvar M, Stone Elander S. Comparison of [($^{11}$)C]flumazenil and [($^{18}$)F]FDG as PET markers of epileptic foci. *J Neurol Neurosurg Psychiatry* 1993; 56: 615-21.

Savic I, Svanborg E, Thorell JO. Cortical benzodiazepine receptor changes are related to frequency of partial seizures: A positron emission tomography study. *Epilepsia* 1996; 37: 236-44.

Savic I, Blomqvist G, Halldin C, et al. Regional increases in [$^{11}$C]flumazenil binding after epilepsy surgery. *Acta Neurol Scand* 1998; 97: 279-86.

Savic I, Lindstrom P, Gulyas B, Halldin C, Andree B, Farde L. Limbic reductions of 5-HT1A receptors in human temporal lobe epilepsy. *Neuroimage* 2004; 62: 1343-51.

Sawrie SM, Martin RC, Gilliam F et al. Nonlinear trends in hippocampal metabolic function and verbal memory: evidence of cognitive reserve in temporal lobe epilepsy. *Epilepsy and Behavior* 2000; 1: 106-11.

Sawrie SM, Martin RC, Gilliam FG, Faught RE, Maton B, Hugg JW, Bush N, Sinclair K, Kuzniecky RI. Visual confrontation naming and hippocampal function: A neural network study using quantitative (1)H magnetic resonance spectroscopy. *Brain* 2000; 123: 770-80.

Sawrie SM, Martin RC, Gilliam F, Knowlton R, Faught E, Kuzniecky R. Verbal retention lateralizes patients with unilateral temporal lobe epilepsy and bilateral hippocampal atrophy. *Epilepsia* 2001; 42: 651-9.

Sawrie SM, Martin RC, Knowlton R, Faught E, Gilliam F, Kuzniecky R. Relationships among hippocampal volumetry, proton magnetic resonance spectroscopy, and verbal memory in temporal lobe epilepsy. *Epilepsia* 2001; 42: 1403-7.

Sette G, Baron JC, Young AR, et al. In vivo mapping of brain benzodiazepine receptor changes by positron emission tomography after focal ischemia in the anesthetized baboon. *Stroke* 1993; 24: 2046-58.

Singer W. Neuronal synchrony: a versatile code for the definition of relations? *Neuron* 1999; 24: 49-65.

Smith ML, Bernal B, Duchowny M, Dunoyer C, Jayakar P, Altman NR. Severity of focal cortical dysplasia and functional organization of the brain. *Epilepsia* 2004; 45: 357.

Sowell ER, Delis D, Stiles J, Jernigan TL. Improved memory functioning and frontal lobe maturation between childhood and adolescence: a structural MRI study. *J Int Neuropsychol Soc* 2001; 7: 312-22.

Sowell ER, Thompson PM, Tessner KD, Toga AW. Mapping continued brain growth and gray matter density reduction in dorsal frontal cortex: Inverse relationships during postadolescent brain maturation. *J Neurosci* 2001; 21: 8819-29.

Sowell ER, Trauner DA, Gamst A, Jernigan TL. Development of cortical and subcortical brain structures in childhood and adolescence: a structural MRI study. *Dev Med Child Neurol* 2002; 44: 4-16.

Sowell ER, Peterson BS, Thompson PM, Welcome SE, Henkenius AL, Toga AW. Mapping cortical change across the human life span. *Nat Neurosci* 2003; 6: 309-15.

Sowell ER, Thompson PM, Leonard CM, Welcome SE, Kan E, Toga AW. Longitudinal mapping of cortical thickness and brain growth in normal children. *J Neurosci* 2004; 24: 8223-31.

Springer JA, Binder JR, Hammeke TA, Swanson SJ, Frost JA, Bellgowan PS, et al. Language dominance in neurologically normal and epilepsy subjects: a functional MRI study. *Brain* 1999; 122 (Pt 11): 2033-46.

Tallon-Baudry C, Bertrand O, Delpuech C, Permier J. Oscillatory gamma-band (30-70 Hz) activity induced by a visual search task in humans. *J Neurosci* 1997; 17: 722-34.

Tallon-Baudry C, Bertrand O. Oscillatory gamma activity in humans and its role in object representation. *Trends Cogn Sci* 1999; 3: 151-62.

Tavitian B, Terrazzino S, Kuhnast B, Marzabal S, Stettler O, Dolle F, Deverre JR, Jobert A, Hinnen F, Bendriem B, Crouzel C, Di Giamberardino L. In vivo imaging of oligonucleotides with positron emission tomography. *Nat Med* 1998; 4: 467-71.

Thivard L, Hombrouck J, Montcel T, Delmaire C, Cohen L, Samson S, et al. Productive and perceptive language reorganization in temporal lobe epilepsy. *Neuroimage* 2005; 24: 841-51.

Toczek MT, Carson RE, Lang L, Ma Y, Spanaki MV, Der MG, Fazilat S, Kopylev L, Herscovitch P, Eckelman WC, Theodore WH. PET imaging of 5-HT1A receptor binding in patients with temporal lobe epilepsy. *Neurology* 2003; 60: 749-56.

Traub RD, Cunningham MO, Gloveli T, LeBeau FE, Bibbig A, Buhl EH, Whittington MA. GABA-enhanced collective behavior in neuronal axons underlies persistent gamma-frequency oscillations. *Proc Natl Acad Sci USA* 2003; 100: 11047-52.

Wendel JD, Trenerry MR, Xu YC, Sencakova D, Cascino GD, Britton JW, Lagerlund TD, Shin C, So EL, Sharbrough FW, Jack CR. The relationship between quantitative T2 relaxometry and memory in nonlesional temporal lobe epilepsy. *Epilepsia* 2001; 42: 863-8.

Woermann FG, Jokeit H, Luerding R, Freitag H, Schulz R, Guertler S, et al. Language lateralization by Wada test and fMRI in 100 patients with epilepsy. *Neurology* 2003; 61: 699-701.

Woolley ML, Marsden CA, Fone KC. 5-ht6 receptors. *Curr Drug Targets CNS Neurol Disord* 2004; 3: 59-79.

Yacoub E, Shmuel A, Pfeuffer J, Van De Moortele PF, Adriany G, Andersen P, Vaughan JT, Merkle H, Ugurbil K, Hu X. Imaging brain function in humans at 7 Tesla. *Magn Reson Med* 2001; 45: 588-94.

Yacoub E, Shmuel A, Pfeuffer J, Van De Moortele PF, Adriany G, Ugurbil K, Hu X. Investigation of the initial dip in fMRI at 7 Tesla. *NMR Biomed* 2001; 14: 408-12.

Zilbovicius M, Boddaert N, Pelin P, et al. Temporal lobe dysfonction in childhood autism: a PET study. *Am J Psychiatry* 2000; 157: 1988-93.

# Age-dependent consequences of seizures and the development of TLE in the rat

## A. Nehlig

*INSERM U666, Université Louis-Pasteur, Strasbourg, France*

---

Temporal lobe epilepsy (TLE) is a common cause of complex partial seizures that most often originate in the mesial temporal structures (Liu *et al.*, 1997). This epilepsy is frequently characterized by lesions in the hippocampus, named hippocampal sclerosis. Retrospective studies have shown that a large proportion of patients with TLE underwent an "initial precipitating injury" (IPI) occurring early in life, most often before 4 years. The IPI is most frequently prolonged complex febrile seizures, status epilepticus (SE), trauma, encephalopathy (Mathern *et al.*, 1997). This early event is followed by a latent phase free of any overt clinical or electroencephalographic (EEG) signs. Spontaneous seizures usually start occurring around 10-15 years and become frequently medically intractable after a few years, thus requiring surgery (Engel, 1995). However, the causal relationship between early seizures and subsequent TLE has not yet been established.

Prospective clinical studies reported that seizures occurring early in life rarely result in hippocampal sclerosis (Shinnar, 1998; Berg *et al.*, 1999). The severity of the epilepsy relates to the earlier age of seizure onset rather than the duration of seizures which is not in favor of early seizures being the cause of later epilepsy (Davies *et al.*, 1996). A recent MRI study performed on children with complex prolonged febrile seizures showed that only a small subset of infants with a preexisting lesion in the hippocampus went on to develop hippocampal sclerosis (VanLandingham *et al.*, 1998). Thus, at the moment it is still not clear whether the IPI could be the sole cause of hippocampal sclerosis or if the IPI needs to be associated to a preexisting factor like a hippocampal lesion, a neuronal migration disorder or a specific genetic background to lead to TLE with hippocampal sclerosis. These issues can more easily be explored by animal research and this chapter will be devoted to animal models of TLE and to what can be learned from these models to clarify the relationship between early seizures and epilepsy.

## ■ Consequences of status epilepticus: the model of temporal lobe epilepsy induced by pilocarpine

### Main age-dependent characteristics

The model of TLE induced in rats by the muscarinic cholinergic agonist, pilocarpine (pilo) alone or combined with lithium (li-pilo) reproduces most clinical, developmental and neuropathological features of human TLE with SE as the initial precipitating injury (Turski et al., 1989; Cavalheiro, 1995; Dubé et al., 2000b). In adult rats, pilo leads to SE followed by a latent seizure-free phase of a mean duration of 14-25 days. During this period, neuronal damage develops mainly in hippocampus, hilus of the dentate gyrus, piriform and entorhinal cortices, amygdala, neocortex and thalamus. Neuronal death leads to the genesis of a new hyperexcitable circuit that will allow the occurrence of spontaneous recurrent seizures (SRS) which characterize the chronic phase. SRS last for the whole animals' life (Turski et al., 1989; Cavalheiro, 1995; Dubé et al., 2000b). In adult rats, TLE can also be triggered by kainic acid injected either systemically (Lothman and Collins, 1981; Ben Ari, 1985), or intracerebrally (Nadler, 1981; Bouilleret et al., 1999). However, epileptogenesis was not studied in immature animals in the latter model.

The consequences of pilo are age-dependent (Dubé et al., 2000b, 2001; Cavalheiro et al., 1987; Priel et al., 1996; Sankar et al., 1998). In PN18-PN24 rats, a pattern of neuronal damage more moderate than in the adult is observed; neuronal death is found mainly in the hilus of the dentate gyrus, entorhinal and piriform cortices, and lateral thalamus. About 30-75% of the rats display SRS after a latent phase of about 37-73 days (Cavalheiro et al., 1987; Priel et al., 1996; Sankar et al., 1998; Dubé et al., 2000b, 2001; Roch et al., 2002b). In PN7-PN11 rats, pilo-induced SE does not lead to neuronal damage or SRS (Dubé et al., 2000b, 2001; Priel et al., 1996; Sankar et al., 1998).

To try to better understand the genesis of epilepsy at the different ages, we used several approaches including the measurement of local cerebral metabolic rates for glucose (LCMRglcs) by the quantitative autoradiographic [$^{14}$C]2-deoxyglucose method, anatomic magnetic resonance imaging (MRI) coupled with the study of neuronal damage during SE, the latent and the chronic phase.

### Functional characteristics of the acute phase of status epilepticus

In PN10 rats, li-pilo SE leads to increases in LCMRglcs in limbic forebrain and cortical areas but not in hypothalamic and thalamic areas. In PN21 and adult rats, increases in local cerebral metabolic rates for glucose are generalized and quite dramatic in the cerebral cortex, mainly entorhinal and piriform, the hippocampus, amygdala, septum and thalamus (Fernandes et al., 1999). In animals aged less than three weeks subjected to kainate-induced seizures, the pattern of brain activation is limited to the hippocampus and septum. In older animals, when the toxin leads to the occurrence of limbic motor seizures, other regions are also activated, namely the amygdaloid complex, thalamus, piriform and entorhinal cortex. At that age, metabolic maps become similar to adult ones and reflect the maturation of limbic circuits allowing the propagation of seizures to extrahippocampal and subcortical sites (Albala et al., 1984; Tremblay et al., 1984).

SE in animals younger than three weeks is followed by none or limited brain damage (Dubé et al., 2001; Fernandes et al., 1999; Priel et al., 1996; Sankar et al., 1998; Albala et al., 1984; Tremblay et al., 1984). In rats aged three weeks or older, kainate, pilo and li-pilo seizures lead to widespread brain damage mainly in hippocampus, amygdala, septum, thalamus, entorhinal and piriform cortex where largest metabolic increases are recorded (Dubé et al., 2001; Fernandes et al., 1999; Sperk, 1994; Tremblay et al., 1984; Turski et al., 1989).

However, given the widespread metabolic increases and lesions recorded in animals that will become epileptic, it is impossible only on the basis of metabolic studies to identify which structures are critical for the genesis of the epilepsy and which ones are secondarily recruited. Therefore, we performed a temporal follow-up of the changes occurring during the acute, latent and chronic phase of the li-pilo model using anatomical magnetic resonance imaging (MRI) in adult and PN21 rats.

## Anatomical MRI follow-up of epileptogenesis

The use of the non-invasive MRI technique allows the temporal follow-up on the same animal of the changes occurring after an insult like SE. We performed a longitudinal study of the MRI signal change starting at 6 h after SE onset and extending through the latent and chronic phase, up to 9 weeks post SE. In adult rats, as soon as 6 h after SE onset, a signal appeared in the piriform and entorhinal cortices (*Figure 1*). This signal intensified and persisted for 2-3 days. Simultaneously, a weaker signal could be recorded in thalamus and amygdala. By 36-48 h post SE, a weak signal started to appear in hippocampus. This signal progressively intensified over time until the end of the measurement period, *i.e.*, 9 weeks. Meanwhile, the signal in the parahippocampal cortices reappeared with the occurrence of SRS, *i.e.* at 2-3 weeks post SE. The early signals reflected edema corresponding to neuronal death while the late damage mainly reflected gliosis. Indeed, in the parahippocampal cortices, the totality of neuronal loss has occurred by 24 h after SE onset while in hippocampus, damage is more progressive. Thus, this study clearly shows that the piriform and entorhinal cortices are activated very rapidly during li-pilo-induced SE and that hippocampal activation appears as a secondary event (Roch et al., 2002a).

In PN21 rats, in which only a subset of animals subjected to li-pilo SE is becoming epileptic, the MRI images obtained were of two different types. In a subset of animals, a clear signal appeared in basal cortices at 24 h after SE onset, as in adult animals. All these rats became epileptic. In another subset of rats, no visible signal could be observed in piriform and entorhinal cortices at 24-48 h after SE. However, in this group, the epileptic development was heterogeneous; some rats went on developing epilepsy and some did not. The quantification of the signal showed that there was a transient, low but measurable increase in piriform and entorhinal cortical signal on the MRI scan of the rats of this subgroup that developed epilepsy. Conversely, the intensity of the MRI signal of PN21 rats that did not become epileptic never showed any measurable change (*Figure 2*). This study in PN21 rats confirms the critical role

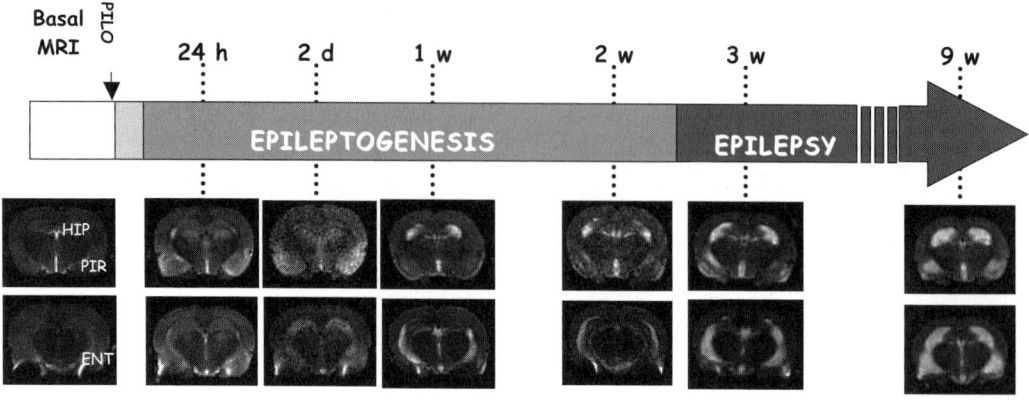

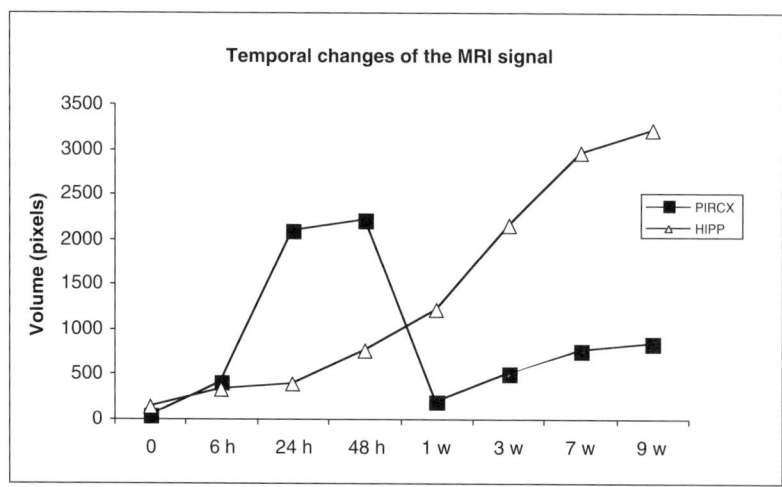

**Figure 1. Time course of anatomical MRI examination and signal quantification in adult rats subjected to li-pilo SE.**
Compared to the basal MRI located on the left of the upper part of the figure, SE induces the rapid appearance of a strong signal in piriform (PIR) and entorhinal (ENT) cortices which is present during 2 days after SE onset. This signal disappears by day 3 and reappears once the animal has become epileptic, here by 3 weeks after SE. A faint hippocampal (HIP) signal is visible by 2 days after SE and this signal constantly increases over time, leading progressively to hippocampal sclerosis. In the piriform and entorhinal cortices, neuronal damage occurs very rapidly and the early signal reflects neuronal necrosis while the late increase in the signal corresponds to gliosis. In the hippocampus, the progressive increase of the signal reflects both neuronal death and gliosis (for more detail, see Roch et al., 2002a).

of the parahippocampal cortices very early in the process of epileptogenesis. Furthermore, at this age, the cortical signal, visible as soon as 24 h after the initial insult is predictive of the epilepsy (Roch et al., 2002b). The hippocampal signal appears later, after about one week post-SE, increases progressively in intensity but is weaker than in adults, reflecting more limited hippocampal damage at that age (Dubé et al., 2001).

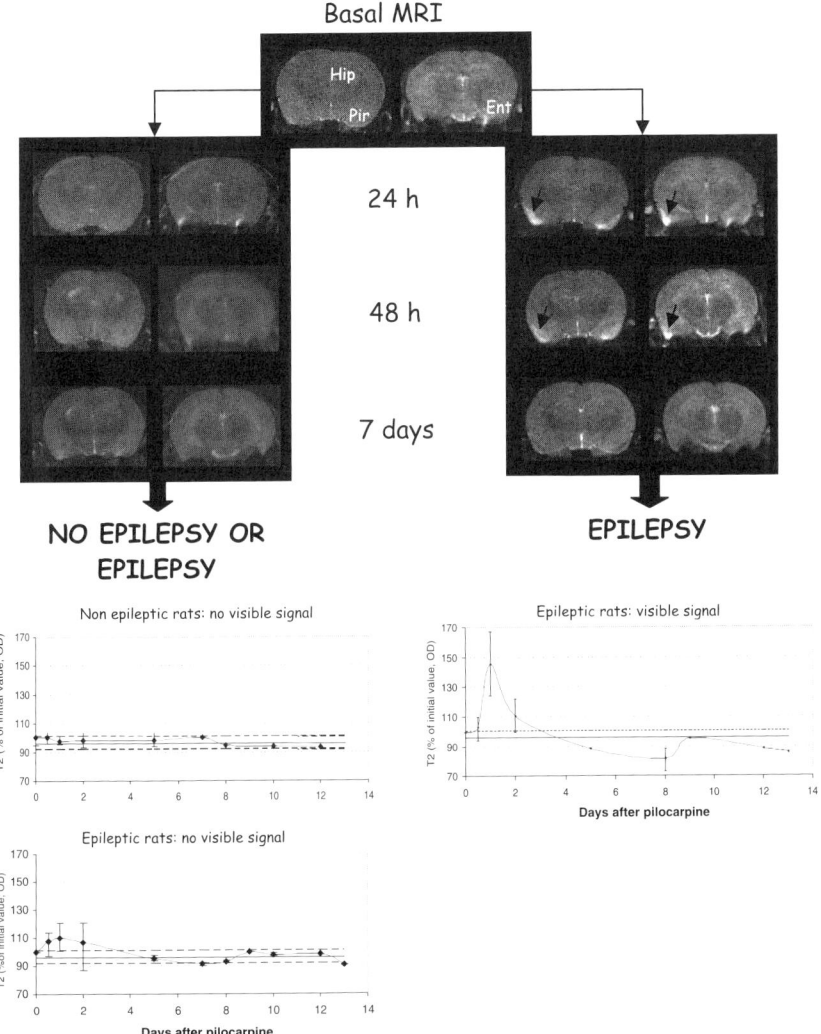

**Figure 2. Early changes in anatomical MRI signal in PN21 rats subjected to li-pilo SE.**
Compared to the basal MRI located on the top of the upper part of the figure, SE induces two distinct profiles in animals of this age. Either, a signal in piriform and entorhinal cortices appears as soon as 24 h and remains visible during 2 days after SE onset. This signal disappears by day 3. All the animals that display this signal will become epileptic. In a second group of animals, no cortical signal could be detected visually on the MRI. Animals with this profile had a heterogeneous outcome, becoming epileptic or not. By quantifying the signal, as shown in the lower part of the figure, in rats with no epilepsy, the signal was never different from the control level while, in rats becoming epileptic in this subgroup, there was a small recordable increase in signal followed by a later decrease. However, the amplitude of these changes were much smaller than in PN21 rats with a visible cortical MRI signal.

Thus, the early activation of piriform and entorhinal cortices appears as the key factor in epileptogenesis while the involvement of the hippocampus is delayed. Moreover, in PN21 rats, the cortical MRI signal is predictive of the occurrence of epilepsy and can be used as a surrogate marker to discriminate as soon as 24 h after SE whether rats will become epileptic or not. The critical involvement of the parahippocampal cortices compared to the hippocampus, early in the epileptogenic process, is further supported by neuroprotection studies. Indeed, we showed that the sole protection of CA1 and/or CA3 is unable to prevent or modify the epileptogenesis (André et al., 2000, 2001; Rigoulot et al., 2003, 2004). The protection of parahippocampal cortices prolongs the latency before SRS but does not prevent their occurrence (André et al., 2003) while the simultaneous protection of Ammon's horn and the cortices delays largely or totally prevents the occurrence of SRS (Rigoulot, François and Nehlig, unpublished data). Thus, in this model, a disease modifying effect requires the protection of basal cortices plus that of CA1 and CA3.

## Functional characteristics of the latent phase

In adult rats; towards the end of the latent phase (at 14 days after SE), local cerebral metabolic rates for glucose levels are decreased in limbic forebrain areas that undergo brain damage while they are increased in brainstem regions like the substantia nigra pars reticulata and the superior colliculus belonging to the remote circuit of control of seizures. In PN21 rats studied at 60 days after SE, local cerebral metabolic rates for glucose are identical to control levels in most forebrain regions and also increased in the regions belonging to the remote circuit of control of seizures (*Figure 3*). In PN10 rats studied at 2 months after SE, metabolic levels are identical in control and li-pilo rats (Dubé et al., 2000a,b). In the adult rat, the most striking feature of this latent period is the relative hypermetabolic rate of the hilus of the dentate gyrus where neuronal death is massive while local cerebral metabolic rates for glucose remain in the normal range. A similar feature can be seen in the piriform cortex and, to a more limited extent, in lateral thalamus. In PN21 rats studied at 60 days after SE, a relative hypermetabolism, less marked than in the adult rat, is also recorded in the hilus of the dentate gyrus. Thus, the hyperactivity of hilar cells, found in both PN21 and adult rats, could represent the secondary key factor necessary to trigger epileptogenesis in this model. Furthermore, the hypermetabolic levels recorded in PN21 and adult rats in the brain areas that are involved in the remote circuit of seizures control may be indicative of a pre-epileptic activity or reflect an activation aimed at the prevention by the brain of the occurrence of the seizures (Dubé et al., 2000a,b).

## Functional characteristics of the chronic phase

Finally, during the interictal period of the chronic phase, in adult rats, most of the forebrain areas that underwent neuronal death are hypometabolic and the relative hypermetabolic level compared to the number of surviving neurons is persisting in the hilus of the dentate gyrus and the piriform cortex. In rats subjected to li-pilo SE at PN21, the relative hypermetabolism of the hilus is still present in animals with SRS while it is not seen in the group of rats that do not become epileptic. The rats that underwent SE at PN10 and were studied about 6 months later exhibit

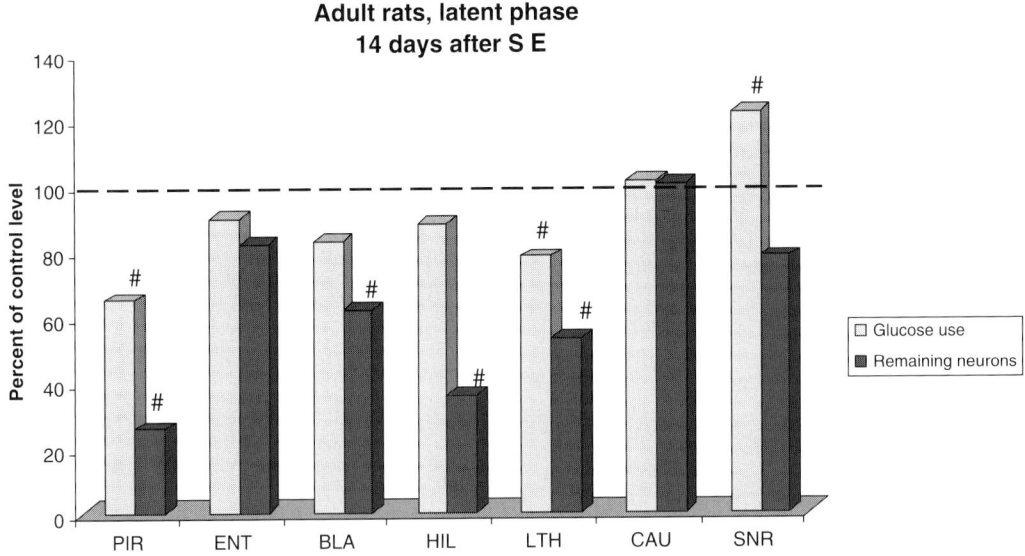
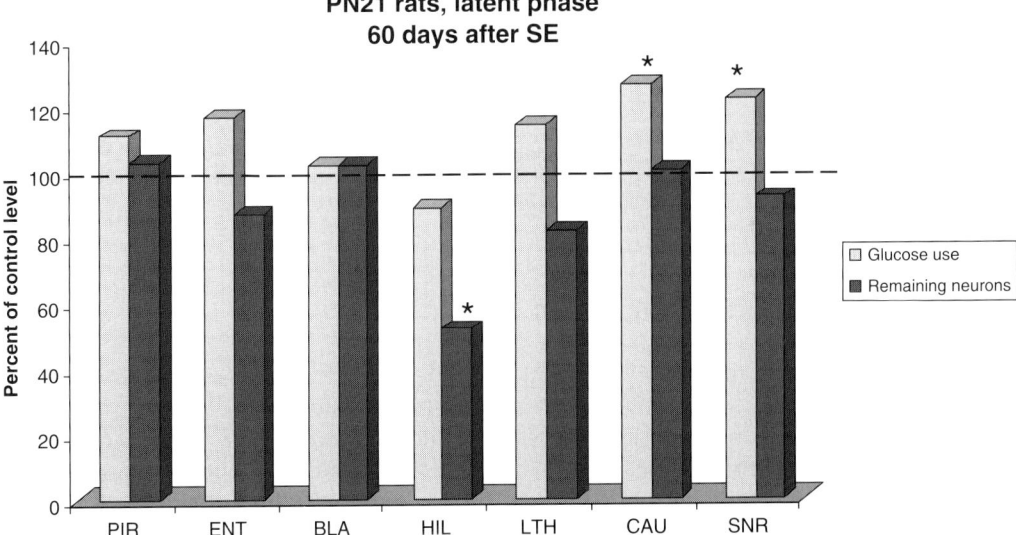

**Figure 3.** Rates of metabolic activity and neuronal loss measured towards the end of the latent phase in adult rats (14 days after SE, upper figure) and PN21 rats (60 days after SE, lower figure) subjected to li-pilo SE. Values are expressed as percentage of control levels in the circuit of the seizures including piriform cortex (PIR), entorhinal cortex (ENT), basolateral amygdala (BLA), hilus of the dentate gyrus (HIL) and lateral thalamus (LTH) and in the part of the remote circuit of seizure control including caudate nucleus (CAU) and substantia nigra pars reticulata (SNR).
\* $p < 0.05$, # $p < 0.01$, statistically significant differences from control.

normometabolic rates in all structures (Dubé et al., 2000b, 2001). Thus, in spontaneously epileptic adult and PN21 rats, the hilus of the dentate gyrus appears as the key structure for the maintenance of the epilepsy.

### Relationship between the initial injury and the occurrence of epilepsy

There is still a debate on whether or not a single initial precipitating injury is sufficient to trigger epileptogenesis in TLE patients. The studies detailed above show that in adult and PN21 rats with SRS, the single initial injury, here SE is able to lead to neuronal death and epilepsy. In that case, the hypothesis according to which one single initial injury may be sufficient to trigger TLE appears valid. However, this is no longer true when one considers the groups of PN21 and PN10 rats that do not become epileptic. In that case, obviously, SE alone is not able to lead to epilepsy. This observation is particularly disturbing when one considers the group of PN10-PN14 rats. Indeed this group has reached a cerebral maturity corresponding to that of the 0-4 year-old human infant (Dobbing and Sands, 1973; Romijn et al., 1991). In humans, this age corresponds to the period of highest susceptibility to the consequences of an initial precipitating injury. To try to understand this apparent contradiction two hypotheses can be raised. First, the lack of consequences may relate to the nature of the initial injury: indeed, most patients with TLE report a history of prolonged febrile seizures and less often SE. Second, it may also be, as shown in the study by VanLandigham et al. (1998) and reviewed by Cendes (2004) that only infants having a preexisting hippocampal lesion or a genetic predisposition and experiencing an acute injury such as prolonged febrile seizures will develop hippocampal sclerosis and TLE. Thus, we will also consider the consequences of prolonged febrile seizures in animals and the possibility that the initial injury may need to be associated to another factor to generate epilepsy.

## ■ Prolonged febrile seizures

Febrile seizures are commonly affecting about 3-5% of infants and young children and their occurrence dramatically decreases with age (Verity et al., 1985; Shinnar, 1990). Retrospective clinical studies report that a large fraction of patients with TLE have a history of prolonged, complex partial febrile seizures (Sagar and Oxbury, 1987; Cendes et al., 1993b; Kuks et al., 1993). Two mechanisms have been suggested to explain the relationship between prolonged complex febrile seizures and later epilepsy. The first one proposed that prolonged seizures injure mesial temporal areas and hence lead to hippocampal sclerosis and TLE (Aicardi and Chevrie, 1976; Maher and McLachlan, 1995). The alternative hypothesis is that there is a preexisting lesion combined or not to a predisposition to febrile convulsions as an inherited trait with a genetic basis that would predispose infants to seizures and later TLE (Cendes et al., 1993a,b; Hernandes et al., 1998). These hypotheses have been partly tested in an animal model of prolonged febrile seizures (Baram et al., 1997).

This model uses PN10-PN11 rats whose cerebral maturity corresponds to the period of high sensitivity to fever-induced seizures in human infants (Dobbing and Sands, 1979; Alling, 1985; Romijn et al., 1991). In this model, core and brain temperature is slowly increased by a stream of heated hair and seizures occur at a threshold temperature of 40.9° C. Hyperthermia is maintained for 30 min and the mean seizure duration is 22 min, corresponding to febrile SE (Jensen and Baram, 2000). The seizures involve primarily the hippocampus but not the neocortex (Baram et al., 1997; Dubé et al., 2000c). Hyperthermia-induced seizures do not lead to any neuronal death although there is clear neuronal suffering expanding over two weeks in the hippocampus and amygdala (Toth et al., 1998).

Adult animals with early febrile seizures become more susceptible than controls to kainate-induced seizures and undergo changes in GABAergic neurotransmission in hippocampal interneurons (Dubé et al., 2000c). Changes in the excitability of the hippocampal circuit can be recorded from one week after the initial insult up to adulthood (Chen et al., 1999). A recent abstract reported spontaneous seizures in 31% of the rats with early febrile seizures (Baram et al., 2004). Moreover, febrile seizures regulate at the transcriptional level the expression of hyperpolarizing-activated, cyclic nucleotide-gated channels (HCNs) in specific populations of hippocampal neurons (Brewster et al., 2002). Thus, early prolonged febrile seizures sensitize the brain to a further insult and may induce epilepsy.

## ■ Nature of the initial insult and temporal lobe epilepsy

The data from the model of prolonged febrile seizures and li-pilo SE confirm the resistance of the very immature rat (PN10-PN11) to seizure-induced neuronal death. However, conversely to febrile seizures (Dubé et al., 2000c), li-pilo SE does not lead to long-term changes in seizure threshold (Nehlig et al., 2002). Thus, the duration of the initial insult may not be the most critical factor, since febrile seizures last for about 22 min while li-pilo SE lasts for about 2-3 h in the PN10 rat. This is in accordance with previous clinical observations (Davies et al., 1996). Conversely, the nature of the initial precipitating injury may be of major importance in the later development of epilepsy. Indeed, 50-60% patients with TLE report a history of complex, prolonged febrile seizures (Sagar and Oxbury, 1987; Cendes et al., 1993a; Kuks et al., 1993; Cendes, 2004). Pilo SE needs to be repeated over 3 consecutive days in PN7, PN8 and PN9 rats to induce long-term consequences. At adulthood, these rats have disturbed EEG recordings including frequent episodes of continuous complex spiking activities and high-voltage ictal discharges with a small percentage of the rats having spontaneous behavioral seizures. These animals suffer from severe cognitive deficits and present *in vitro* persistent hyperexcitability in CA1 hippocampal area. These changes are not accompanied by any major long-term pathological change (Santos et al., 2000). This experimental paradigm supports the hypothesis that recurrent seizures occurring early are harmful to the immature brain.

At the moment most studies on immature animals are still unable to answer the issue of whether or not the initial insult, SE or febrile seizures need to be associated to a preexisting lesion or a genetic factor to lead to hippocampal sclerosis and TLE. The study by VanLandigham et al. (1998) reported that only the subset of children with a preexisting hippocampal lesion developed hippocampal sclerosis after an episode of complex, prolonged febrile seizures. Likewise, Shinnar et al. (1992) reported that the presence of a preexisting neurological abnormality or a history of febrile seizures was a significant risk factor for recurrent SE. Similarly, a history of febrile seizures increased the risk of unprovoked seizures and the development of epilepsy in a group of 283 neurologically compromised children followed prospectively (Shinnar et al., 1990). This last study is in accordance with the higher susceptibility to seizures found after prolonged febrile seizures in immature rats (Dubé et al., 2000c). However, at the moment neither experimental nor clinical studies allow to distinguish between the possibility that febrile seizures may be more likely to produce neuronal injury or that seizure threshold may be reduced in infants with neurological abnormalities.

Recent studies addressed the latter issue in a neuronal model induced by the administration of methylazoxymethanol (MAM) to pregnant dams. MAM crosses the placental barrier and induces a variety of dysplasias including cortical heterotopias (Baraban and Schwartzkroin, 1996; Germano and Sperber, 1998; Chevassus-au-Louis et al., 1999). The offspring of MAM-treated dams have a lower threshold to hyperthermia- (Germano et al., 1996a), kainate- (Germano et al., 1996b), kindling (Germano et al., 1998) or flurothyl-induced seizures than control offspring (Baraban and Schwartzkroin, 1998). Furthermore, these seizures induce neuronal damage which is never seen in normal animals of the same age (Germano et al., 1996a,b, 1998). In the same model of MAM-induced dysplasias, immature offspring needed a lower dose of pilocarpine to seize but were unable to survive li-pilo SE (Dubé and Nehlig, unpublished data). Thus, in the animal model of MAM-induced neuronal migration disorders, the dysplasias render the immature brain more sensitive to a further episode of seizures which is in line with the hypothesis raised in clinical studies according to which a preexisting factor (including a lesion) favors the development of hippocampal sclerosis and hence TLE (VanLandigham et al., 1998; Shinnar et al., 1990, 1992).

However, the issue concerning the nature of the factors underlying the genesis of TLE still remains to be clarified. It seems most likely that animal research on this issue will not really progress as long as we persist using "normal" animals that correspond to the normal human population of infants that can experience prolonged febrile seizures without any sequelae (VanLandigham et al., 1998). The aim would rather be to try to identify whether or not it is necessary to combine several insults, either a preexisting lesion – MAM studies favor that hypothesis (Germano et al., 1996a,b, 1998; Baraban and Schwartzkroin, 1998) – or repeated seizure events like in the pilocarpine model (Santos et al., 2000). The role of other factors should be studied as well and in this respect the genetic issue needs to be addressed. A recent human study showed that the overexpression of homozygotes for interleukin (IL)-1B-511*2 leading to a high production of IL-1β a proinflammatory cytokine involved in seizure-induced neuronal death (Vezzani et al., 2004; Voutsinos-Porche et al., 2004), favors a cascade of events connecting minor events such as febrile seizures to hippocampal sclerosis (Kanemoto et al., 2000). Likewise, when li-pilo SE was induced in GAERS (Genetic Absence Epilepsy Rat from Strasbourg), PN10 and PN21 animals developed SE with a much lower dose of pilo and damage was induced in the lateral thalamus of PN10 rats which is never seen in normal control rats (Dubé and Nehlig, unpublished data). Thus, this recent data suggest that subtle anomalies linked to lesions or genetic predisposition could render the immature brain more

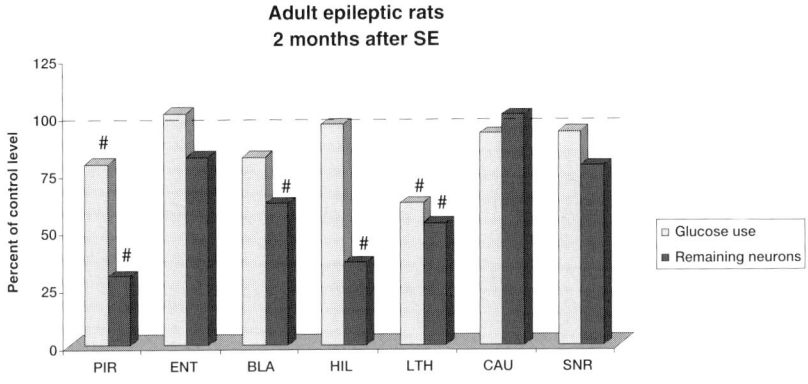
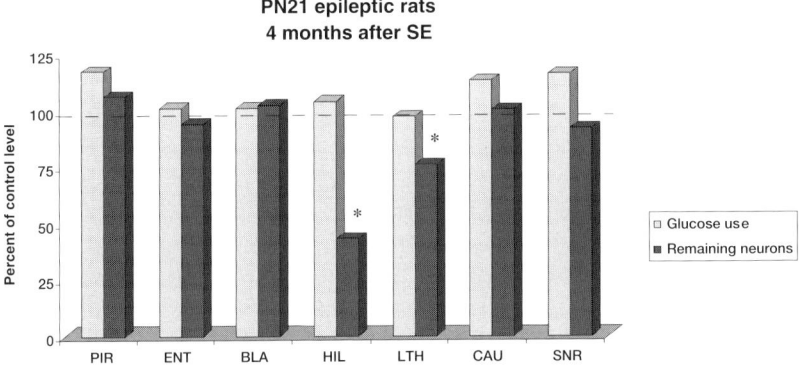
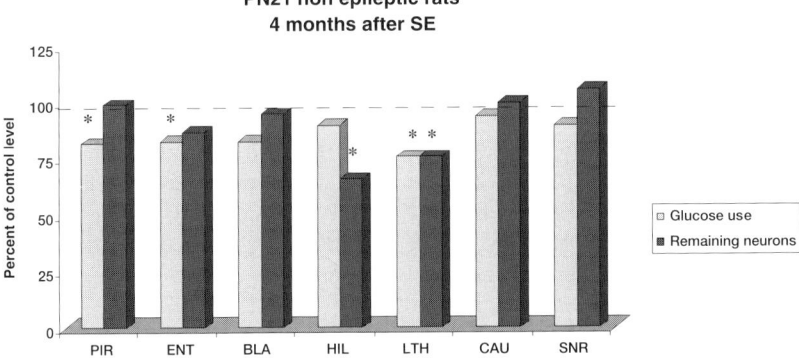

**Figure 4.** Rates of metabolic activity and neuronal loss measured during the chronic phase in adult rats (2 months after SE, upper figure) and PN21 epileptic and non epileptic rats (4 months after SE, middle and lower figure, respectively) subjected to li-pilo SE.
Values are expressed as percentage of control levels in the circuit of the seizures including piriform cortex (PIR), entorhinal cortex (ENT), basolateral amygdala (BLA), hilus of the dentate gyrus (HIL) and lateral thalamus (LTH) and in the part of the remote circuit of seizure control including caudate nucleus (CAU) and substantia nigra pars reticulata (SNR).
* $p < 0.05$, # $p < 0.01$, statistically significant differences from control.

susceptible to the cascade of events leading to hippocampal sclerosis and open new avenues to the clarification of the nature of the factors involved in the genesis of hippocampal sclerosis and TLE and hence to the genesis of better prevention strategies.

## ■ Cognitive deficits and age-dependent epileptogenesis

The lesions and plasticity phenomena induced by SE and leading to circuit reorganization and epileptogenesis are accompanied by behavioral and cognitive deficits. Their severity depends on the age of the animals at the time of SE (for review see Lado et al., 2000; Majak and Pitkänen, 2004). Most studies reported that there is none or only minor functional impairment in spatial memory tested in a radial arm maze or Morris water maze paradigm when rats are subjected to SE earlier than PN10-PN14 (Sarkisian et al., 1997; Lynch et al., 2000; Lai et al., 2002; Cilio et al., 2003; Kubova et al., 2004). Conversely, all rats undergoing SE after PN14 develop behavioral impairment, mainly in spatial memory tasks, visuo-spatial learning and emotional behavior (Sarkisian et al., 1997; Mikati et al., 2001; Wu et al., 2001; Faverjon et al., 2002; Rutten et al., 2002; Cilio et al., 2003; Kubova et al., 2004). This age-related difference most likely reflects a more limited spread of seizure activity and the resistance of the very immature brain to seizure-induced neuronal death. However, the repetition of pilo-induced SE in PN7, 8 and 9 rats leads to learning impairments and increased spontaneous exploration in rats tested at PN60-PN70 (Santos et al., 2000), which shows that cognitive deficits may occur even the seizures unable to spread given the immaturity of limbic circuits at this young age are repeated. These cognitive deficits are accompanied by persisting hyperexcitability in CA1 (dos Santos et al., 2000). Likewise, repeated seizures performed between PN0 and PN5 (5 fluorothyl seizures per day) also lead to impaired visuo-spatial learning and decreased activity levels when rats were tested as adults. These deficits correlate with sprouting of mossy fibers in CA3 and the supragranular region but not with hyperexcitability in the hippocampus (Holmes et al., 1998). In the same line, several laboratories reported recently neurodegeneration in various regions, namely hippocampus and thalamus in animals subjected to SE as early as PN12 (Sankar et al., 1998; Kubova et al., 2001); this neuronal damage induced long-term memory deficits and enhanced anxiety and fear (Lado et al., 2000; Stafstrom and Sasaki-Adams, 2003; Kubova et al., 2004).

Although it has been shown that seizure-induced plasticity during development influences cognitive function in adulthood, the contribution of a lesion to learning impairment is difficult to assess in our current models of SE because of the multifocal injury. However, from kindling studies, it seems that rats develop spatial memory deficits after approximately 35 seizures which corresponds to 13% reduction in the density of hippocampal areas (Sutula et al., 1995; Kotloski et al., 2002). Moreover, a few studies reported that the degree of CA3 mossy fiber sprouting inversely correlates with learning and animals with more CA3 mossy fiber terminals perform less well than animals with fewer terminals (Lipp et al., 1988; Holmes et al., 1998; Huang *et al.*, 1999). Thus, the relation between the extent of neuronal loss and reorganization and the occurrence of cognitive deficits in the developing brain should receive more attention.

*In conclusion*, it appears that the sequence of events leading to epileptogenesis involves first the piriform and entorhinal cortices very early in the process. The hippocampus is only involved later and the hilus of the dentate gyrus appears to be a key structure in the genesis and maintenance of spontaneous seizures. The use of anatomical MRI allows to discriminate very early in the process whether a rat pup will become chronically epileptic or not. This opens new avenues for the understanding of the regional, cellular and molecular changes that are critical to the genesis of TLE and should allow to develop new strategies of prevention. Finally, there might be a correlation between neuronal reorganization in the hippocampus, especially mossy fiber sprouting and cognitive deficits in animals subjected to SE in infancy but this issue needs further clarification.

# References

Aicardi J, Chevrie JJ. Febrile convulsions: neurological sequelae and mental retardation. In: Brazier MAB, Coceani F, eds. *Brain Dysfunction in Infantile Febrile Convulsions*. New York: Raven Press, 1976: 247-57.

Albala BJ, Moshé SL, Okada R. Kainic-acid seizures: a developmental study. *Brain Res* 1984; 315: 139-48.

Alling C. Biochemical maturation of the brain and the concept of vulnerable periods. In: Rydberg U *et al.*, ed. *Alcohol and the Developing Brain*. New York: Raven Press, 1985: 5-10.

André V, Ferrandon A, Marescaux C, Nehlig A. The lesional and epileptic consequences of lithium-pilocarpine-induced status epilepticus are affected by previous exposure to isolated seizures: effects of amygdala kindling and maximal electroshocks. *Neuroscience* 2000; 99: 469-81.

André V, Ferrandon A, Marescaux C, Nehlig A. Vigabatrin protects against hippocampal damage but is not antiepileptogenic in the lithium-pilocarpine model of temporal lobe epilepsy. *Epilepsy Res* 2001; 47: 99-117.

André V, Rigoulot MA, Koning E, Ferrandon A, Nehlig A. Long-term pregabalin treatment protects basal cortices and delays the occurrence of spontaneous seizures in the lithium-pilocarpine model in the rat. *Epilepsia* 2003; 44: 893-903.

Baraban SC, Schwartzkroin PA. Flurothyl seizure susceptibility in rats following prenatal methylazoxymethanol treatment. *Epilepsy Res* 1996; 23: 189-94.

Baram TZ, Gerth A, Schultz L. Febrile seizures: an age appropriate model. *Dev Brain Res* 1997; 246: 134-43.

Baram TZ, Dubé CM, Chung G, Akthar F. Prolonged experimental febrile seizures in immature rat cause spontaneous behavioral and electrophysiological seizures during adulthood. *Epilepsia* 2004; 45 (suppl 7): 6 (Abstract).

Ben-Ari Y. Limbic seizures and brain damage produced by kainic acid: mechanisms and relevance to human temporal lobe epilepsy. *Neuroscience* 1985; 13: 312-8.

Berg AT, Shinnar S, Levy SR, Testa FM. Childhood-onset epilepsy with and without preceding febrile seizures. *Neurology* 1999; 53: 1742-8.

Brewster A, Bender RA, Chen Y, Dubé C, Eghbal-Ahmadi M, Baram TZ. Developmental febrile seizures modulate hippocampal gene expression of hyperpolarization-activated channels in an isoform- and cell-specific manner. *J Neurosci* 2002; 22: 4591-9.

Bouilleret V, Ridoux V, Depaulis A, Marescaux C, Nehlig A, Le Gal La Salle G. Recurrent seizures and hippocampal sclerosis following intrahippocampal kainate injection in adult mice: EEG, histopathology and synaptic reorganization similar to mesial temporal lobe epilepsy. *Neuroscience* 1999; 89: 717-29.

Cavalheiro EA, Silva DF, Turski WA, Calderazzo-Filho LS, Bortolotto ZA, Turski L. The susceptibility of rats to pilocarpine-induced seizures is age-dependent. *Dev Brain Res* 1987; 37: 43-58.

Cavalheiro EA. The pilocarpine model of epilepsy. *Ital J Neurol Sci* 1995; 16: 33-7.

Cendes F. Febrile seizures and mesial temporal sclerosis. *Curr Opin Neurol* 2004; 17: 161-4.

Cendes F, Andermann F, Dubeau F, Gloor P, Evans A, Jones-Gotman M, et al. Early childhood prolonged febrile convulsions, atrophy and sclerosis of mesial structures, and temporal lobe epilepsy: a MRI volumetric study. *Neurology* 1993a; 43: 1083-7.

Cendes F, Andermann F, Gloor P, Lopes-Cendes I, Andermann E, Melanson D, et al. Atrophy of mesial temporal structures in patients with temporal lobe epilepsy: cause or consequence of repeated seizures? *Ann Neurol* 1993b; 34: 795-801.

Chen K, Baram TZ, Soltesz I. Febrile seizures in the immature brain result in persistent modification of neuronal excitability in limbic circuits. *Nature Med* 1999; 5: 888-94.

Chevassus-au-Louis N, Baraban SC, Gaiarsa JL, et al. Cortical malforamtions and epilepsy: new insights from animal models. *Epilepsia* 1998; 40: 811-21.

Cilio MR, Sogawa Y, Cha BH, Liu X, Huang LT, Holmes GL. Long-term effects of status epilepticus in the immature brain are specific for age and model. *Epilepsia* 2003; 44: 518-28.

Davies KG, Hermann BP, Dohan FJ, et al. Relationship of hippocampal sclerosis to duration and age of onset of epilepsy, and childhood febrile seizures in temporal lobectomy patients. *Epilepsy Res* 1996; 24: 119-26.

Dobbing J, Sands J. Comparative aspects of the brain growth spurt. *Early Hum Dev* 1979; 3: 79-83.

dos Santos NF, Arida RM, Filho EM, Priel MR, Cavalheiro EA. Epileptogenesis in immature rats following recurrent status epilepticus. *Brain Res Rev* 2000; 32: 269-76.

Dubé C, Boyet S, Marescaux C, Nehlig A. Progressive metabolic changes underlying the chronic reorganization of brain circuits during the silent phase of the lithium-pilocarpine model of epilepsy in the immature and adult rat. *Exp Neurol* 2000a; 162: 146-57.

Dubé C, Marescaux C, Nehlig A. A metabolic and neuropathological approach to the understanding of plastic changes occurring in the immature and adult rat brain during lithium-pilocarpine induced epileptogenesis. *Epilepsia* 2000b; 41 (suppl 6): S36-S43.

Dubé C, Chen K, Eghbal-Ahmadi M, Brunson K, Soltesz I, Baram TZ. Prolonged febrile seizures in the immature rat model enhance hippocampal excitability long term. *Ann Neurol* 2000c; 47: 336-44.

Dubé C, Boyet S, Marescaux C, Nehlig A. Relationship between neuronal loss and interictal glucose metabolism during the chronic phase of the lithium-pilocarpine model of epilepsy in the immature and adult rat. *Exp Neurol* 2001; 167: 227-41.

Engel J Jr. Critical evaluation of animal models for localization-related epilepsy. *Ital J Neurol Sci* 1995; 16: 9-16.

Faverjon S, Silveira DC, Fu DD, Cha BH, Akman C, Hu Y, et al. Beneficial effects of enriched environment following status epilepticus in immature rats. *Neurology* 2002; 59: 1356-64.

Fernandes MJS, Dubé C, Boyet S, Marescaux C, Nehlig A. Correlation between hypermetabolism and neuronal damage during status epilepticus induced by lithium and pilocarpine in immature and adult rats. *J Cereb Blood Flow Metab* 1999; 19: 195-209.

Germano IM, Zhang YF, Sperber EF, Moshé SL. Neuronal migration disorders increase seizure susceptibility to febrile seizures. *Epilepsia* 1996a; 37: 902-10.

Germano IM, Sperber EF, Moshé SL. Molecular and experimental aspects of neuronal migration disorders. In: Guerrini R, Andermann F, Canapichi R *et al.*, ed. *Dysplasias of cerebral cortex and epilepsy.* New York: Lippincott-Raven, 1996b: 22-34.

Germano IM, Sperber EF. Transplacentally induced neuronal migration disorders: an animal model for the study of the epilepsies. *J Neurosci Res* 1998; 51: 473-88.

Germano IM, Sperber EF, Ahuja S, Moshé SL. Evidence of enhanced kindling and hippocampal neuronal injury in immature rats with neuronal migration disorders. *Epilepsia* 1998; 39: 1253-60.

Hernandes G, Effenberger O, Vinz B, *et al.* Hippocampal malformation as a cause of familial febrile convulsions and subsequent hippocampal sclerosis. *Neurology* 1998; 50: 909-17.

Holmes GL, Gairsa JL, Chevassus-Au-Louis N, Ben-Ari Y. Consequences of neonatal seizures in the rat: morphological and behavioral effects. *Ann Neurol* 1998; 44: 845-57.

Huang LT, Cilio MR, Silveira DC, McCabe BK, Sogawa Y, Stafstrom CE, *et al.* Long-term effects of neonatal seizures: a behavioral, electrophysiological, and histological study. *Dev Brain Res* 1999; 118: 99-107.

Jensen FE, Baram TZ. Developmental seizures induced by common early-life insults: short- and long-term effects on seizure susceptibility. *Mental Retard Dev Dis Res Rev* 2000; 6: 253-7.

Kanemoto K, Kawasaki J, Miyamaoto T, Obayashi H, Nishimura M. Interleukin (IL)-1β, IL-1α, and IL-1 receptor antagonist gene polymorphisms in patients with temporal lobe epilepsy. *Ann Neurol* 2000; 47: 571-4.

Kotloski R, Lynch M, Lauersdorf S, Sutula T. Repeated brief seizures induce progressive hippocampal neuron loss and memory deficits. *Prog Brain Res* 2002; 135: 95-110.

Kubova H, Druga R, Lukasiuk K, Suchomelova L, Haugvicova R, Jirmanova I, *et al.* Status epilepticus causes necrotic damage in the mediodorsal nucleus of the thalamus in immature rats. *J Neurosci* 2001; 21: 3593-9.

Kubova H, Mares P, Suchomelova L, Brozek G, Druga R, Pitkänen A. Status epilepticus in immature rats leads to behavioural and cognitive impairment and epileptogenesis. *Eur J Neurosci* 2004; 19: 3255-65.

Kuks JBM, Cook MJ, Fish DR, Stevens JM, Shorvon SD. Hippocampal sclerosis in epilepsy and childhood febrile seizures. *Lancet* 1993; 342: 1391-4.

Lado FA, Sankar R, Lowenstein D, Moshé SL. Age-dependent consequences of seizures: relationship to seizure frequency, brain damage, and circuitry reorganization. *Ment Retard Dev Disabil Res Rev* 2000; 6: 242-52.

Lai MC, Liou CW, Yang SN, Wang CL, Hung PL, Wu Cl, *et al.* Recurrent bicuculline-induced seizures in rat pups cause long-term motor deficits and increase vulnerability to a subsequent insult. *Epilepsy Behav* 2002; 3: 60-6.

Lipp HP, Schwegler H, Heimrich B, Driscoll P. Infrapyramidal mossy fibers and two-way avoidance learning: developmental modification of hippocampal circuitry and adult behavior of rats and mice. *J Neurosci* 1988; 8: 1905-21.

Liu Z, Mikati M, Holmes G. Mesial temporal sclerosis: pathogenesis and significance. *Pediatr Neurol* 1997; 12: 5-16.

Lothman EW, Collins RC. Kainic acid induced limbic seizures: metabolic, behavioral, electroencephalographic and neuropathological correlates. *Brain Res* 1981; 218: 299-318.

Lothman EW, Bertram EH, Beckenstein JW, Perlin JB. Self-sustaining limbic status epilepticus induced by "continuous" hippocampal stimulation: electrographic and behavioral characteristics. *Epilepsy Res* 1989; 3: 107-19.

Lynch M, Sayin U, Bownds J, Janumpalli S, Sutula T. Long-term consequences of early postnatal seizures on hippocampal learning and plasticity. *Eur J Neurosci* 2000; 12: 2252-64.

Maher J, McLachlan RS. Febrile convulsions: is seizure duration the most important predictor of temporal lobe epilepsy? *Brain* 1995; 118: 1521-8.

Majak K, Pitkänen A. Do seizures cause irreversible cognitive damage? Evidence from animal studies. *Epilepsy Behav* 2004; 5 (suppl 1): S35-S44.

Mathern G, Babb T, Armstrong D. Mesial temporal lobe epilepsy. In: Engel J, Jr, Pedley T, eds. *Epilepsy: a Comprehensive Textbook*. New York: Lippincott-Raven, 1997: 133-55.

Mikati MA, Tarif S, Lteif L, Jawad MA. Time sequence and types of memory deficits after experimental status epilepticus. *Epilepsy Res* 2001; 43: 97-101.

Nadler JV. Minireview: kainic acid as a tool for the study of temporal lobe epilepsy. *Life Sci* 1981; 29: 2031-42.

Nehlig A, Dubé C, Koning E. Status epilepticus induced by lithium-pilocarpine in the immature rat does not change the long-term susceptibility to seizures. *Epilepsy Res* 2002, 51: 189-97.

Priel MR, Ferreira dos Santos N, Cavalheiro EA. Developmental aspects of the pilocarpine model of epilepsy. *Epilepsy Res* 1996; 26: 115-21.

Rigoulot MA, Leroy C, Koning E, Ferrandon A, Nehlig A. A chronic low-dose caffeine exposure protects against hippocampal damage but not against the occurrence of epilepsy in the lithium-pilocarpine model in the rat. *Epilepsia* 2003; 44: 529-35.

Rigoulot MA, Koning E, Ferrandon A, Nehlig A Neuroprotective effect of topiramate in the lithium-pilocarpine model of epilepsy. *J Pharmacol Exp Ther* 2004; 308: 787-95.

Roch C, Leroy C, Nehlig A, Namer IJ. Contribution of magnetic resonance imaging to the study of the lithium-pilocarpine model of temporal lobe epilepsy in adult rats. *Epilepsia* 2002a; 43: 325-35.

Roch C, Leroy C, Nehlig A, Namer IJ. Predictive value of cortical injury for the development of temporal lobe epilepsy in 21-day-old rats: a MRI approach using the lithium-pilocarpine model. *Epilepsia* 2002b; 43: 1129-36.

Romijn HJ, Hofman MA, Gransberger A. At what age is the developing cerebral cortex of the rat comparable to that of the full-term newborn baby? *Early Hum Dev* 1991; 26: 61-7.

Rutten A, van Albada M, Silveira DC, Cha BH, Liu X, Hu YN, et al. Memory impairment following status epilepticus in immature rats: time-course and environmental effects. *Eur J Neurosci* 2002; 16: 501-13.

Sagar HJ, Oxbury JM. Hippocampal neuron loss in temporal lobe epilepsy: correlation with early childhood convulsions. *Ann Neurol* 1987; 22: 334-40.

Sankar R, Shin DH, Liu H, Mazarati A, Pereira de Vasconcelos A, Wasterlain CG. Patterns of status epilepticus-induced neuronal injury during development and long-term consequences. *J Neurosci* 1998; 18: 8382-93.

Santos NF, Marques RH, Correia L, Sinigaglia-Coimbra R, Calderazzo L, Sanabria ER, et al. Multiple pilocarpine-induced status epilepticus in developing rats: a long-term behavioral and electrophysiological study. *Epilepsia* 2000; 41 (suppl 6): S57-S63.

Sarkisian MR, Tandon P, Liu Z, Yang Y, Hori A, Holmes GL, et al. Multiple kainic acid seizures in the immature and adult brain: ictal manifestations and long-term effects on learning and memory. *Epilepsia* 1997; 38: 1157-66.

Shinnar S, Berg AT, Moshé SL, Petix M, Maytal J, Kang H, et al. Risk of seizure recurrence following a first unprovoked seizure in childhood: a prospective study. *Pediatrics* 1990; 85: 1076-85.

Shinnar S, Maytal J, Krasnoff L, Moshé SL. Recurrent status epilepticus in children. *Ann Neurol* 1992; 31: 598-604.

Shinnar S. Febrile seizures. In: Johnson RT, ed. *Current therapy in Neurological Disease*. Philadelphia: Decker. 1990: 28-45.

Shinnar S. Prolonged febrile seizures and medial temporal sclerosis. *Ann Neurol* 1998; 43: 411-2.

Sperk G. Kainic acid seizures in the rat. *Prog Neurobiol* 1994; 42: 1-32.

Stafstrom CE, Sasaki-Adams DM. NMDA-induced seizures in developing rats cause long-term learning impairment and increased seizure susceptibility. *Epilepsy Res* 2003; 53: 129-37.

Sutula TP, Cavazos JE, Woodard AR. Long-term structural and functional alterations induced in the hippocampus by kindling: implications for memory dysfunction and the development of epilepsy. *Hippocampus* 1994; 4: 254-8.

Toth Z, Yan XX, Haftoglou S, Ribak CE, Baram TZ. Seizure-induced neuronal injury: vulnerability to febrile seizures in immature rat model. *J Neurosci* 1998; 18: 4285-94.

Tremblay E, Nitecka L, Berger ML, Ben-Ari Y. Maturation of kainic acid seizure-brain damage syndrome in the rat. I. Clinical, electrographic and metabolic observations. *Neuroscience* 1984; 13: 1051-72.

Turski L, Ikonomidou C, Turski WA, Bortolotto ZA, Cavalheiro EA. Review: Cholinergic mechanisms and epileptogenesis. The seizures induced by pilocarpine: a novel experimental model of intractable epilepsy. *Synapse* 1989; 3: 154-71.

VanLandingham KE, Heinz ER, Cavazos JE, Lewis DV. Magnetic resonance imaging evidence of hippocampal injury after prolonged focal febrile convulsions. *Ann Neurol* 1998; 43: 413-26.

Verity CM, Butler NR, Golding J. Febrile convulsions in a national cohort followed up from birth. I. Prevalence and recurrence in the first years of life. *Br Med J* 1985; 290: 1307-10.

Vezzani A, Moneta D, Richichi C, Perego C, De Simoni MG. Functional role of proinflammatory and anti-inflammatory cytokines in seizures. *Adv Exp Med Biol* 2004; 548: 123-33.

Voutsinos-Porche B, Koning E, Kaplan H, Ferrandon A, Guenounou M, Nehlig A, *et al.* Temporal patterns of the cerebral inflammatory response in the rat lithium-pilocarpine model of temporal lobe epilepsy. *Neurobiol Dis* 2004; 17: 385-402.

Wu CL, Huang LT, Liou CW, Wang TJ, Tung YR, Hsu HY, *et al.* Lithium-pilocarpine-induced status epilepticus in immature rats result in long-term deficits in spatial learning and hippocampal cell loss. *Neurosci Lett* 2001; 312: 113-7.

# Maturation of synchronised activities and epileptogenesis: *when* is as important as *what*!

## Y. Ben-Ari

*INMED/INSERM, Parc Scientifique de Luminy, Marseille, France*

The fundamental challenge that we face when trying to understand the mechanisms at work during brain development and how they are affected by insults is the heterogeneity. At any given point in time, adjacent neurons are in very different developmental stages. Some are undeveloped with few or no functional synapses, others have already many synapses and operate as if they are in a mature functional network. In addition, there are many developmental gradients that cover almost all the molecular and cellular signals that govern the behaviour of the neuron.

The principal transmitter gated receptors and synapses have a sequential maturation with GABAergic synapses preceding glutamate synapses and dendritic targeted GABAergic synapses preceding somatic innervating interneurons (Ben-Ari, 2002; Tyzio et al., 1999). Similarly, GABA inhibits adult neurons but excites immature ones – because of a different chloride gradient that leads to an accumulation of chloride in the neuron and thus an efflux when GABA receptors are activated (Ben-Ari et al., 1989; Tyzio et al., 2003). These gradients have been observed in all species and brain structures studied indicating that they have been kept throughout evolution. They are also observed in primate neurons *in utero* and are thus valid for human foetuses and pre-term babies (Khazipov et al., 2001). The obvious implications of these gradients are that drugs targeted to a given molecular species will have complex unexpected actions: they will exert no action on some neurons endowed with different molecular species and act only on that proportion of neurons that have shifted to adult types of molecular species. In addition, the gradient of heterogeneity will depend notably on the species: animals that have an extended period of brain development – such as primates – will offer a picture of heterogeneity for an extended period of time thus allowing extrinsic factors to exert a stronger influence than animals in which this period is restricted to a few days.

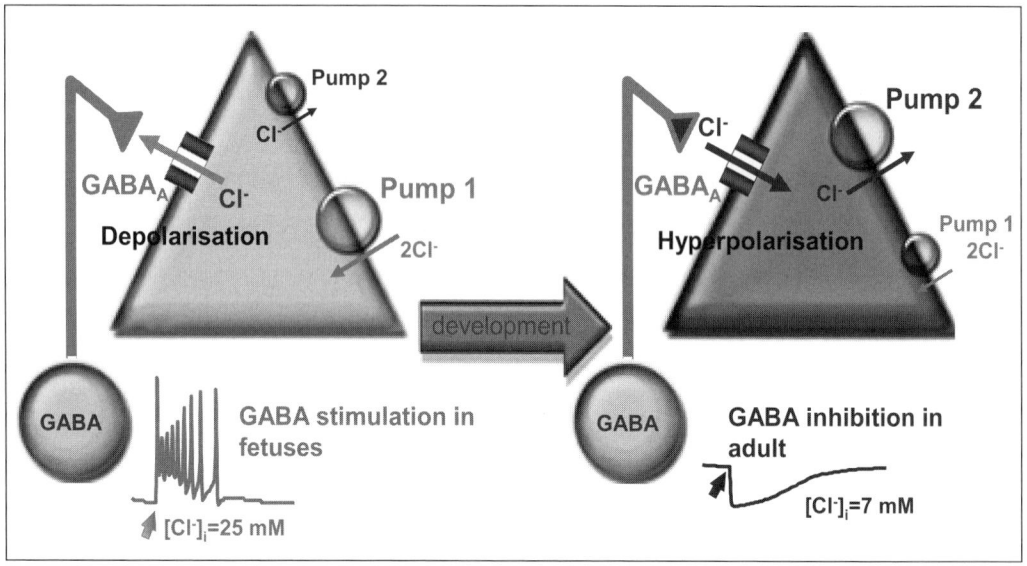

**Figure 1.** Schematic diagram depicting the alterations of the intracellular concentration of chloride during maturation. In immature neurons, this concentration is high because of a delayed maturation of the KCC2 co-transporter that extrudes chloride and an early maturation of another pump that intrudes chloride.

One of the consequences of this developmentally programmed heterogeneity is that the generators of behaviourally relevant patterns and oscillations will not operate as long as a minimal density of mature neurons and synapses is operative. It is possible that the occurrence of a minimal pioneering network may modulate other immature neuronal populations that at that stage are "in another trip". Therefore, patterns and oscillations may only concern local networks and will not have necessarily the same significance as in more adult networks.

The net consequence of this ensemble of sequences and heterogeneity is that the *generation of oscillations* and *of seizures* will strongly depend on the time of occurrence and not only the intrinsic aetiology of the seizures. In fact, the conditions required for the transformation by seizures of a naive network to an epileptogenic one will also depend on the timing: some seizures may not be deleterious at a given developmental stage and severely handicapping at another. In this brief review, we shall raise some of these issues and speculate – at least for some aspects consequently to the lack of data – on their implications to the clinician point of view. The central issue is to determine whether the signature notably in electrographic terms of seizures gives an indication of both the developmental stage of the various populations of neurons but also of the expected severity of the seizures. This type of information may also enable to determine the pharmacological developmental stage and thus the type of therapy that may fit best to treat the epilepsies.

One point deserves emphasis form the start: basic mechanisms that operate in rodents also operate in humans and their consequences in term of epileptogenesis are not dissimilar. The most important limitations that we have are not so much the species barrier as the lack of compelling data occasionally from animal data and more frequently from humans because of obvious limitations. Almost all our present knowledge on the mechanisms of human epilepsies is derived from animal models and the therapeutic tools that are in use have their origin in basic mechanisms discovered in animal networks. Most importantly, the sequence of events and pathological alterations that occurs after seizures is quite similar in human and animal models of epilepsies. The argument that a given mechanism or observation is only valid in rodents or other animal species than humans is usually infirmed once a better understanding of its operation become available.

## Basic developmental sequences: the background

In the adult brain, glutamatergic neurons constitute the vast majority of neurons and provide the main source of the excitatory drive whereas the dense network of GABAergic interneurons that constitute 10-15% of the neurons provide the source of the inhibitory drive. In spite of this apparent imbalance, interneurons play a crucial role in the generation of behaviourally relevant patterns (Freund and Buszaki, 1996). Various types of interneurons control the fine discharge of the principal cells and the patterns that networks will generate. In the absence of functional GABAergic neurons and synapses, cortical networks seize and do not generate behaviourally relevant patterns. Therefore, determining the functional maturation of interneurons will provide interesting information on the state of maturation of the network. Since, GABAergic inhibition also plays a central role in seizure generation, understanding the mechanisms that lead to the transformation of an ensemble of immature unconnected neurons to an emerging functional network is crucial to better understand the relation between an epileptogenic event and its consequences in the developing brain.

## GABA interneurons and synapses set the tune already at a very early stage

In the developing hippocampus, interneurons do not develop hand in hand with the pyramidal neurons: GABAergic interneurons and synapses mature first and are operative at a stage when the principal cells are silent (Ben-Ari et al., 2004, also see Gao et al., 2001 for other brain structures). Interneurons divide prior to glutamatergic neurons, extend their axons and dendrites prior to the principal cells, establish functional synapses before principal neurons and can generate patterns when principal neurons are essentially inert. Most interestingly, the rules for establishing functional GABA or glutamate synapses between an axon and its dendritic target are not identical: GABA synapses are established once the contact is established whereas glutamate synapses can only be formed when the target neuron has reached a certain degree of maturation. Therefore, in spite of a rather long journey – interneurons are not generated in the close vicinity of the principal neurons but in the distal ganglionic eminence – interneurons must for some reason be at work at an early stage.

We also discovered the reasons for this early requirement. In all developing brain structures and species, GABAergic synapses are excitatory because of a higher intracellular concentration of chloride. The consequence is that when GABA receptors are activated there is an efflux of chloride instead of the usual influx and a depolarisation that will generate action potentials, remove the voltage dependent Magnesium blockade leading to an influx of calcium (Ben-Ari et al., 1997). This early action of GABA reverses subsequently with the delayed activation of a chloride co-transporter that will export chloride from the inside to the outside and install the adult concentration of chloride. We elsewhere suggested that this sequence provides a solution to the problem of how to maintain an equilibrium between excitation and inhibition during brain maturation. The excitatory drive provided by GABAergic synapses – that is always closer to the resting membrane potential than glutamate even when excitatory is not toxic and enables to excite enough to increase calcium intracellularly and facilitate developmental processes that require that rise without danger. Also, the longer kinetics of GABAergic currents – than glutamate AMPA receptor mediated ones – enable to summate synaptic currents in neurons that possess but few synapses. An obvious consequence of this early expression of functional GABAergic synapses is that GABA mimetic agents and anti epileptic drugs will exert a particularly strong action on the activity dependent formation of the network (Repesa and Ben-Ari, 2005). Interestingly, there is a night/day cycle in the suprachiasmatic nucleus associated with a shift from depolarisation to hyperpolarisation of GABA actions suggesting that the shift may apply not only during maturation but also in relation to fundamental biological processes (Wagner et al., 1997). In human epileptic neurons, there is a similar shift suggesting that the depolarisation produced by GABA is also associated with seizures: it can be triggered (see below) and permanently altered in epileptic neurons (Cohen et al., 2002). The explanation for these shifts have now been extensively investigated and include the late activation of a co-transporter that removes chloride (Rivera et al., 1999; Hubner et al., 2001; Stein et al., 2004).

## ■ Developing networks talk only one language

We discovered some time ago that the developing hippocampal network has a single pattern – to which we referred as Giant Depolarising Potentials (GDPs) (Ben-Ari et al., 1989; Ben-Ari, 2001). This pattern is characterised by recurrent bursts with large polysynaptic currents mediated by GABA and glutamate receptors. Subsequent studies revealed that a similar pattern is present in all developing networks, in all species including the developing primate hippocampus *in utero*. GDPs provide almost all the activity as long as GABAergic synapses are present. The shift from excitatory to inhibitory GABA signals the end of GDPs and the expression of more adult patterns; it is at that stage that a network is sufficiently complex that it can generate behaviourally relevant patterns.

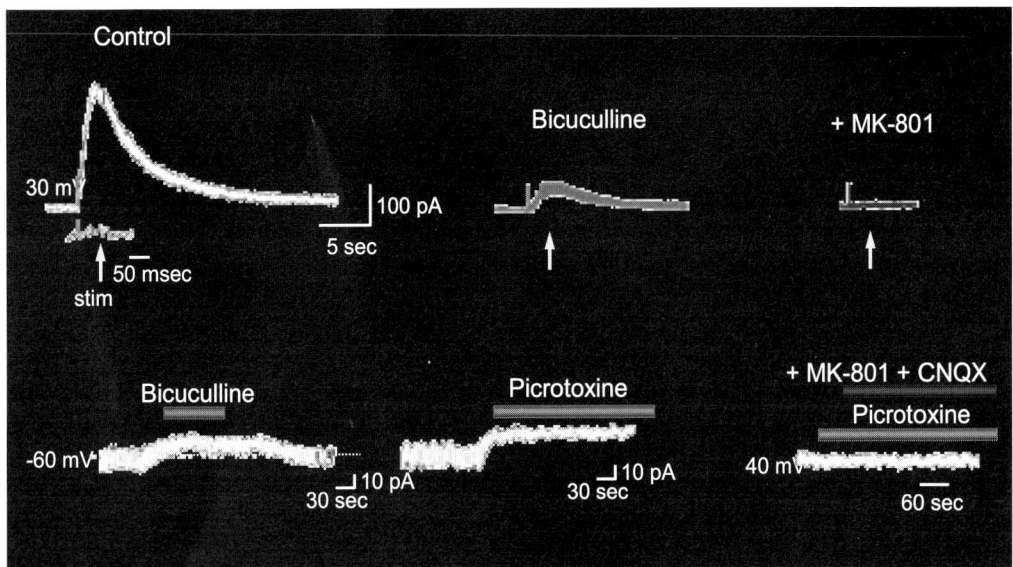

**Figure 2.** Prior to synapse formation, neurons communicate by means of a non vesicular release of GABA and to a lesser extent glutamate. An electrical stimulation generates a large current mediated primarily by GABA as it is largely blocked by a GABA receptor antagonist. The remaining current is blocked by an antagonist of NMDA receptors. The electrical stimulation does not generate a synaptic response (Demarques *et al.*, *Neuron*).

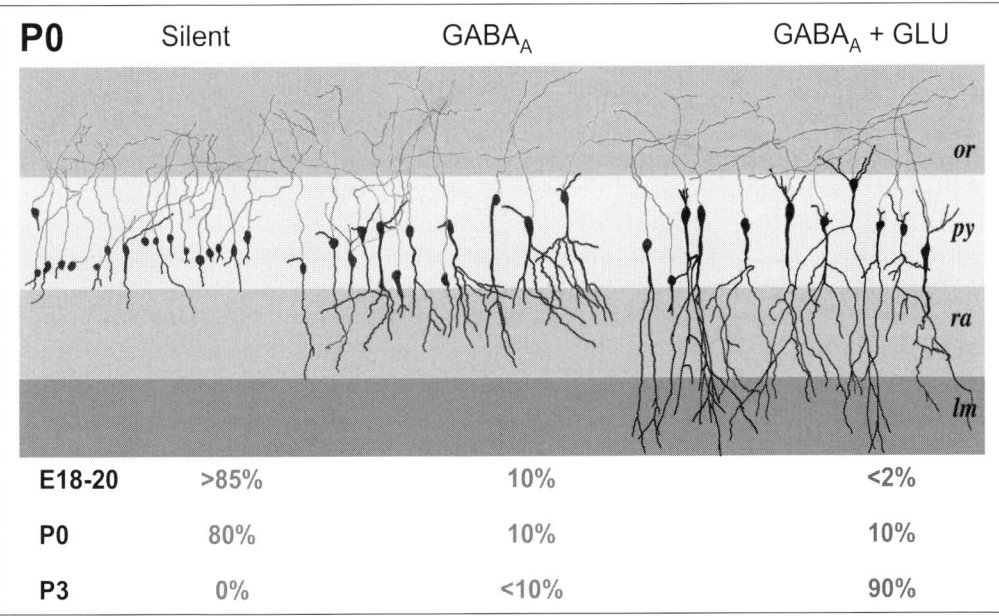

**Figure 3.** GABAergic synapses are established prior to glutamatergic ones. Pyramidal neurons were patch clamped in a hippocampal slice at birth (P0). Small cells (80%) have no synaptic currents, larger ones (10%) that have a small apical dentrite have GABA but not glutamate synapses and the largest ones at that stage (10%) that have apical dendrites that reach the distal molecular layer have GABA and glutamate synapses (Tyzio *et al.*, *J Neuroscience*).

GDPs are generated by the combined action of excitatory GABA synapses and large NMDA receptor mediated synaptic currents. The latter are of particularly long duration in the developing brain consequently to the presence of a subunit of NMDA receptors that confer to immature neurons a very long kinetic. The synergistic actions of GABA and NMDA receptors is the core of this pattern, the small depolarisation produced by GABA is sufficient to remove the blockade from NMDA receptors and generate the long poly-synaptic currents notably *via* the activation of an excitatory recurrent loop – the activation of interneurons leading in return to an enhancement of the excitation on principal cells and the generation of large synaptic currents. GDPs have now been recorded in a plethora of techniques – including cell attached and whole cell recordings as well as fields and surface recordings – and preparations including slices but also cultures and *in vivo*. In the intact hippocampus *in vitro* – a preparation developed in the laboratory that have major advantages in comparison to slices – GDPs can be generated by a wide range of sites but they propagate along the developmental gradient – from rostral to caudal sites – indicating a developmental gradient of activity (Khalilov et al., 1997, 2003). GDPs can be considered as a type of a primitive pattern with little information content that is here to signal activity in developing connections and promote synapse formation and possibly provide initial signals for the construction of operating functional units on the basis of neurons that fire together wire together.

## ■ Spindles and sharp waves are present early and go from the periphery to the centre

Recordings in chronically implanted pups revealed the presence of sharp waves and tails that are reminiscent of GDPs (Leinekugel et al., 2002; Khazipov et al., 2004). These patterns are generated by GABA and glutamatergic synaptic currents as revealed by whole cell recordings in un-anaesthetised restrained pups. Most importantly, when these events are recorded in both the periphery and the cortical centre – the sensori-motor cortex – the spindles in the periphery precedes those in the centre. Lesions of the spinal cord reveal a large reduction of spontaneous spindles suggesting that the peripherally generated spindles are the generators of those in the cortical sites. These and other similar observations are in line with the concepts that developing circuits in the periphery and centres communicate *via* a single pattern and that peripheral structures can provide a strong source of modulation of the centres. In a wider perspective, these studies raise the possibility that the programming of the construction of central cortical organisations including cortical maps and other functional entities are controlled or at least modulated by peripheral activity. In this perspective, a unified pattern of activity in developing structures is perfectly capable to supply a signature of space rather than specific content and thus contribute to the wiring of distant structures. The alterations produced by aberrant activities such as seizures would produce their deleterious sequelae merely by interrupting these patterns rather than by more specific information containing signals.

## Seizures beget seizures

That seizures can lead to long-term consequences including quasi-permanent alterations of the network including a reduced treshold for the generation of additional seizures has been considered as a basic mechanism of epilepsies and a basic property of the developing and adult brains for several decades. But this has never been directly demonstrated. We recently developed a unique preparation in which this property can be tested readily *in vitro* in conditions that can provide a definitive test of this property (*Figure 4*). The preparation consists of a triple chamber that can accommodate the two intact hippocampi and their connecting commissures in three independent compartments. It becomes possible to apply a convulsive agent to one hippocampus and let a given number of seizures to propagate to the other hippocampus, then interrupt the connections and determine whether the hippocampus has been transformed by the seizures and generate more readily seizures (Khalivo et al., 2003). We found that a series of brief seizures generated by the application of kainate to one hippocampus generate seizures that propagate to the other site and lead to a transformation of the naive hippocampus to an epileptic one that generates spontaneous and evoked seizures. This transformation requires functional NMDA receptors in the naive hippocampus: applications of kainate to one hippocampus and an antagonist of NMDA receptors to the other blocks the transformation: seizures can take place repeatedly without any long lasting consequence. The transformation is thus analogous to a form of long-term plasticity – an alteration of synaptic plasticity. Seizures do beget seizures and the induction mechanism has been clarified in this preparation. We also use this approach to investigate the properties of networks that have become epileptic. Patching neurons from the epileptic hippocampus, we found that GABA excites again neurons: the seizures induced a long term transformation of the inhibitory actions of GABA from inhibitory to excitatory most likely because of a loss of the capacity to remove and regulate chloride *via* co-transporters. To some extent, epileptogenesis recapitulates ontogenesis and seizures re-induce a return to immature neurons with an excitatory GABA – except that now the high density of glutamate synapses, seizures will be generated in these conditions. Interesting the crucial role of GABAergic synapses in synchronisations is also observed *in vivo* in patch clamp recordings (Khazipov and Holmes, 2003).

## A Paracrine release of GABA and glutamate prior to synapse formation

In a wide range of systems, receptors develop before synapses and the obvious question is whether they exert a function. Or in other terms, does the modulation by neuronal activity starts with synapse formation or does it occur at an earlier stage thanks to other actions that can be identified already in immature neurons that are devoid of synaptic connections. In the neuromuscular junction, receptors do play a major role in the formation of the neuromuscular junction.

We examined whether they are also operative at a very early stage in the hippocampus (E18-P0). We found that there is a tonic release of GABA and glutamate at an early stage, since a GABA receptor antagonist generates a tonic current indicating an

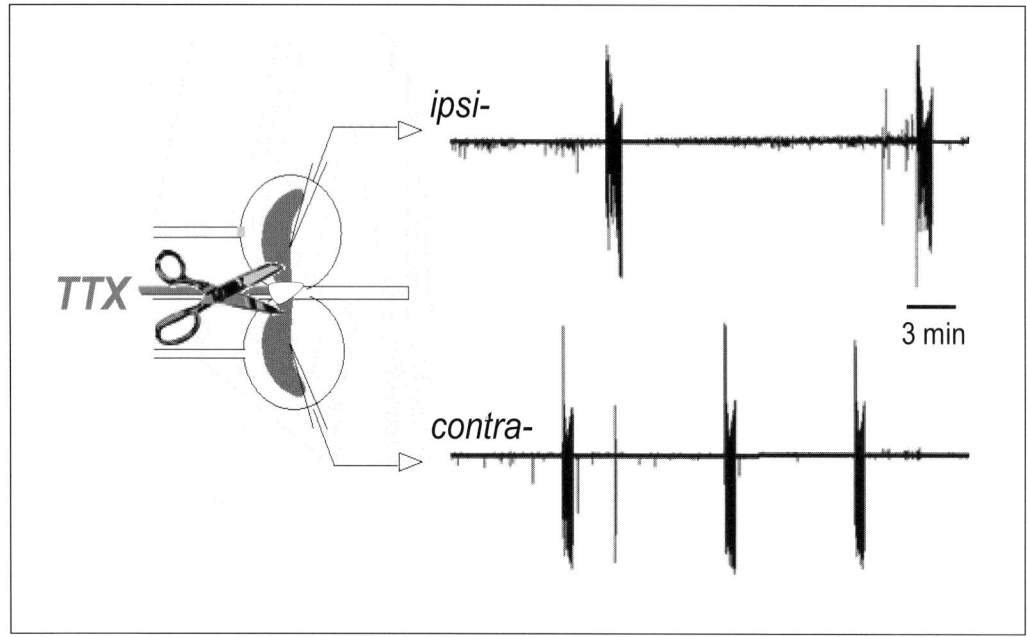

**Figure 4. Seizures beget seizures.**
Using the triple chamber, the convulsive agent kainate was applied to one hippocampus generating seizures that propagate to the other side – the naive – hippocampus. After a few applications, the naive side became epileptic even though it never received a convulsive agent (Khalilov et al., Nature Neuroscience).

ongoing release of GABA. In addition, electrical stimuli of the vicinity of the recorded neuron generate a large long lasting current generated by GABA and NMDA receptors – but not AMPA receptors (Demarque et al., 2002). The release mechanisms are quite unique in the sense that they do not require the classical release mechanisms including calcium and the release machinery – they can be even generated in animals in which the release machinery has been knocked out. This paracrinic release of GABA acts on distal neurons to generate large currents prior to synapse formation. At a later stage, this system disappears and is replaced by the more conventional focal action of transmitters. We also tested the possible role of this mechanism and found that blocking GABA receptors alters neuronal migration indicating that this activity dependent process is modulated by a non focal paracrinic action of transmitters most notably GABA. These and other observations are in line with the extensive indication that GABA is a morphogenic agent at an early stage and that it modulated neuronal migration in addition to synapse formation and neuronal growth and differentiation. Again agents acting on GABA receptors are expected to act on neurons that possess few or no synapses at all. This type of mechanism could be involved in the formation of heterotopic masses and other migration disorders. Thus, transmitters notably GABA can modulate early developmental processes by means of actions on receptors that are in essence extrasynaptic as synapses do not exist at that stage (also see Owens et al., 1999, 2002; Represa and Ben-Ari, 2005).

## In adults seizures beget seizures via a very different mechanism

Animal models of temporal lobe epilepsies have been instrumental in providing a general view of the events that following a status lead to long lasting alterations of the network including the transformation by seizures of a naive network to one that seizes. The basic events have been described first with the kainate model of epilepsies and confirmed with the pilocarpine one developed subsequently.

In essence, these studies performed in the late seventies, indicate that kainate generates a status – by a mechanism that has now been almost fully determined – which is often associated with cell death. The most vulnerable neurons – the CA3 pyramidal neurons and somatostatin containing interneurons – degenerate leading to a significant loss of dendritic GABAergic inhibition, recently directly determined by the first recordings from dendrites of epileptic neurons. This is followed during the so called silent period – two weeks that follow the status – by the activation of a cascade of genes – over 1,500 according to the studies of the late Yoav Citri in Israel (Nedivi et al., 1993) – that represents an obvious cascade of events that will lead to sprouting of glutamatergic mossy fibres and establishment of novel aberrant synapses. This includes first immediate early genes triggered by the calcium rise, growth factor genes a few hours later, genes coding for cytoskeletal proteins that signals important rearrangement within surviving neurons and lastly genes coding for extracellular matrix signalling guidings signals that will direct the growing axons to their targets. The functionality of the newly established synapses is now compellingly established following recordings from the various actors of this scenario. There is a five fold increase of glutamatergic EPSCs in dendrites and somata of neurons including pyramidal neurons and surviving interneurons that are receiving these aberrant synapses. The consequence is that more seizures will be generated because of the enhanced glutamatergic drive and the loss of dendritic inhibition. But, because many interneurons notably those that innervate the somata of the principal cells survive and are overexcited by the newly formed glutamatergic synapses, seizures will not occur continuously, there is a second defence line that is operative in the epileptic tissue (reviewed in Cossart et al., 2001, 2005).

A general difference between these long lasting actions and those described above for younger networks is that here the cascade includes a period of silence in general and cell death most frequently. This is not the case in early immature networks since neurons are at that stage more resistant to the pathogenic – cell death inducing actions of kainate and other epileptogenic drugs. Therefore, seizures can beget seizures but via different mechanisms in adults and immature neurons and alos with very different consequences since in the developing brain, this will affect processes that are unique to that stage.

# Conclusions

The deleterious consequences of an insult in a developing brain will be necessarily dependent on the state of maturation of the network.

A very early insult coming at a stage when most neurons are still migrating and have no functional synapses can affect migration – that is strongly dependent on activity, calcium currents and NMDA receptor mediated currents. This action will not involve synaptic mechanisms of toxicity as these are absent but other mechanisms that can be receptor dependent. Alterations of the paracrine release of transmitters can modulate the speed of migration, the development of neurites and axonal elongation or other essential functions (cell division, differentiation, etc.).

An insult coming later when neurons start having a significant number of synapses will progressively use synapse and activity dependent forms of toxicity and impede the operation of the newly formed network. It is at that stage that the more conventional forms of seizure induced alterations are expected to occur.

Initially, the disturbance occurs because of an alteration by the insult of the dominating GDP pattern and its associated mechanisms. Interruption of this pattern leads to malformation of the connections and the construction of the network without necessarily producing cell death – immature neurons are relatively resistant to that pathogenic mechanism. For instance, abnormal activity can lead to malformation of the cortical maps and other functional units somewhat in accordance with the widely recognised sensory disturbances produced by seizures in developing sensory structures of the visual or auditory systems (viz the Landau-Kleffner syndrome or the critical phases of visual development). The conclusions of this postulated sequence is that at all these stages, epileptogenic mechanisms will differ and strongly depend on the state of maturation of network driven patterns. A better understanding of these time and developmental stage dependent seizures will enable to define in a more rationale manner seizures and have better predictions of their deleterious consequences.

# References

Ben-Ari Y. Excitatory actions of GABA during development: the nature of the nurture. *Nat Rev Neurosci* 2002; 3 (9): 728-39.

Ben-Ari Y, Cherubini E, Corradetti R, Gaiarsa JL. Giant synaptic potentials in immature rat CA3 hippocampal neurones. *J Physiol* 1989; 416: 303-25.

Ben-Ari Y, Khalilov I, Represa A, Gozlan H. Interneurons set the tune of developing networks. *Trends Neurosci* 2004; 27 (7): 422-7.

Ben-Ari Y, Khazipov R, Caillard O, Leinekugel X, Gaiarsa JL. GABAA, NMDA and AMPA receptors: a developmentally regulated "ménage à trois". *Trends Neurosci* 1997; 20 (11): 523-9.

Ben-Ari Y. Developing networks play a similar melody. *Trends Neurosci* 2001; 24 (6): 353-60.

Cohen I, Navarro V, Clemenceau S, Baulac M, Miles R. On the origin of interictal activity in human temporal lobe epilepsy *in vitro*. *Science* 2002; 298 (5597): 1418-21.

Cossart R, Bernard C, Ben-Ari Y. Multiple facets of GABAergic neurons and synapses: multiple fates of GABA signalling in epilepsies. *Trends Neurosci* 2005; in press.

Cossart R, Dinocourt C, Hirsch JC, Merchan-Perez A, De Felipe J, Ben-Ari Y, Esclapez M, Bernard C. Dendritic but not somatic GABAergic inhibition is decreased in experimental epilepsy. *Nat Neurosci* 2001; 4 (1): 52-62.

Demarque M, Represa A, Becq H, Khalilov I, Ben-Ari Y, Aniksztejn L. Paracrine intercellular communication by a Ca2+- and SNARE-independent release of GABA and glutamate prior to synapse formation. *Neuron* 2002; 36 (6): 1051-61.

Freund T, Buszaki G. Interneurons of the hippocampus. *Hippocampus* 1996; 6 (4): 347-470.

Gao XB, van den Pol AN. GABA, not glutamate, a primary transmitter driving action potentials in developing hypothalamic neurons. *J Neurophysiol* 2001; 85 (1): 425-34.

Hauser WA. Epidemiology of epilepsy in children. *Neurosurg Clin North Am* 1995; 6: 419-29.

Holmes GL, Ben-Ari Y. Seizures in the developing brain: perhaps not so benign after all. *Neuron* 1998; 21 (6): 1231-4.

Hubner CA, Stein V, Hermans-Borgmeyer I, Meyer T, Ballanyi K, Jentsch TJ. Disruption of KCC2 reveals an essential role of K-Cl transport already in early synaptic inhibition. *Neuron* 2001; 30 (2): 515-24.

Khalilov I, Esclapez M, Medina I, Aggoun D, Lamsa K, Leinekugel X, Khazipov R, Ben-Ari Y. A novel *in vitro* preparation: the intact hippocampal formation. *Neuron* 1997; 19 (4): 743-9.

Khalilov I, Holmes GL, Ben-Ari Y. *In vitro* formation of a secondary epiletogenic mirror focus by interhippocampal propagation of seizures. *Nat Neurosci* 2003; 6 (10): 1079-85.

Khazipov R, Esclapez M, Caillard O, Bernard C, Khalilov I, Tyzio R, Hirsch R, Dzhala Y, Berger B, Ben-Ari Y. Early development of neuronal activity in the primate hippocampus *in utero*. *J Neurosci* 2001; 21 (24): 9770-81.

Khazipov R, Holmes GL. Synchronization of kainate-induced epileptic activity via GABAergic inhibition in the superfused rat hippocampus *in vivo*. *J Neurosci* 2003; 23 (12): 5337-41.

Khazipov R, Sirota A, Leinekugel X, Holmes GL, Ben-Ari Y, Buzsaki G. Early motor activity drives spindle bursts in the developing somatosensory cortex. *Nature* 2004; 432 (7018): 758-61.

Leinekugel X, Khazipov R, Cannon R, Hirase H, Ben-Ari Y, Buzsaki G. Correlated bursts of activity in the neonatal hippocampus *in vivo*. *Science* 2002; 296 (5575): 2049-52.

Nedivi E, Hevroni D, Naot D, Israeli D, Citri Y. Numerous candidate plasticity-related genes revealed by differential cDNA cloning. *Nature* 1993; 363 (6431): 718-22.

Owens DF, Kriegstein AR. Is there more to GABA than synaptic inhibition? *Nat Rev Neurosci* 2002; 3 (9): 715-27.

Owens DF, Liu X, Kriegstein AR. Changing properties of GABA(A) receptor-mediated signaling during early neocortical development. *J Neurophysiol* 1999; 82 (2): 570-83.

Represa A, Ben-Ari Y. Trophic actions of GABA in neuronal development. *Trends Neurosci* 2005, in press.

Rivera C, Voipio J, Payne JA, Ruusuvuori E, Lahtinen H, Lamsa K, Pirvola U, Saarma M, Kaila K. The k+/Cl- co-transporter KCC2 renders GABA hyperpolarizing during neuronal maturation. *Nature* 1999; 397 (6716): 251-5.

Stein V, Hermans-Bormeyer I, Jentsch TJ, Hubner CA. Expression of the KCl co-transporter KCC2 parallels neuronal maturation and the emergence of low intracellular chloride. *J Comp Neurol* 2004; 468 (1): 57-64.

Tyzio R, Ivanov A, Bernard C, Holmes GL, Ben-Ari Y, Khazipov R. Membrane potential of CA3 hippocampal pyramidal cells during postnatal development. *J Neurophysiol* 2003; 90 (5): 2964-72.

Tyzio R, Represa A, Jorquera I, Ben-Ari Y, Gozlan H, Aniksztejn L. The establishment of GABAergic and glutamatergic synapses on CA1 pyramidal neurons is sequential and correlates with the development of the apical dendrite. *J Neurosci* 1999; 19 (23): 10372-82.

Wagner S, Castel M, Gainer H, Yarom Y. GABA in the mammalian suprachiasmatic nucleus and its role in diurnal rhythmicity. *Nature* 1997; 387 (6633): 554-5.

# Temporal lobe epileptogenesis and epilepsy in the developing brain: bridging the gap between the laboratory and the clinic

H.J. Hasson[1], J. Veliskova[1,2,4], S.R. Haut[1,4], S. Shinnar[1,3,4], S.L. Moshé[1-4]

[1] Departments of Neurology, [2] Neuroscience and [3] Pediatrics, [4] Laboratory of Developmental Epilepsy and the Comprehensive Epilepsy Management Center, Montefiore Medical Center, Albert Einstein College of Medicine, New York, USA

Epileptic seizures may be brief or prolonged, focal or generalized, and occur as single or repetitive events. Seizures can cause both morphological and functional changes as well as cognitive and neuropsychological alterations. The short and long term consequences can be influenced by several factors including age, seizure type and its cause, seizure frequency, epilepsy syndrome, genetic background, sex and the neurological status of the individual. It should be pointed out that the notion that all identified changes resulting from seizures are detrimental to brain function has not been validated. Often, the observed change is transient or may not affect an individual's function in a significant way. Additional studies aimed at identifying the spectrum and meaning of seizure-induced alterations must be pursued.

Many studies identify various changes that occur after seizures. The conclusion is frequently reached that these changes affect the brain negatively, just because the changes are there. The next step showing that the changes indeed alter the long term outcome is frequently missing. The majority of the published studies are concerned with seizure-induced hippocampal changes. One reason the hippocampus is focused on is because one of the common forms of epilepsy, mesial temporal lobe epilepsy (MTLE), is the epilepsy syndrome most remedial to surgery, and is defined by neuropathological and imaging changes of the hippocampus. The hippocampus is an excellent anatomic landmark for neuroimaging, with protocols developed to quantify structural injury including volume and biochemical alterations including changes in bioenergetics. The hippocampus is also an excellent target for *in vitro* electrophysiology due to its well-defined anatomy and physiology.

In relation to seizure-induced neuronal damage, the prevailing hypothesis is that the cell loss, especially in the hippocampus, may contribute to further seizure genesis due to structural reorganization (Blumcke et al., 2002; Engel Jr. et al., 1997; Mathern et al., 2002; Sutula et al., 2003; Thom et al., 2002). MTLE is often associated with an atrophied hippocampus demonstrating high gradient-echo signal on magnetic resonance imaging (MRI), indicative of Mesial Temporal Sclerosis (MTS). Anatomically, MTS is defined as neuronal cell loss and gliosis at CA1 and end-folium with relative sparing of transitional cortex measured at the mid-body of the anterior-posterior axis. Structural and functional glial changes, synaptic reorganization and dentate granule cell dispersion are present. Extrahippocampal temporal and extratemporal pathology (termed "dual pathology") is often noted (Wieser, 2004). On MRI, MTS is defined as hippocampal atrophy together with increased T2 signal in the hippocampus. In surgical series, this has an excellent but not perfect correlation with anatomically defined MTS (Wieser, 2004).

Because of a relative lack of prospective human data, it is difficult to resolve issues related to the cause and consequences observed after seizures in humans. One of the difficulties is that patients cannot be identified prior to their first seizure. Therefore causation is difficult to prove as no pre-seizure testing had been done. One technique that is starting to be used is MRI and other advanced imaging modalities very soon after the first seizure. With the exception of the most acute changes that may take place, the imaging can be used to demonstrate the state of the pre-seizure brain. However, even this approach is limited for several reasons. Imaging may be not easily obtainable after the initial seizure unless the seizure is prolonged. In children, it may not be possible to perform timely or often serial imaging, as seizures recur, because of safety issues, ethical and financial constraints, especially in children that may require sedation. Validation of the meaning of the identified changes in relation to the development of a permanent epileptic disorder or other functional (neuropsychological) alterations has not yet been achieved.

Animal models of seizures have provided significant information towards the understanding of seizure-related sequelae and offer the opportunity to explore cellular, molecular and functional changes following seizures as a function of age and sex. In models, the pre-existing substrate is known, and thus changes occurring following seizures can be considered causally related to the seizure per se, although the means by which the seizures were induced may have an impact as well. Combining different data sets may reveal common findings transcending the model. Animal models in rodents show a variety of changes. Seizures produce unique gene expression patterns, cell injury or loss, interfere with neo-neurogenesis, induce synaptic remodeling, activate glia, and produce inflammatory-like reactions.

Despite the apparent neuropathologic similarities between experimental and human epilepsies, caution must be used when generalizing conclusions from animal data to humans. Nevertheless, the rigorous experimental data, together with clinical advances in anatomic and functional imaging and data from surgical resective series have produced significant new insights into the understanding of seizure-induced alterations in children. In this review (which complements the recent review published in *Lancet Neurology* (Haut et al., 2004), we will attempt to bridge the gap between the laboratory and the clinic as it pertains to the consequences of either status epilepticus (SE) or one or multiple brief seizures on the normal and abnormal brain in children and developing rodents (mostly rats). To obtain a complete picture, the reader is referred to the chapter authored by Nehlig in this volume which focuses on age-dependent features of the consequences of seizures early in life in experimental models based on imaging techniques and behavioral approaches.

To understand translational animal and human studies, it is important to translate the development of neural events from the rodent to the human brain (Holmes, 1986; Moshé, 1987). Factors that must be considered include brain growth, rate of protein synthesis, myelinization, structural connectivity, synaptic density, or cerebral glucose utilization rate. The rat is born at a relatively premature state. Nevertheless, based on these factors, it has been proposed that rats at postnatal day (P) 8-10 roughly correspond to full-term human newborns (Avishai-Eliner et al., 2002; Dobbing and Sands, 1979; Gottlieb et al., 1977; Moshé, 1987; Nehlig, 1997). The 2-3 week old rats seem to be equivalent to human infants to toddlers (Nehlig, 1997; Velisek and Moshe, 2002). The 3-5 week old rats correspond to a peripubertal child (Nehlig, 1997; Velisek and Moshe, 2002) as puberty starts at P32-38 (Ojeda and Urbanski, 1994).

## ■ Consequences of SE in the setting of a normal brain

### Clinical studies

In children presenting either as a first unprovoked seizure or newly diagnosed epilepsy, 10-12% present with SE (Hauser et al., 1982; Shinnar et al., 1996; Shinnar et al., 2001a). If one excludes acute symptomatic cases, then the morbidity and mortality of SE in children is very low (Maytal et al., 1989; Shinnar and Babb, 1997). New neurological deficits are rare. In children with acute symptomatic SE, there is significant morbidity and mortality but it is difficult to separate this from the known morbidity and mortality of the underlying acute insult (e.g. meningitis, head trauma, stroke). Children with a prolonged first seizure have the same recurrence risk as those with a brief initial seizure. However, if the first episode is prolonged then there is a higher risk that future episodes would be prolonged as well. (Shinnar et al., 1996; Shinnar et al., 2001a). This argues for a predisposition to prolonged seizures in specific children rather than the seizure causing damage as otherwise, one would have expected a higher recurrence risk following a prolonged seizure (Shinnar et al., 2001a). The same phenomenon is seen in children with febrile seizures where a prolonged initial febrile seizure does not increase the recurrence risk of another febrile seizure but if another one does occur it is likely to be prolonged (Berg and Shinnar, 1996).

There are limited pathologic data following SE. Biochemical or imaging surrogate markers of neuronal injury have not been identified. For example, neuron specific enolase (NSE, a marker of neuronal injury) has not been found to be a reliable measure in children (Gurnett et al., 2003). There are reports of increases in diffusion weighted imaging (DWI) signal after convulsive (Hisano et al., 2000) and nonconvulsive (Kassem-Moussa et al., 2000) SE but their significance remains unclear.

Magnetic resonance spectroscopy (MRS) studies have identified decreased N-acetyl-aspartate (NAA)/creatine ratio, suggesting that acute neuronal dysfunction may occur in partial SE but the long term consequences of this remain uncertain (Park et al., 2000).

## Animal studies

The immature hippocampus is relatively resistant to SE-induced morphological damage, although the immature brain is very susceptible in general to acute epileptogenic insults (Cavalheiro et al., 1987; Swann and Moshé, 1997; Velísková et al., 1988). Even long-lasting SE regardless of seizure origin (non-limbic or limbic) induced by flurothyl (Sperber et al., 1999; Wasterlain, 1978), pentylenetetrazol (Nehlig and de Vasconselos, 1996) NMDA (Stafstrom and Sasaki-Adams, 2003) or kainic acid (Albala et al., 1984; Ben-Ari et al., 1984; Haas et al., 2001; Stafstrom et al., 1992) and pilocarpine (Cavalheiro et al., 1987) showed little or no neuronal damage in the hippocampus or extrahippocampal regions in rats younger than three weeks, although the hippocampus and other cortical structures exhibited prolonged electrographic discharges (Albala et al., 1984; Sperber et al., 1999; Tremblay et al., 1984). Synaptic reorganization in the supraganular layer of the dentate gyrus of the hippocampus does not occur following SE before the third postnatal week (Haas et al., 2001; Sankar et al., 1998; Sperber et al., 1991; Yang et al., 1998). Many factors may contribute to the relative resistance of immature hippocampus to SE-induced damage (Haut et al., 2004). With maturation, the extent of hippocampal damage increases (Albala et al., 1984; Sankar et al., 1998).

There are few reports suggesting that a degree of hippocampal or extrahippocampal injury may occur during early development. Occasional hippocampal damage can be detected in rats from the second postnatal week (Avishai-Eliner et al., 2002; Baram and Ribak, 1995; Baram and Schultz, 1991; de Feo et al., 1986; Haas et al., 2001; Kubova et al., 2001; Ribak and Baram, 1996; Sankar et al., 1999; Sankar et al., 1998; Stafstrom et al., 1992; Thompson et al., 1998; Watts et al., 1995). However, the implications of these data are not fully understood. In a recent report, Da Silva et al. showed that three episodes of pilocarpine-induced SE during the perinatal period (P7-P9) resulted in abnormal distribution of neocortical and hippocampal interneurons and reduction of natural apoptosis in P35 rats suggesting that recurrent episodes of SE may produce long-term changes in inhibitory circuitry (Da Silva et al., 2003). There was no structural neocortical or hippocampal damage.

Thus, developmental studies demonstrate that the immature brain is relatively resistant to SE-induced morphological damage and compared to the mature brain (Haut et al., 2004). Although some studies strike and show that under specific circumstances, SE-induced damage may occur in immature brain, the extent of damage is far less prominent compared to SE-induced changes in adulthood. The variability in the results may provide an important clue as to why different epileptogenic insults produce variable results. SE early in life may also prime the brain to the effects of subsequent insults (Giorgi et al., 2004; Koh et al., 1999). The consequences may be either detrimental to the brain or in some cases beneficial. Deleterious effects were reported by Koh (Koh et al., 1999). SE at P15 increased the sensitivity to SE-induced damage later in life. These data suggest that SE early in life could constitute a priming condition for some type of brain injury without producing detectable morphological changes or increasing seizure susceptibility. This observation is supported in part by the data reported by Giorgi et al. (Giorgi et al., 2004). These investigators reported strike both that SE induced in P15 rats can alter the outcome of a subsequent focal ischemic insult later in life. KA-induced SE increased the size of the infarct and this may be partly related to the long duration of the SE. Interestingly, an hour-long flurothyl-induced SE had a neuroprotective effect.

*What is the relationship of SE to subsequent development of epilepsy in normal immature brain?* There is ample evidence that epileptogenesis is age- and model-dependent (Albala et al., 1984; Sperber et al., 1991; Wasterlain et al., 2002). Up to the age P21, spontaneous seizures do not occur following KA, and are rarely observed following lithium/pilocarpine SE (Sankar et al., 1998). At P21 rats, depending on the seizure model used, spontaneous seizures occur irregularly in 10-73% of animals (Priel et al., 1996; Roch et al., 2002; Stafstrom et al., 1992; Wasterlain et al., 2002). For rats exposed to SE in adulthood, the incidence of seizures reaches almost 100%, within 2-3 months (Stafstrom et al., 1992; Wasterlain et al., 2002). Also, P15 rats exposed to KA-SE are not more prone to develop amygdala kindled seizures as adults than controls (Okada et al., 1984). MRI has been used to identify epilepsy prone animals following SE at P21 {Roch, 2002 #9997, see also Nehlig in this volume}. Rats with no MRI abnormalities and no changes in T2 relation time, which did not develop spontaneous seizures. Rats with visible structural MRI strike the coma abnormalities or without visible abnormalities, but with changes in T2 relation time, developed spontaneous seizures. Not all rats with epilepsy showed hippocampal damage, suggesting that other factors may be responsible. In contrast, induction of three episodes of pilocarpine SE in P7-P9 rats produced long term changes in epileptogenesis, documented by electrographic epileptiform discharges and *in vitro* hyperexcitability of hippocampal networks (Santos et al., 2000).

The neuropsychologic/cognitive consequences are also age specific and much less prominent than those seen following seizures in adult animals. SE induced by systemic administration of KA in infant rats resulted in an impaired ability of the rats to acquire conditioned avoidance responses later in life (de Feo et al., 1986). This impairment was specific to KA and not to other agents. One possible explanation may be that it was not the seizure that caused the impairment but the direct chemical damage to the brain from the KA. Another possibility is that the type of seizure caused by KA is different than that caused by other convulsants, and the difference in outcome may be secondary to the specific seizure type and location. Prolonged KA-induced seizures on P1-P14 also altered performance of the affected rats in the radial maze in adulthood. While the rats treated with KA on P1-P14 required significantly more trials to reach criterion and displayed more reference and working errors, their impairment was significantly smaller than the impairment induced by KA in adult rats (Lynch et al., 2000).

The cognitive impairment from SE is dependent on the developmental age of the rat at the time of SE. P16 rats with lithium-pilocarpine induced SE and subsequently tested for spatial learning and memory tasks at P55 were slower in finding the platform in the water maze than were controls (Cilio et al., 2003). P20 rats demonstrated more severe memory impairment and no significant differences were noted between rats subjected to SE at P12 and controls (Cilio et al., 2003). Similarly, SE induced at P20 causes spatial memory deficits that persist into adulthood. The pattern of poor water maze performance that was observed indicates that these rats suffer a permanent deficit in navigational memory. The cognitive deficits correlate with abnormal place cells at the network level and abnormal connectivity at the structural level (Liu et al., 2003). Repeated bouts of pilocarpine induced SE at P7, P8 and P9 produce permanent cognitive deficits (Santos et al., 2000).

As with anatomical consequences, Koh et al. exposed P15 rats to KA SE and when the rats reached P45, tested their ability to navigate a water maze. They found that the rats that experienced SE performed equally well as controls. However, when the rats experienced a second episode of KA SE as adults there was a significant impairment in water maze ability compared to animals who experienced a single episode of SE (Koh et al., 1999). In this case, the manifestations of symptomatic damage and behavioral effects required a second insult to manifest themselves. Furthermore, the timing of the second insult may be important, as rats exposed repeatedly to KA-SE between ages 20-26 days (Sarkisian et al., 1997) did not develop deficits as were seen in rats exposed to KA SE at age 15 days and again at age 45 days (Koh et al., 1999).

Food deprivation does not appear to be a significant factor in cognitive outcome but maternal deprivation may be (Akman et al., 2004; Huang et al., 2002). Interestingly, although malnutrition does not decrease the seizure threshold to KA SE, it further promotes neurogenesis in the hippocampal dentate gyrus induced by SE itself in P15 rats (Nunes et al., 2000).

## ■ The role of the cause of SE in inducing injury

### Clinical studies

The cause of the episode of SE is the most important determinant of outcome (Maytal et al., 1989; Shinnar and Babb, 1997). In acute symptomatic SE, the common causes are hypoxia/ischemia, trauma, meningitis/encephalitis, and metabolic derangements (DeLorenzo et al., 1995; Maytal et al., 1989) all of which may cause neuronal injury. Determining the additive effects of SE may be challenging. In acute symptomatic SE, unlike in unprovoked SE, prolonged duration of seizure during the initial seizure is associated with a higher risk of epilepsy, however it is also known that a more severe insult will result in SE, and therefore it is difficult to assess whether the increased incidence of epilepsy is secondary to the SE or to the more severe insult that caused the SE (Shinnar and Babb, 1997). DeLorenzo et al. suggests that SE does induce damage independent of the cause of the SE in adults, but this was seen in SE only greater than 2 hours (DeLorenzo et al., 1995).

In children with underlying brain abnormalities, SE is more likely to occur than in those who are neurologically normal (Berg et al., 1999; Berg et al., 2004; Sillanpaa and Shinnar, 2002). However, SE appears to be a marker for neurological abnormality and appears to only modestly affect long term outcome after controlling for etiology (Sillanpaa and Shinnar, 2002).

Genetic factors may influence both the predisposition to SE (Corey et al., 1998) and the occurrence of seizure-induced damage. As previously discussed, it is clear that certain children have a predisposition to SE. In twin studies there is an increased concordance of SE in monozygotic vs dizygotic twins (Corey et al., 1998). In this study if one twin had SE, the other was more likely not just to have seizures but to have SE. Homozygosity for dynorphin is significantly associated with SE (Stogmann et al., 2002) and heterozygosity is associated with the presence of familial temporal lobe epilepsy (TLE). One study (Kanemoto et al., 2000) found that individuals homozygous for alleles regulating production of interleukin-1β (a pro-inflammatory molecule produced during SE) were more likely to develop MTS following febrile SE but other studies have not replicated this finding. This report is of particular interest as interleukin-1β interacts with NMDA receptors and in animal models is both proconvulsant and mediates seizure induced injury (Vezzani et al., 2000).

## Animal studies

There are limited studies determining whether SE-induced neuronal damage may be enhanced in the setting of a compromised brain in developing rats. Hypoxia induced during the first two postnatal weeks may lead to acute seizures (Jensen et al., 1991) and increased seizure susceptibility persisting till adulthood (Jensen et al., 1992; Jensen and Wang, 1996; Olson et al., 1985). Also, rats exposed to hypoxia at P10, demonstrate enhanced neuronal injury to KA-induced SE at P21 or older age groups (Koh et al., 2001). However, other studies showed that hypoxia/ischemia or mechanical injury had no effect on seizure susceptibility later in life (Holmes and Weber, 1985; Moshé and Albala, 1985; Setkowicz and Janeczko, 2003). These differences may be strain specific, suggesting a genetic influence. The neurobehavioral consequences may also be strain specific: hypoxia-induced seizures in P10 Long-Evans rats have no significant long term impairment in water maze performance (Jensen et al., 1992) but in P10 Sprague-Dawley rats there is impairment of spatial learning at P45 (Yang et al., 2004). The basis for this variability and the mechanisms of possible long term learning impairment await further study.

Hypoxia/ischemia obtained by combining unilateral carotid ligation in combination with hypoxia in P10 rats showed a high number of rats with acute seizures (Jensen et al., 1994). Although, the long-term consequences have not been studied in this model, Williams et al., using a model of hypoxia/ischemia in neonatal rats that did not produce acute seizures, reported that 40% of the rats become spontaneously epileptic later on (Williams et al., 2004). Although these rats have significant hippocampal lesions ipsilaterally to the ligation, the frequency of the spontaneous seizures does not correlate with the extent of the hippocampal lesion. Also, in P10 rats, the occurrence of KA SE on top of hypoxia/ischemia exacerbates the damage induced by neonatal hypoxia-ischemia alone (Wirrell et al., 2001; Yager et al., 2002). On the other hand, seizures that may occur prior to hypoxia-ischemia in P7 and P13 rats may have a modest neuroprotective effect, especially in P13 rats (Towfighi et al., 1999).

Hippocampal damage was detected following KA-induced SE in P17 rats pretreated with lipopolysaccharide, which mimics CNS inflammatory processes by inducing proinflammatory cytokines (Lee et al., 2000). Pittman et al. found that a neuroimmune challenge with lipopolysaccharide and its associated fever reduce seizure threshold (Heida et al., 2004). At this age, KA-induced SE itself does not produce significant hippocampal damage and only limited glia activation and cytokine induction (Rizzi et al., 2003).

The consequences of SE in the setting of an already, chronically abnormal brain may be different. Prenatal exposure to DNA alkylating agent methylazoxymethanol acetate (MAM) at embryonic day (E) 15, results in moderate to severe heterotopias within the cortex and hippocampus (Germano and Sperber, 1998). MAM-treated rats had significantly increased seizure susceptibility at P15 (Chevassus-au-Louis et al., 1998; de Feo et al., 1995; Germano and Sperber, 1998; Germano et al., 1998; Germano et al., 1996). Moreover, kindling in a P15 NMD rats produced acute neuronal damage in the CA3 hippocampal region (Germano et al., 1998), which does not occur at this age in normal rats (Haas et al., 2001).

Differences in seizure susceptibility among distinct rat strains have been identified in developing rats (Golden et al., 1995). However, there are no studies on genetic influence contributing to SE-induced neuronal damage during development, besides the differences in the outcome of hypoxic-induced seizures discussed earlier. As mentioned above, there is conflicting evidence whether hypoxia early in life has an effect on seizure susceptibility later in life. The paucity of data begs for additional studies to determine the effects of SE in animals with different genetic backgrounds.

The role of cognitive reserve as a variable in effecting cognitive outcomes following seizures has not been fully elucidated. One study using fast and slow learning rats that experienced lithium pilocarpine SE at P21 did not find any significant differences between the fast and slow learners when the rats were tested in the water maze 23 days later (Akman et al., 2003).

## ■ Consequences of febrile SE

### Clinical studies

A febrile seizure is a seizure in a child older than 1 month, in the presence of a febrile illness without a CNS infection, metabolic imbalance, or other acute neurological injury. Children with prior afebrile seizures are excluded. Febrile SE is a seizure that meets criteria for both SE and febrile seizure and represents the extreme end of the complex febrile seizure spectrum (Proceedings AES course, 1993; Recommendations of the EFA working group, 1993). While febrile SE represents approximately 5% of children with febrile seizures (Berg and Shinnar, 1996), these are so common that febrile SE accounts for 25% of all childhood SE and more than two thirds of SE in the second year of life (Shinnar et al., 1997). Prolonged febrile seizures and febrile SE are associated with a substantially elevated risk for future epilepsy (Annegers et al., 1987; Nelson and Ellenberg, 1978; Shinnar et al., 1996). Many but not all retrospective studies link febrile SE and later MTLE (Abou-Khalil et al., 1993; Berg et al., 1999), whereas prospective studies of febrile seizures have not found such an association (Shinnar, 2002; Shinnar, 2003). Part of the problem is the rarity of febrile SE in these epidemiological studies and the relative short follow-up in most as well as the lack of imaging studies. Recent data show that MRIs performed within 72 hours after febrile SE do demonstrate acute hippocampal edema and swelling in some cases (VanLandingham et al., 1998). In a few cases progression to MTS has been demonstrated. The initial degree of T2 abnormality may predict subsequent hippocampal atrophy (Lewis et al., 2002). While it is clear that this phenomenon exists, it is unclear how often and in which situations this happens. An ongoing prospective multicenter study is attempting to address this question in a definitive fashion.

## Animal studies

Along the line of strong age-dependent occurrence of febrile seizures in infants and young children, animal studies suggest higher susceptibility to hyperthermia-induced seizures during early development compared to adult rats (Holtzman et al., 1981; Liebregts et al., 2002; McCaughran and Schechter, 1982). An *in vitro* study shows that hyperthermic epileptiform activity can be induced in hippocampal slices only during a discrete developmental period (P5-P20) (Tancredi et al., 1992). Prolonged hyperthermic seizures early in life result in transient acute neuronal damage in the hippocampus and amygdala, which are detectable up to 2 weeks later but do not lead to long-term decrease in neuronal number (Toth et al., 1998), neither to neo-neurogenesis (Bender et al., 2003). On the other hand, mossy fiber density was increased after 3 months following hyperthermic seizures, suggesting changes in hippocampal synaptic connectivity(Bender et al., 2003) along with increases in excitability of the network (Chen et al., 1999). Brain MRI studies have shown that experimental febrile seizures increase T2 signal in limbic structures in 75% at 24 hours and in 87.5% of the rats a week later. Enhanced seizure susceptibility following hyperthermic seizures persists into adulthood (Dube et al., 2000).

One determinant in hyperthermic-induced seizure outcome is a preexisting localized cortical lesion. Scantlebury et al, have shown that 86% of rats with focal lesions and hyperthermic seizures at P10 develop spontaneous seizures in adulthood. These rats also demonstrate some relatively minor impairment in the Morris water maze (Scantlebury et al., 2004).

## ■ Effects of single or multiple short duration seizures

### Clinical studies

There are no clinical data that a single brief seizure is associated with brain damage (Shinnar and Hauser, 2002). Children with even one seizure have a significant rate of preexisting abnormalities on imaging studies (Hirtz et al., 2000; Shinnar et al., 2001b). Functional imaging studies have shown no MRS differences in NAA/creatine values in temporal lobes following complex partial seizures (Cendes et al., 1997).

The long-term effects of recurrent seizures are difficult to assess as chronic changes may be due to the underlying pathology and anticonvulsant use. The results of studies attempting to document progressive neuronal loss from recurrent seizures are mixed. There is some evidence that progressive volume loss can occur following recurrent seizures that may correlate with generalized tonic-clonic seizure burden. Examination of resected hippocampal tissue in intractable TLE reveals neuronal loss, the extent of which has been correlated with duration of epilepsy and seizure burden (Sutula et al., 2003). However this may be specific to the syndrome rather than the number or type of seizures, as this has only been demonstrated in TLE not in frontal lobe epilepsy. The best evidence to date is that long term damage, anatomical or functional, is most likely related to the specific epilepsy syndrome rather than to seizures per se, though frequent or prolonged seizures may also play a role. The lack of apparent neuronal injury associated with "benign" epilepsies also supports this concept as full remittance of seizures appears to be independent of pre-remission seizure frequency and anti-epileptic treatment usage (Ambrosetto and Tassinari, 1990). As stated repeatedly, the results of retrospective studies must be interpreted with caution.

Children with epilepsy have a high rate of cognitive and behavioral abnormalities. These are more common in children with epilepsy of long duration and there is some evidence for progressive decline (Sutula and Hermann, 1999). But other epidemiological studies have not found such evidence (Ellenberg et al., 1986). Once again the underlying syndrome appears to be most important. Patients with MTLE do show progressive memory loss but those with other epilepsies such as frontal lobe do not appear to. The cognitive and behavioral changes seen with the Landau Kleffner Syndrome and the syndrome of Continuous Spike and Wave in Slow Wave Sleep appear to be independent of the number of seizures or even of whether seizures occur at all (Holmes et al., 1981). More recent work has shown a high rate of preexisting cognitive and behavioral abnormalities in children with newly diagnosed epilepsy (Austin et al., 2004; Fastenau et al., 2004; Oostrom et al., 2003). Thus more work is required to elucidate the relative contributions of preexisting disorder, the specific epilepsy syndrome, the effect of medications, the social and family setting and the contributions of seizures per se to the cognitive and behavioral problems that are being increasingly recognized as part and parcel of childhood epilepsy.

## Animal studies

A single brief hyperthermic seizure at P10-12 did not produce mossy fiber sprouting and did not increase seizure susceptibility later in life (Chang et al., 2003). A single brief hyperthermic seizure at P22 is associated with mossy fiber sprouting but does not lead to neurodegeneration (Jiang et al., 1999) or to increases in seizure susceptibility later in life (Gulec and Noyan, 2001).

Compared to the adult brain, the immature brain also seems to be more resistant to the effects of repeated brief seizures. Haas et al. (Haas et al., 2001) showed that amygdala kindling results in more severe behavioral seizure expression in P16 rats including tonic-clonic phase, not observed in adults (Haas et al., 2001). Spontaneous seizures were also observed after 30 stimulations; this is much earlier than in adults. But acute neuronal damage, cell loss or mossy fiber sprouting was not detected (Haas et al., 2001). Nevertheless, in these rats kindling persists (Moshé and Albala, 1982). Lack of neuronal loss was also found following recurrent seizures induced by injections of tetanus toxin into the hippocampus (Lee et al., 2001), although loss of dendritic spines, changes in neuronal excitability and spontaneous seizures develop in adulthood in this model (Anderson et al., 1999; Jiang et al., 1998; Lee et al., 1995; Smith et al., 1998). Recurrent seizures during the first week of life do not lead to immediate cell damage (Riviello et al., 2002) and in contrast to adults, neo-neurogenesis in hippocampus is decreased (McCabe et al., 2001). When examined in adulthood, rats with neonatal seizures had decreased seizure threshold and mossy fiber sprouting in the CA3 and subgranular region (Holmes et al., 1998; Holmes et al., 1999). In another study, repeated brief hyperthermic seizures between P5-20 increased seizure susceptibility in adulthood (McCaughran and Schechter, 1982). Recurrent flurothyl seizures in immature rats do not lead to spontaneous recurrent seizures. However, animals subjected to multiple flurothyl-induced seizures demonstrate a kindling phenomenon with decreased latency to forelimb clonus (Liu et al., 1999). In addition, recurrent flurothyl seizures are associated with a reduced seizure threshold when examined at an older age (Holmes et al., 1998; Sogawa et al., 2001).

The basis for the reduced seizure threshold following recurrent flurothyl seizures has been addressed using in vitro recordings (Villeneuve et al., 2000). Intracellular recordings of CA1 and CA3 pyramidal neurons from neonatal flurothyl-induced seizures revealed impairment in spike frequency adaptation. In addition, the after hyperpolarizing potentials following a spike train were markedly reduced when compared with controls. In contrast, no significant alterations in the firing properties of CA3 pyramidal neurons were found. It was concluded that neonatal seizures lead to persistent changes in intrinsic membrane properties of CA1 pyramidal neurons. These alterations are consistent with an increase in neuronal excitability and may contribute to the behavioral deficit and epileptogenic predisposition observed in rats that experienced repeated neonatal seizures.

These data suggest that early in life, repeated seizures can produce a kindling effect and increase the epileptic potential of the brain permanently. This increase in seizure susceptibility is associated with relative minor hippocampal changes compared to the effects of similar seizures in the adult brain. However, this is not universal. Repeated brief hyperthermic seizures at P10-12 neither produce mossy fiber sprouting, nor increase seizure susceptibility later in life (Chang et al., 2003).

In animal models, recurrent seizures during the first few weeks of life cause cognitive impairment in adolescence and adulthood. There is impairment of visual spatial memory following neonatal seizures induced by flurothyl, in rats tested using the Morris water maze (Bo et al., 2004; Holmes et al., 1998; Huang et al., 2002; Liu et al., 1999; Neill et al., 1996). The cognitive impairment was found in adulthood following recurrent neonatal seizures but not following a single seizure at P6 (Bo et al., 2004). Animals subjected to recurrent flurothyl seizures between P15-20 have also been shown to have impairment of auditory discrimination (Neill et al., 1996). Many studies have been done showing the cognitive effects of seizures in PTZ kindled animals. The cognitive and memory impairments are age dependent. Older rats are more sensitive to the same stimulus than young adult rats (Grecksch et al., 1997). Swann et al. have shown that recurrent seizures caused by intrahippocampal injection of tetanus toxin, beginning in early life can lead to a significant deficiency in spatial learning. These findings were even in the absence of hippocampal synchronized network discharging or a substantial loss of hippocampal pyramidal cells (Lee et al., 2001). Once again, it should be emphasized that the effects observed in adults are more severe (Mellanby and George, 1979).

## ■ Concluding remarks

Seizures occur more frequently early in life reflecting both the increased predisposition of the immature brain to experience a seizure in response to a stimulus that may be trivial in adulthood and the higher incidence of epileptogenic insults (Hauser, 1994). It is established that a seizure can induce a variety of structural and functional changes especially in the hippocampus, an area of active investigation and the focus of this review. However, other brain regions can be modulated by seizures including cortical and subcortical structures such as the substantia nigra (Moshé, 1989; Moshé et al., 1995). Some of the changes are in terms of neuronal loss and subsequent structural reorganization and are believed to play a role in further epileptogenesis. The significance of other changes is unclear and may not necessarily be detrimental. Indeed, in some cases seizures have been reported to have beneficial effects on certain brain functions (Andre et al., 2000; Goddard et al., 1969; Hernandez and Warner, 1995; Kelly and McIntyre, 1994; Kondratyev et al., 2001; Pagnin et al., 2004; Zhang et al., 2002). The picture is further complicated by the role played by other important elements such as the underlying state of the brain, the cause of the epilepsy, genetic predisposition and the potential detrimental effects of antiepileptic treatments.

Animal studies show that the immature brain is more resistant to seizure and SE-induced damage than adults. Determination of the spectrum of age-related seizure-induced changes and their significance are an important first step for development of new effective neuroprotective and antiepileptic therapies. These studies must be carried in humans and animal models of epilepsy, a true translational undertaking.

Seizures in patients with abnormal brain or specific genetic susceptibilities can be more harmful than in those without additional abnormalities. Neuroimaging has identified that malformations of cortical development are one of the main causes of refractory epilepsies (Sisodiya, 2004). To better understand the pathophysiology of these conditions it is imperative, once again, to develop appropriate animal models. These experimental models would be expected to meet certain minimum criteria as partially outlined at the recently concluded AES paediatric epilepsy workshop held under the aegis of NINDS in May 2004. These would include spontaneous recurrent seizures that occur within a developmental window corresponding to that seen in humans; lack of responsiveness to conventional treatments identified by earlier screening paradigms; and in the long-term, untreated animals should be likely to develop neurocognitive deficits and spontaneous recurrent seizures or reduced seizure thresholds as seen in human populations. Genetic models with spontaneous seizures and low mortality rates must also be identified.

Treatments should be designed to eliminate co-morbidities associated with epileptic seizures. Neuropsychological and neuropsychiatric disturbances are two important comorbidities that require special attention. The second step will be to identify early predictive surrogate markers that can be modified by the treatments; otherwise the discovery process will be very slow as the full complement of the epileptic condition may take years to emerge. Along the same lines, there are many lessons to be learned from the "benign" epileptic syndromes, in which the seizures do not appear to harm the brain and the individual's lifestyle.

Together, these approaches will allow the design of appropriate therapeutic strategies including early and aggressive treatments to control all seizures without producing any treatment-related side effects. Nevertheless, this may not always be possible. The risk/benefit ratio of the current or future antiepileptic treatments is one of the biggest challenges in seizure management. Enhanced understanding of the spectrum of seizure-related changes as a function of age and as it is modified by the developmental/aging process will lead to the development of specific treatments to the individual needs.

**Acknowledgments: Supported by grants NS-20253, NS-43209, NS-02192, NS-45160, K12 NS048856 (NSADA) from NINDS, a CURE Foundation Research Grant and the Heffer Family Medical Foundation. SS and SLM are the recipients of the Martin A. and Emily L. Fisher fellowship in Neurology and Pediatrics. HH is an NSADA trainee.**

# References

Abou-Khalil B, Andermann E, Andermann F, Olivier A, Quesney LF. Temporal lobe epilepsy after prolonged febrile convulsions: excellent outcome after surgical treatment. *Epilepsia* 1993; 34: 878-83.

Akman C, Zhao Q, Liu X, Holmes GL. Effect of food deprivation during early development on cognition and neurogenesis in the rat. *Epilepsy Behav* 2004; 5: 446-54.

Akman CI, Hu Y, Fu DD, Holmes GL. The influence of cognitive reserve on seizure-induced injury. *Epilepsy Behav* 2003; 4: 435-40.

Albala BJ, Moshé SL, Okada R. Kainic-acid-induced seizures: a developmental study. *Dev Brain Res* 1984; 13: 139-48.

Ambrosetto G, Tassinari CA. Antiepileptic drug treatment of benign childhood epilepsy with rolandic spikes: is it necessary? *Epilepsia* 1990; 31: 802-5.

Anderson AE, Hrachovy RA, Antalffy BA, Armstrong DL, Swann JW. A chronic focal epilepsy with mossy fiber sprouting follows recurrent seizures induced by intrahippocampal tetanus toxin injection in infant rats. *Neuroscience* 1999; 92: 73-82.

Andre V, Ferrandon A, Marescaux C, Nehlig A. Electroshocks delay seizures and subsequent epileptogenesis but do not prevent neuronal damage in the lithium-pilocarpine model of epilepsy. *Epilepsy Res* 2000; 42: 7-22.

Annegers JF, Hauser WA, Shirts SB, Kurland LT. Factors prognostic of unprovoked seizures after febrile convulsions. *N Engl J Med* 1987; 316: 493-8.

Austin JK, Dunn DW, Johnson CS, Perkins SM. Behavioral issues involving children and adolescents with epilepsy and the impact of their families: recent research data. *Epilepsy Behav* 2004; 5 (suppl 3): S33-41.

Avishai-Eliner S, Brunson KL, Sandman CA, Baram TZ. Stressed-out, or in (utero)? *Trends Neurosci* 2002; 25: 518-24.

Baram TZ, Ribak CE. Peptide-induced infant status epilepticus causes neuronal death and synaptic reorganization. *Neuroreport* 1995; 6: 277-80.

Baram TZ, Schultz L. Corticotropin-releasing hormone is a rapid and potent convulsant in the infant rat. *Brain Res Dev Brain Res* 1991; 61: 97-101.

Ben-Ari Y, Tremblay E, Berger M, Nitecka L. Kainic acid seizure syndrome and binding sites in developing rats. *Brain Res* 1984; 316: 284-8.

Bender RA, Dube C, Gonzalez-Vega R, Mina EW, Baram TZ. Mossy fiber plasticity and enhanced hippocampal excitability, without hippocampal cell loss or altered neurogenesis, in an animal model of prolonged febrile seizures. *Hippocampus* 2003; 13: 399-412.

Berg AT, Shinnar S. Complex febrile seizures. *Epilepsia* 1996; 37: 126-33.

Berg AT, Shinnar S, Levy SR, Testa FM. Childhood-onset epilepsy with and without preceding febrile seizures. *Neurology* 1999; 53: 1742-8.

Berg AT, Shinnar S, Testa FM, Levy SR, Frobish D, Smith SN, et al. Status epilepticus after the initial diagnosis of epilepsy in children. *Neurology* 2004; 63: 1027-34.

Blumcke I, Thom M, Wiestler OD. Ammon's horn sclerosis: a maldevelopmental disorder associated with temporal lobe epilepsy. *Brain Pathol* 2002; 12: 199-211.

Bo T, Jiang Y, Cao H, Wang J, Wu X. Long-term effects of seizures in neonatal rats on spatial learning ability and N-methyl-d-aspartate receptor expression in the brain. *Brain Res Dev Brain Res* 2004; 152: 137-42.

Cavalheiro EA, Silva DF, Turski WA, Calderazzo-Filho LS, Bortolotto ZA, Turski L. The susceptibility of rats to pilocarpine-induced seizures is age-dependent. *Dev Brain Res* 1987; 465: 43-58.

Cendes F, Andermann F, Dubeau F, Matthews PM, Arnold DL. Normalization of neuronal metabolic dysfunction after surgery for temporal lobe epilepsy. Evidence from proton MR spectroscopic imaging. *Neurology* 1997; 49: 1525-33.

Chang YC, Huang AM, Kuo YM, Wang ST, Chang YY, Huang CC. Febrile seizures impair memory and cAMP response-element binding protein activation. *Ann Neurol* 2003; 54: 706-18.

Chen K, Baram TZ, Soltesz I. Febrile seizures in the developing brain result in persistent modification of neuronal excitability in limbic circuits. *Nat Med* 1999; 5: 888-94.

Chevassus-au-Louis N, Ben-Ari Y, Vergnes M. Decreased seizure threshold and more rapid rate of kindling in rats with cortical malformation induced by prenatal treatment with methylazoxymethanol. *Brain Res* 1998; 812: 252-5.

Cilio MR, Sogawa Y, Cha BH, Liu X, Huang LT, Holmes GL. Long-term effects of status epilepticus in the immature brain are specific for age and model. *Epilepsia* 2003; 44: 518-28.

Corey LA, Pellock JM, Boggs JG, Miller LL, DeLorenzo RJ. Evidence for a genetic predisposition for status epilepticus. *Neurology* 1998; 50: 558-60.

Da Silva AV, Regondi MC, Spreafico R, Cavalheiro EA. *Neocortical changes induced by repetitive episodes of pilocarpine-induced status epilepticus during postnatal development.* 7th Workshop on the Neurobiology of Epilepsy, 2003.

de Feo MR, Mecarelli O, Palladini G, Ricci GF. Long-term effects of early status epilepticus on the acquisition of conditioned avoidance behavior in rats. *Epilepsia* 1986; 27: 476-82.

de Feo MR, Mecarelli O, Ricci GF. Seizure susceptibility in immature rats with microencephaly induced by prenatal exposure to methylazoxymethanol acetate. *Pharmacol Res* 1995; 31: 109-14.

DeLorenzo RJ, Pellock JM, Towne AR, Boggs JG. Epidemiology of status epilepticus. *J Clin Neurophysiol* 1995; 12: 316-25.

Dobbing J, Sands J. Comparative aspects of the brain growth spurt. *Early Hum Dev* 1979; 3: 79-83.

Dube C, Chen K, Eghbal-Ahmadi M, Brunson K, Soltesz I, Baram TZ. Prolonged febrile seizures in the immature rat model enhance hippocampal excitability long term. *Ann Neurol* 2000; 47: 336-44.

Ellenberg JH, Hirtz DG, Nelson KB. Do seizures in children cause intellectual deterioration? *N Engl J Med* 1986; 314: 1085-8.

Engel Jr. J, Williamson PD, Wieser H-G. Mesial temporal lobe epilepsy. In: Engel Jr. J and Pedley TA, editors. *Epilepsy: A Comprehensive Textbook.* Philadelphia: Lippincot-Raven Publishers, 1997: 2417-26.

Fastenau PS, Shen J, Dunn DW, Perkins SM, Hermann BP, Austin JK. Neuropsychological predictors of academic underachievement in pediatric epilepsy: moderating roles of demographic, seizure, and psychosocial variables. *Epilepsia* 2004; 45: 1261-72.

Germano IM, Sperber EF. Transplacentally induced neuronal migration disorders: an animal model for the study of the epilepsies. *J Neurosci Res* 1998; 51: 473-88.

Germano IM, Sperber EF, Ahuja S, Moshe SL. Evidence of enhanced kindling and hippocampal neuronal injury in immature rats with neuronal migration disorders. *Epilepsia* 1998; 39: 1253-60.

Germano IM, Zhang YF, Sperber EF, Moshe SL. Neuronal migration disorders increase susceptibility to hyperthermia-induced seizures in developing rats. *Epilepsia* 1996; 37: 902-10.

Giorgi FS, Malhotra S, Rosenbaum DM, Moshé SL. Effects of status epilepticus early in life on susceptibility to ischemic injury in adulthood. *Neurology* 2004; 62: A254; abstract # S26.006.

Goddard GV, McIntyre DC, Leech CK. A permanent change in brain function resulting from daily electrical stimulation. *Exp Neurol* 1969; 25: 295-330.

Golden GT, Smith GG, Ferraro TN, Reyes PF. Rat strain and age differences in kainic acid induced seizures. *Epilepsy Res* 1995; 20: 151-9.

Gottlieb A, Keydar I, Epstein HT. Rodent brain growth stages: an analytical review. *Biol Neonate* 1977; 32: 166-76.

Grecksch G, Becker A, Rauca C. Effect of age on pentylenetetrazol-kindling and kindling-induced impairments of learning performance. *Pharmacol Biochem Behav* 1997; 56: 595-601.

Gulec G, Noyan B. Do recurrent febrile convulsions decrease the threshold for pilocarpine-induced seizures? Effects of nitric oxide. *Brain Res Dev Brain Res* 2001; 126: 223-8.

Gurnett CA, Landt M, Wong M. Analysis of cerebrospinal fluid glial fibrillary acidic protein after seizures in children. *Epilepsia* 2003; 44: 1455-8.

Haas KZ, Sperber EF, Opanashuk LA, Stanton PK, Moshe SL. Resistance of immature hippocampus to morphologic and physiologic alterations following status epilepticus or kindling. *Hippocampus* 2001; 11: 615-25.

Hauser W. The prevalence and incidence of convulsive disorders in children. *Epilepsia* 1994; 35: 1-6.

Hauser WA, Anderson VE, Loewenson RB, McRoberts SM. Seizure recurrence after a first unprovoked seizure. *N England J Med* 1982; 307: 522-8.

Haut SR, Veliskova J, Moshe SL. Susceptibility of immature and adult brains to seizure effects. *Lancet Neurol* 2004; 3: 608-17.

Heida JG, Boisse L, Pittman QJ. Lipopolysaccharide-induced febrile convulsions in the rat: short-term sequelae. *Epilepsia* 2004; 45: 1317-29.

Hernandez TD, Warner LA. Kindled seizures during a critical post-lesion period exert a lasting impact on behavioral recovery. *Brain Res* 1995; 673: 208-16.

Hirtz D, Ashwal S, Berg A, Bettis D, Camfield C, Camfield P, *et al*. *Practice parameter: evaluating a first nonfebrile seizure in children*. Report of the quality standards subcommittee of the American Academy of Neurology, The Child Neurology Society, and The American Epilepsy Society. *Neurology* 2000; 55: 616-23.

Hisano T, Ohno M, Egawa T, Takano T, Shimada M. Changes in diffusion-weighted MRI after status epilepticus. *Pediatr Neurol* 2000; 22: 327-9.

Holmes GL. Morphological and physiological maturation of the brain in the neonate and young child. *J Clin Neurophysiol* 1986; 3: 209-38.

Holmes GL, Gairsa JL, Chevassus-Au-Louis N, Ben-Ari Y. Consequences of neonatal seizures in the rat: morphological and behavioral effects. *Ann Neurol* 1998; 44: 845-57.

Holmes GL, McKeever M, Saunders Z. Epileptiform activity in aphasia of childhood: an epiphenomenon? *Epilepsia* 1981; 22: 631-9.

Holmes GL, Sarkisian M, Ben-Ari Y, Chevassus-Au-Louis N. Mossy fiber sprouting after recurrent seizures during early development in rats. *J Comp Neurol* 1999; 404: 537-53.

Holmes GL, Weber DA. Effects of hypoxic-ischemic encephalopathies on kindling in developing animals. *Exp Neurol* 1985; 90: 194-203.

Holtzman D, Obana K, Olson J. Hyperthermia-induced seizures in the rat pup: a model for febrile convulsions in children. *Science* 1981; 213: 1034-6.

Huang LT, Holmes GL, Lai MC, Hung PL, Wang CL, Wang TJ, et al. Maternal deprivation stress exacerbates cognitive deficits in immature rats with recurrent seizures. *Epilepsia* 2002; 43: 1141-8.

Jensen FE, Applegate CD, Holtzman D, Belin TR, Burchfiel JL. Epileptogenic effect of hypoxia in the immature rodent brain. *Ann Neurol* 1991; 29: 629-37.

Jensen FE, Gardner GJ, Williams AP, Gallop PM, Aizenman E, Rosenberg PA. The putative essential nutrient pyrroloquinoline quinone is neuroprotective in a rodent model of hypoxic/ischemic brain injury. *Neuroscience* 1994; 62: 399-406.

Jensen FE, Holmes GL, Lombroso CT, Blume HK, Firkusny IR. Age-dependent changes in long-term seizure susceptibility and behavior after hypoxia in rats. *Epilepsia* 1992; 33: 971-80.

Jensen FE, Wang C. Hypoxia-induced hyperexcitability *in vivo* and *in vitro* in the immature hippocampus. *Epilepsy Res* 1996; 26: 131-40.

Jiang M, Lee CL, Smith KL, Swann JW. Spine loss and other persistent alterations of hippocampal pyramidal cell dendrites in a model of early-onset epilepsy. *J Neurosci* 1998; 18: 8356-68.

Jiang W, Duong TM, de Lanerolle NC. The neuropathology of hyperthermic seizures in the rat. *Epilepsia* 1999; 40: 5-19.

Kanemoto K, Kawasaki J, Miyamoto T, Obayashi H, Nishimura M. Interleukin (IL)1beta, IL-1alpha, and IL-1 receptor antagonist gene polymorphisms in patients with temporal lobe epilepsy. *Ann Neurol* 2000; 47: 571-4.

Kassem-Moussa H, Provenzale JM, Petrella JR, Lewis DV. Early diffusion-weighted MR imaging abnormalities in sustained seizure activity. *AJR Am J Roentgenol* 2000; 174: 1304-6.

Kelly ME, McIntyre DC. Hippocampal kindling protects several structures from the neuronal damage resulting from kainic acid-induced status epilepticus. *Brain Res* 1994; 634: 245-56.

Koh S, Storey TW, Santos TC, Mian AY, Cole AJ. Early-life seizures in rats increase susceptibility to seizure-induced brain injury in adulthood. *Neurology* 1999; 53: 915-21.

Koh S, Storey TW, Santos TC, Mian AY, Cole AJ. Early-life seizures in rats increase susceptibility to seizure-induced brain injury in adulthood. 1999. *Neurology* 2001; 57: S22-8.

Kondratyev A, Sahibzada N, Gale K. Electroconvulsive shock exposure prevents neuronal apoptosis after kainic acid-evoked status epilepticus. *Brain Res Mol Brain Res* 2001; 91: 1-13.

Kubova H, Druga R, Lukasiuk K, Suchomelova L, Haugvicova R, Jirmanova I, et al. Status epilepticus causes necrotic damage in the mediodorsal nucleus of the thalamus in immature rats. *J Neurosci* 2001; 21: 3593-9.

Lee CL, Hannay J, Hrachovy R, Rashid S, Antalffy B, Swann JW. Spatial learning deficits without hippocampal neuronal loss in a model of early-onset epilepsy. *Neuroscience* 2001; 107: 71-84.

Lee CL, Hrachovy RA, Smith KL, Frost JD, Jr., Swann JW. Tetanus toxin-induced seizures in infant rats and their effects on hippocampal excitability in adulthood. *Brain Res* 1995; 677: 97-109.

Lee SH, Han SH, Lee KW. Kainic acid-induced seizures cause neuronal death in infant rats pretreated with lipopolysaccharide. *Neuroreport* 2000; 11: 507-10.

Lewis DV, Barboriak DP, MacFall JR, Provenzale JM, Mitchell TV, VanLandingham KE. Do prolonged febrile seizures produce medial temporal sclerosis? Hypotheses, MRI evidence and unanswered questions. *Prog Brain Res* 2002; 135: 263-78.

Liebregts MT, McLachlan RS, Leung LS. Hyperthermia induces age-dependent changes in rat hippocampal excitability. *Ann Neurol* 2002; 52: 318-26.

Liu X, Muller RU, Huang LT, Kubie JL, Rotenberg A, Rivard B, et al. Seizure-induced changes in place cell physiology: relationship to spatial memory. *J Neurosci* 2003; 23: 11505-15.

Liu Z, Yang Y, Silveira DC, Sarkisian MR, Tandon P, Huang LT, et al. Consequences of recurrent seizures during early brain development. *Neuroscience* 1999; 92: 1443-54.

Lynch M, Sayin U, Bownds J, Janumpalli S, Sutula T. Long-term consequences of early postnatal seizures on hippocampal learning and plasticity. *Eur J Neurosci* 2000; 12: 2252-64.

Mathern GW, Adelson PD, Cahan LD, Leite JP. Hippocampal neuron damage in human epilepsy: Meyer's hypothesis revisited. *Prog Brain Res* 2002; 135: 237-51.

Maytal J, Shinnar S, Moshe SL, Alvarez LA. Low morbidity and mortality of status epilepticus in children. *Pediatrics* 1989; 83: 323-31.

McCabe BK, Silveira DC, Cilio MR, Cha BH, Liu X, Sogawa Y, et al. Reduced neurogenesis after neonatal seizures. *J Neurosci* 2001; 21: 2094-103.

McCaughran JA, Jr., Schechter N. Experimental febrile convulsions: long-term effects of hyperthermia-induced convulsions in the developing rat. *Epilepsia* 1982; 23: 173-83.

Mellanby J, George G. Tetanus toxin and experimental epilepsy in rats. *Adv Cytopharmacol* 1979; 3: 401-8.

Moshé SL. Epileptogenesis and the immature brain. *Epilepsia* 1987; 28 (suppl): S3-S15.

Moshé SL. Ontogeny of seizures and substantia nigra modulation. In: Kellaway P and Noebels JF, eds. *Problems and concepts in developmental neurophysiology*. Baltimore: Johns Hopkins Press, 1989: 247-62.

Moshé SL, Albala BJ. Kindling in developing rats: persistence of seizures into adulthood. *Dev Brain Res* 1982; 4: 67-71.

Moshé SL, Albala BJ. Perinatal hypoxia and subsequent development of seizures. *Physiol Behav* 1985; 35: 819-23.

Moshé SL, Garant DS, Sperber EF, Velísková J, Kubová H, Brown LL. Ontogeny and topography of seizure regulation by the substantia nigra. *Brain & Development* 1995.

Nehlig A. Cerebral energy metabolism, glucose transport and blood flow: changes with maturation and adaptation to hypoglycaemia. *Diabetes Metab* 1997; 23: 18-29.

Nehlig A, de Vasconselos AP. The model of pentylenetetrazol-induced status epilepticus in the immature rat: short- and long-term effects. *Epilepsy Res.* 1996; 26: 93-103.

Neill JC, Liu Z, Sarkisian M, Tandon P, Yang Y, Stafstrom CE, et al. Recurrent seizures in immature rats: effect on auditory and visual discrimination. *Brain Res Dev Brain Res* 1996; 95: 283-92.

Nelson KB, Ellenberg JH. Prognosis in children with febrile seizures. *Pediatrics* 1978; 61: 720-7.

Nunes ML, Liptakova S, Veliskova J, Sperber EF, Moshe SL. Malnutrition increases dentate granule cell proliferation in immature rats after status epilepticus. *Epilepsia* 2000; 41 (suppl 6): S48-52.

Ojeda SR, Urbanski HF. Puberty in the rat. In: Knobil E and Neil J, ed. *The Physiology of Reproduction*. Vol. 2. New York: Raven Press, Ltd., 1994: 363-409.

Okada R, Moshé SL, Albala BJ. Infantile status epilepticus and future seizure susceptibility in the rat. *Dev Brain Res* 1984; 15: 177-83.

Olson JE, Horne DS, Holtzman D, Miller M. Hyperthermia-induced seizures in rat pups with preexisting ischemic brain injury. *Epilepsia* 1985; 26: 360-4.

Oostrom KJ, Smeets-Schouten A, Kruitwagen CL, Peters AC, Jennekens-Schinkel A. Not only a matter of epilepsy: early problems of cognition and behavior in children with "epilepsy only" – a prospective, longitudinal, controlled study starting at diagnosis. *Pediatrics* 2003; 112: 1338-44.

Pagnin D, de Queiroz V, Pini S, Cassano GB. Efficacy of ECT in depression: a meta-analytic review. *J Ect* 2004; 20: 13-20.

Park YD, Allison JD, Weiss KL, Smith JR, Lee MR, King DW. Proton magnetic resonance spectroscopic observations of epilepsia partialis continua in children. *J Child Neurol* 2000; 15: 729-33.

Priel MR, dos Santos NF, Cavalheiro EA. Developmental aspects of the pilocarpine model of epilepsy. *Epilepsy Res* 1996; 26: 115-21.

Proceedings of the American Epilepsy Society Course. Status epilepticus. Philadelphia, Pennsylvania, December 1991. *Epilepsia* 1993; 34 (suppl 1): S1-81.

Recommendations of the Epilepsy Foundation of America's Working Group on Status Epilepticus. Treatment of convulsive status epilepticus. JAMA 1993b; 270: 854-9.

Ribak CE, Baram TZ. Selective death of hippocampal CA3 pyramidal cells with mossy fiber afferents after CRH-induced status epilepticus in infant rats. *Brain Res Dev Brain Res* 1996; 91: 245-51.

Riviello P, de Rogalski Landrot I, Holmes GL. Lack of cell loss following recurrent neonatal seizures. *Dev Brain Res* 2002; 135: 101-4.

Rizzi M, Perego C, Aliprandi M, Richichi C, Ravizza T, Colella D, et al. Glia activation and cytokine increase in rat hippocampus by kainic acid-induced status epilepticus during postnatal development. *Neurobiol Dis* 2003; 14: 494-503.

Roch C, Leroy C, Nehlig A, Namer IJ. Predictive value of cortical injury for the development of temporal lobe epilepsy in 21-day-old rats: an MRI approach using the lithium-pilocarpine model. *Epilepsia* 2002; 43: 1129-36.

Sankar R, Shin D, Mazarati AM, Liu H, Wasterlain CG. Ontogeny of self-sustaining status epilepticus. *Developmental Neuroscience* 1999; 21: 345-51.

Sankar R, Shin DH, Liu H, Mazarati A, Pereira de Vasconcelos A, Wasterlain CG. Patterns of status epilepticus-induced neuronal injury during development and long-term consequences. *J Neurosci* 1998; 18: 8382-93.

Santos NF, Marques RH, Correia L, Sinigaglia-Coimbra R, Calderazzo L, Sanabria ER, et al. Multiple pilocarpine-induced status epilepticus in developing rats: a long-term behavioral and electrophysiological study. *Epilepsia* 2000; 41 (suppl 6): S57-63.

Sarkisian MR, Tandon P, Liu Z, Yang Y, Hori A, Holmes GL, et al. Multiple kainic acid seizures in the immature and adult brain: ictal manifestations and long-term effects on learning and memory. *Epilepsia* 1997; 38: 1157-66.

Scantlebury MH, Ouellet PL, Psarropoulou C, Carmant L. Freeze lesion-induced focal cortical dysplasia predisposes to atypical hyperthermic seizures in the immature rat. *Epilepsia* 2004; 45: 592-600.

Setkowicz Z, Janeczko K. Long-term changes in susceptibility to pilocarpine-induced status epilepticus following neocortical injuries in the rat at different developmental stages. *Epilepsy Res* 2003; 53: 216-24.

Shinnar S. Do febrile seizures lead to temporal lobe epilepsy? Prospective and epidemiological studies. *Febrile seizures*. San Diego: Academic Press, 2002: xxiii, 337.

Shinnar S. Febrile Seizures and Mesial Temporal Sclerosis. *Epilepsy Curr* 2003; 3: 115-8.

Shinnar S, Babb T. Long-term sequelae of status epilepticus. Engel J Jr, Pedley TA ed. *Epilepsy: a comprehensive textbook*. Philadelphia: Lippincott-Raven, 1997: 755-63.

Shinnar S, Berg AT, Moshe SL, O'Dell C, Alemany M, Newstein D, et al. The risk of seizure recurrence after a first unprovoked afebrile seizure in childhood: an extended follow-up. *Pediatrics* 1996; 98: 216-25.

Shinnar S, Berg AT, Moshe SL, Shinnar R. How long do new-onset seizures in children last? *Ann Neurol* 2001a; 49: 659-64.

Shinnar S, Hauser W. Do occasional brief seizures cause detectable clinical consequences? Vol. 135, 2002.

Shinnar S, O'Dell C, Mitnick R, Berg AT, Moshe SL. Neuroimaging abnormalities in children with an apparent first unprovoked seizure. *Epilepsy Res* 2001b; 43: 261-9.

Shinnar S, Pellock JM, Moshe SL, Maytal J, O'Dell C, Driscoll SM, et al. In whom does status epilepticus occur: age-related differences in children. *Epilepsia* 1997; 38: 907-14.

Sillanpaa M, Shinnar S. Status epilepticus in a population-based cohort with childhood-onset epilepsy in Finland. *Ann Neurol* 2002; 52: 303-10.

Sisodiya SM. Malformations of cortical development: burdens and insights from important causes of human epilepsy. *Lancet Neurol* 2004; 3: 29-38.

Smith KL, Lee CL, Swann JW. Local circuit abnormalities in chronically epileptic rats after intrahippocampal tetanus toxin injection in infancy. *J Neurophysiol* 1998; 79: 106-16.

Sogawa Y, Monokoshi M, Silveira DC, Cha BH, Cilio MR, McCabe BK, *et al.* Timing of cognitive deficits following neonatal seizures: relationship to histological changes in the hippocampus. *Brain Res Dev Brain Res* 2001; 131: 73-83.

Sperber EF, Haas KZ, Romero MT, Stanton PK. Flurothyl status epilepticus in developing rats: behavioral, electrographic histological and electrophysiological studies. *Brain Res Dev Brain Res* 1999; 116: 59-68.

Sperber EF, Haas KZ, Stanton PK, Moshe SL. Resistance of the immature hippocampus to seizure-induced synaptic reorganization. *Dev Brain Res* 1991; 60: 88-93.

Stafstrom CE, Sasaki-Adams DM. NMDA-induced seizures in developing rats cause long-term learning impairment and increased seizure susceptibility. *Epilepsy Res* 2003; 53: 129-37.

Stafstrom CE, Thompson JL, Holmes GL. Kainic acid seizures in the developing brain: status epilepticus and spontaneous recurrent seizures. *Dev Brain Res* 1992; 65: 227-36.

Stogmann E, Zimprich A, Baumgartner C, Aull-Watschinger S, Hollt V, Zimprich F. A functional polymorphism in the prodynorphin gene promotor is associated with temporal lobe epilepsy. *Ann Neurol* 2002; 51: 260-3.

Sutula TP, Hagen J, Pitkanen A. Do epileptic seizures damage the brain? *Curr Opin Neurol* 2003; 16: 189-95.

Sutula TP, Hermann B. Progression in mesial temporal lobe epilepsy. *Ann Neurol* 1999; 45: 553-6.

Swann JW, Moshé SL. Developmental issues in animal models. In: Engel Jr. J and Pedley TA, ed. *Epilepsy: A Comprehensive Textbook*. Philadelphia: Lippincott-Raven Publishers, 1997: 467-80.

Tancredi V, D'Arcangelo G, Zona C, Siniscalchi A, Avoli M. Induction of epileptiform activity by temperature elevation in hippocampal slices from young rats: an *in vitro* model for febrile seizures? *Epilepsia* 1992; 33: 228-34.

Thom M, Sisodiya SM, Beckett A, Martinian L, Lin WR, Harkness W, *et al.* Cytoarchitectural abnormalities in hippocampal sclerosis. *J Neuropathol Exp Neurol* 2002; 61: 510-9.

Thompson K, Holm AM, Schousboe A, Popper P, Micevych P, Wasterlain C. Hippocampal stimulation produces neuronal death in the immature brain. *Neuroscience* 1998; 82: 337-48.

Toth Z, Yan XX, Haftoglou S, Ribak CE, Baram TZ. Seizure-induced neuronal injury: vulnerability to febrile seizures in an immature rat model. *J Neurosci* 1998; 18: 4285-94.

Towfighi J, Housman C, Mauger D, Vannucci RC. Effect of seizures on cerebral hypoxic-ischemic lesions in immature rats. *Brain Res Dev Brain Res* 1999; 113: 83-95.

Tremblay E, Nitecka L, Berger ML, Ben-Ari Y. Maturation of kainic acid seizure-brain damage syndrome in the rat. I. Clinical, electrographic and metabolic observations. *Neuroscience* 1984; 13: 1051-72.

VanLandingham KE, Heinz ER, Cavazos JE, Lewis DV. Magnetic resonance imaging evidence of hippocampal injury after prolonged focal febrile convulsions. *Ann Neurol* 1998; 43: 413-26.

Velisek L, Moshe SL. Effects of brief seizures during development. *Prog Brain Res* 2002; 135: 355-64.

Velísková J, Velísek L, Mares P. Epileptic phenomena produced by kainic acid in laboratory rats during ontogenesis. *Physiol Bohemoslov* 1988; 37: 395-405.

Vezzani A, Moneta D, Conti M, Richichi C, Ravizza T, De Luigi A, *et al.* Powerful anticonvulsant action of IL-1 receptor antagonist on intracerebral injection and astrocytic overexpression in mice. *Proc Natl Acad Sci USA* 2000; 97: 11534-9.

Villeneuve N, Ben-Ari Y, Holmes GL, Gaiarsa JL. Neonatal seizures induced persistent changes in intrinsic properties of CA1 rat hippocampal cells. *Ann Neurol* 2000; 47: 729-38.

Wasterlain CG. Neonatal seizures and brain growth. *Neuropadiatrie* 1978; 9: 213-28.

Wasterlain CG, Niquet J, Thompson KW, Baldwin R, Liu H, Sankar R, *et al.* Seizure-induced neuronal death in the immature brain. *Prog Brain Res* 2002; 135: 335-53.

Watts AE, Hicks GA, Henderson G. Putative pre- and postsynaptic ATP-sensitive potassium channels in the rat substantia nigra *in vitro*. *J Neurosci* 1995; 15: 3065-74.

Wieser HG. ILAE Commission Report. Mesial temporal lobe epilepsy with hippocampal sclerosis. *Epilepsia* 2004; 45: 695-714.

Williams PA, Dou P, Dudek FE. Epilepsy and synaptic reorganization in a perinatal rat model of hypoxia-ischemia. *Epilepsia* 2004; 45: 1210-8.

Wirrell EC, Armstrong EA, Osman LD, Yager JY. Prolonged seizures exacerbate perinatal hypoxic-ischemic brain damage. *Pediatr Res* 2001; 50: 445-54.

Yager JY, Armstrong EA, Miyashita H, Wirrell EC. Prolonged neonatal seizures exacerbate hypoxic-ischemic brain damage: correlation with cerebral energy metabolism and excitatory amino acid release. *Dev Neurosci* 2002; 24: 367-81.

Yang SN, Huang CB, Yang CH, Lai MC, Chen WF, Wang CL, et al. Impaired SynGAP expression and long-term spatial learning and memory in hippocampal CA1 area from rats previously exposed to perinatal hypoxia-induced insults: beneficial effects of A68930. *Neurosci Lett* 2004; 371: 73-8.

Yang Y, Tandon P, Liu Z, Sarkisian MR, Stafstrom CE, Holmes GL. Synaptic reorganization following kainic acid-induced seizures during development. *Dev Brain Res* 1998; 107: 169-77.

Zhang X, Cui SS, Wallace AE, Hannesson DK, Schmued LC, Saucier DM, et al. Relations between brain pathology and temporal lobe epilepsy. *J Neurosci* 2002; 22: 6052-61.

# Does epileptic activity influence speech organization in temporal lobe epilepsy?

J. Janszky[1,2], A. Ebner[2], M. Mertens[2], C. Gyimesi[1], H. Jokeit[2], F.G. Woermann[2]

[1] *Department of Neurology, University of Pécs, Pécs, Hungary*
[2] *Epilepsy Center Bethel, Bielefeld, Germany*

## ■ Two types of epileptic activity: interictal and ictal epileptic activity

The term "epileptic activity" is not a well-defined entity. Epilepsy is characterized by interictal and ictal epileptic disturbances. For many years it has been hypothesized that the temporal summation and spatial spread of *interictal* epileptiform discharges (IED) may evolve to *ictal* discharges resulting in electroclinical seizure (Ralston et al., 1958). Recent studies, however, indicate that there is no such causal relationship between IED and seizures and interictal spiking does not increase prior to seizures (Katz et al., 1991). IED may represent decreased seizure susceptibility (Engel and Ackermann, 1980), and may inhibit the expression of seizures (Librizzi and de Curtis, 2003). Moreover, IED frequency is the highest immediately after the seizures (Gotman and Marciani, 1985). The region of the seizure activity is mirrored to the following IED activity (Janszky et al., 2001). These data indicate a negative feedback mechanism between IED and seizures: seizures induce the IED, while IED inhibit the seizures (Janszky and Ebner, 2002).

## ■ The effect of epileptic activity on cognitive functions

Cognitive disturbances in epilepsy are multicausal. The etiological factors, for example underlying genetic disorders or the underlying epileptogenic lesion obviously have an influence on the neuropsychological performance of epileptic patients (Helmstedter and Kurthen, 2001). Antiepileptic drugs and concomitant psychiatric complications may also interfere with the cognitive performance (see corresponding chapters in this volume). Thus, the investigation of the cognitive effect of epileptic activity itself independent of other disturbing factors may prove difficult. The acute effect of seizures or interictal activity on memory or speech functions can be more easily investigated than the long-term neuropsychological consequences. A more accurate investigation of the chronic effects of epileptic activities on cognition requires longitudinal studies over decades and should also consider that the effect of drugs and some epileptic lesions (for example the hippocampal sclerosis), as well as psychiatric disorders may also undergo progression over time. Thus, until now only cross-sectional, retrospective studies have been available, having investigated the chronic cognitive effects of epileptic activity.

## Effect of ictal activity on the cognitive functions

Experimentally evoked repeated seizures induce a long-term spatial memory deficit in rats (Lynch et al., 2000). Some data concerning human epilepsy suggests that temporal lobe seizures had short-term, and probably also long-term, effects on human memory functions (Kapur et al., 1989). In a prospective study, Jokeit et al. (2001b) tested patients with intractable temporal lobe epilepsy (TLE) by giving them verbal memory tasks every 24 hours during video-EEG monitoring. The retrieval performance was tested 30 minutes and 24 hours after the initial learning phase. Patients who had left-sided seizures between the initial learning phase and the 24-hour retrieval had significantly impaired performance. Another study investigated the role of ictal activity in a simple short-term memory test: whether patients can remember their auras during the video-EEG monitoring. This study found that patients who forget their auras usually have bilateral seizure activity, thus, we can suppose that bilateral epileptiform activity impairs memory production not only ipsilaterally but also contralaterally to the seizure onset (Schulz et al., 2001).

Not just the memory functions, but even the speech functions and their brain representation may directly be influenced by seizures. Left temporal lobe seizures cause ictal and postictal speech disturbances in 75% of patients (Gabr et al., 1989), suggesting that temporal-lobe seizures at least transiently disturb speech production. Jayakar et al. (2002) reported the case of a 14-year-old child in whom, after a cluster of left temporal lobe seizures, the language-activated functional magnetic resonance imaging (fMRI) using four different tasks suggested a right temporal receptive speech area. At the time of the investigation the patient showed no aphasic symptoms. Two weeks later when the patient had an usual seizure frequency, the fMRI using the same tasks was repeated and revealed a left temporal receptive speech area.

## Effect of interictal activity on the cognitive functions

As we pointed out, seizures and the interictal activity are two different pathophysiological phenomena. Not only the seizures, however, but also the interictal epileptiform activity may disturb higher cognitive functions. Frequent interictal activity propagating to the speech centers may cause speech disturbances as seen in acquired epileptic aphasia (Landau-Kleffner syndrome) where continuous bilateral epileptic activity results in perceptive speech disturbance or even in complete aphasia in those children who have already developed speech before the onset of the disorder (Landau and Kleffner, 1957). In this syndrome, language deterioration occurs despite good seizure control and is thought to be related to the interictal epileptiform activity involving the posterior part of temporal lobes (Shinnar and Hauser, 2002). Aarts et al. (1984) found that frequent IED resulted in transient cognitive impairment (TCI) in epilepsy patients, while such impairment was not present in those periods when no interictal epileptiform activity appeared during neuropsychological testing. Moreover, impairment of non-verbal spatial task performance was demonstrated during right-sided interictal discharges, while during left-sided paroxysms, the verbal cognitive performance was disturbed. This suggests that the cognitive impairment caused by IED is specific and reflects the functional disturbance of the area where the spikes originate. Some patients are clearly handicapped by TCI and their functioning improves when the IED were suppressed by medication (Aarts et al., 1984). Thus, it is reasonable to assume that chronic, frequent IED may cause long-term localized neuropsychological deficits. Conversely, in another study, Aldenkamp and coworkers (1996) analyzed the relationship between focal or generalized IED and cognitive functions and found that neither in patients with seizures under antiepileptic treatment nor in seizure-free patients having IED could any TCI be detected. They assume that the TCI occurs infrequently in epilepsy.

We suggest that wether TCI plays a crucial role in cognitive deficit of epilepsy or not, the interictal epileptic disturbance may influence the organization of cognitive functions even if they are not detectable by clinical testing. The interictal PET shows a hypometabolism around the epileptic focus which extends beyond the epileptogenic lesion or the epileptic region. Recent studies indicate that this hypometabolism may be related to a disturbance caused by ictal (Savic et al., 1997; Schlaug et al., 1997, Chassoux et al., 2004) or interictal epileptic activity (Hong et al., 2002). Thus, it is reasonable to assume that the cognitive functions linked to hypofunctional areas may undergo a long-term contralateral reorganization.

In recent studies we investigated patients with TLE by memory-activated fMRI. We found that the fMRI-lateralization of mesiotemporal visuospatial memory functions in MTLE-HS patients is asymmetric: the larger activation usually appears contralateral to the side of the epileptogenic region, suggesting that the representation of certain memory functions may undergo a reorganization in the presence of unilateral epileptic activity (Jokeit et al., 2001a). On the other hand, in patients with *bilateral* independent epileptiform discharges, this type of asymmetry was significantly less frequent (Janszky et al., 2004). Similar to our findings, in patients with bilateral epileptiform (ictal or interictal) activity, the Wada test does not show lateralization of the epileptogenic region (Benbadis et al., 1995). This data suggests that bilateral interictal and ictal activity may influence the memory functions and their organization, or they can prevent the contralateral reorganization of memory (Janszky et al., 2004).

## Lateralization of speech functions

The lateralization of speech functions is the most conspicuous phenomenon indicating that the two hemispheres of our brain are not equivalent and have different functions. There is a lot of data showing that this lateralization difference is prepogammed and already starts in the postnatal period. Both the executive speech region

(Broca's area) (Foundas et al., 1996) and perceptive secondary auditory centres (planum temporale) (Geschwind and Levitsky, 1968) show a morphological asymmetry in comparison with the contralateral homologous brain regions in favour of the left side. This asymmetry is already present in the last gestational trimester (Wada et al., 1975) and shows no change with increasing age, suggesting that the left-right functional differentiation follows a structural asymmetry that is already "preset" (Geschwind and Levitsky, 1968). Human non-speech sounds, e.g. baby babbling (Holowka and Petitto, 2002) or non-verbal vocalizations in frontal lobe seizures (Janszky et al., 2000) may also be related to the left hemisphere, suggesting that not only speech, but vocalization at a subverbal level independent of age is also a product of the left hemisphere in humans. Moreover, the lateralization of sound production is not a human-specific phenomenon; subhuman vertebrates appear to have left-hemisphere dominance of vocal productions (Walker, 1980). Others suggest that the left-right functional asymmetry is already present at the prelanguage age in infants, i.e. the left hemisphere is specialised in the temporal modality of a given stimulus while the right hemisphere in the spatial modality, which difference is the functional basis as to why language becomes confined to the left hemisphere (Witelson, 1987). Indeed, Dehaene-Lambertz et al. (2002) found that precursors of adult cortical language areas are already active in infants well before the onset of speech production. They investigated 3-month-old infants by using fMRI activated by speech perception. They found that, similar to those of adults, the left-lateralised brain regions, including the superior temporal and angular gyri, were already active in infants during speech perception.

Despite this strong left-sided predispostion of the brain morphology and function, Chiron et al. (1997) suggested that the right hemisphere might be still the dominant one until age 3 considering the Broca and Broca-homologous areas, sensomotor cortex and the temporoposterior regions; after age 3 a shift towards left hemispheric dominance begins (Rasmussen and Milner, 1977; Marcotte and Morere, 1990). Most studies suggest that this process may be completed at age 4-8 (Rasmussen and Milner, 1977; Hecaen, 1976; Balsamo et al., 2002). However, Gaillard et al. (2000) found that even children aged 8-12 years showed significantly more right-hemispheric participation in speech production than adults. Thus, the participation of the right hemisphere in speech functions gradually decreases over time, but the role of the right hemispheric homologue brain areas is unclear in adolescence or adulthood because the fMRI studies revealed that a significant right-sided activity is present during speech functions even in normal adults (Springer et al., 1999).

## ■ The effect of lesion on speech lateralization

Left-sided lesions may cause contralateral speech reorganization (Rasmussen and Milner, 1977). In the past years, many studies investigated speech lateralization in epilepsy patients (Rasmussen and Milner, 1977; Rausch and Walsh, 1984; Woods et al., 1988; Rey et al., 1988; Helmstaedter et al., 1997; Springer et al., 1999). The drawback of all these studies is that they included a mixed population of epileptic patients and not a circumscribed epilepsy syndrome. Consequently, in such populations, the different type of disturbances cannot be adequately investigated and separated from each other, *i.e.* the influence of age, localization, lateralization of the lesion and the epileptic activity itself. Investigating a "mixed" population may strongly influence our thinking regarding speech organization in a false direction. For many years, *e.g.* it was believed that men had a stronger left-sided speech lateralization than women (McGlone, 1977). However, Kertész and Sheppard (1981) pointed out that this belief was due to the investigation of non-homogeneous populations. Indeed, most recent studies have not confirmed that men and women have a significant difference in speech lateralization (Frost *et al.*, 1999; Springer *et al.*, 1999).

Although some memory disturbances caused by epilepsy can be experimentally modelled in animals (Kotloski *et al.*, 2002), it is impossible to investigate speech in experimental models, as language is a unique human ability, the main basis for communication, human thinking and self-consciousness (Popper and Eccles, 1977). For this reason, we should look for an epilepsy population which is as homogenous as possible with the same lesions in the same structure where the time at the occurrence of the lesion and the onset of epilepsy is not different, in order to investigate not only the lesional factors but also the influence of epileptic activity.

## ■ Mesial temporal lobe epilepsy with hippocampal sclerosis: the "human model" for focal epilepsy

Concerning the most frequent epileptogenic lesions, only three such "natural human epilepsy" models could be considered: a homogenous population with childhood head traumatic or ischemic lesions in a common localization or the syndrome of mesial TLE with hippocampal sclerosis (MTLE-HS). Since patients of the first two kinds of populations are relatively rare and are often not drug-resistant, such patients rarely undergo presurgical evaluation. To create a "natural model" from posttraumatic or post-stroke epilepsy with an adequate number of patients is almost impossible. For these reasons, in our studies assessing the role of epileptic activity in speech lateralization described below, we investigated patients with video-EEG proved MTLE and HS based on MRI findings. In MTLE-HS, the seizure onset region is localised to the mesiotemporal structures, thus, it is a unique, homogenous epilepsy syndrome (Wieser *et al.*, 2004). Moreover it is the most frequent chronic focal epilepsy. Human and experimental data suggest that the cause of hippocampal sclerosis (HS) is due to an initial precipitating injury (IPI) occurring in early childhood or infancy, which induces functional and structural damage to the hippocampus gradually evolving to HS (Mathern *et al.*, 1995; Maher *et al.*, 1995; Toth *et al.*, 1998; Chen *et al.*, 1999). The factors that influence speech reorganization can be investigated in MTLE-HS since these patients have the same pathology in the same location and this pathology is located far away from the eloquent speech areas. In addition, the influence of the timing of the brain damage (*i.e.* IPI) can also be evaluated separately from the other timing factors, *e.g.* onset of non-febrile seizures. By evaluating a homogenous epilepsy population, we were able to investigate the effect of epileptic activity on speech organization separately from the lesion effects.

## Investigating the chronic effect of epileptic activity on language lateralization in MTLE-HS

In order to investigate the chronic effect of interictal and ictal activity on speech representation, we have recently conducted two cross-sectional studies.

In the first study we investigated 100 patients with MTLE-HS. All patients underwent comprehensive presurgical evaluation. Of 100 patients, left-sided speech occurred in 76% of the left-sided and in 100% of the right-sided MTLE-HS patients ($p < 0.05$). For further evaluation, we included only the 83 left-sided MTLE-HS patients. Based on the Wada test, we categorized patients into two groups: patients with left-sided and patients with atypical (right-sided or bilateral) speech representation. Left-sided speech was present in 63 patients, while in 20 (24%) patients the Wada test revealed atypical speech dominance. In this study, we found that atypical speech representation in left MTLE-HS was associated with higher spiking frequency ($p < 0.05$) (*Figure 1*). Spikes in MTLE-HS are generated in the mesiotemporal structures. However, 10-50% of them propagate to the lateral temporal neocortex (Niedermeyer and Rocca, 1972; Alarcon et al., 1994; Clemens et al., 2003). Since we did not use intracranial electrodes in this study, the spike frequency was related to the degree of the interictal epileptic involvement of the temporal neocortex. Thus, our findings indicate that even the interictal epileptic activity may interfere with the functions of the temporal speech receptive areas.

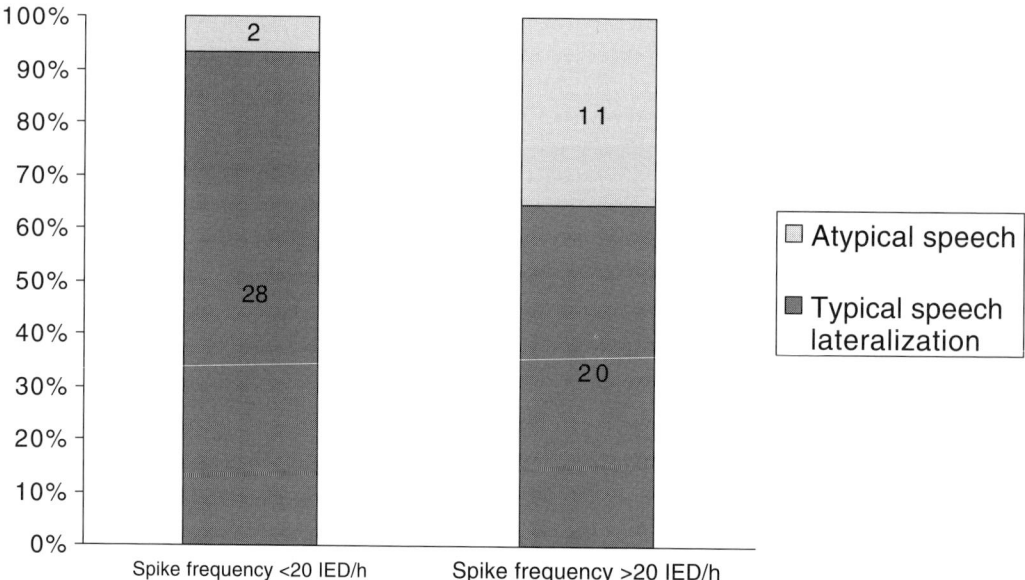

**Figure 1. Wada test study.**
Patients below *vs* above the median spike frequency: higher spike frequency is associated with atypical speech confirmed by Wada test (considering the categorization represented on this figure, this difference was highly significant ($p < 0.01$)

Another result of this study was that seizure spread had an influence on speech organization in epilepsy. Namely, sensory auras typically representing a temporo-posterior seizure involvement (Ebner, 1994; Wunderlich et al., 2000) were associated with atypical speech in left MTLE-HS (p < 0.01), indicating that seizures may cause a long-term functional disturbance in the left auditory/speech receptive region and may induce contralateral speech reorganization. On the other hand, seizure spread probably not involving the lateral neocortical regions, but rather limbic structures (complex partial seizures with psychic auras, such as affective or mnestic auras), was associated with left-sided speech (p < 0.05). *Figure 2* represents the differences for speech representation in patients with psychic or sensory auras.

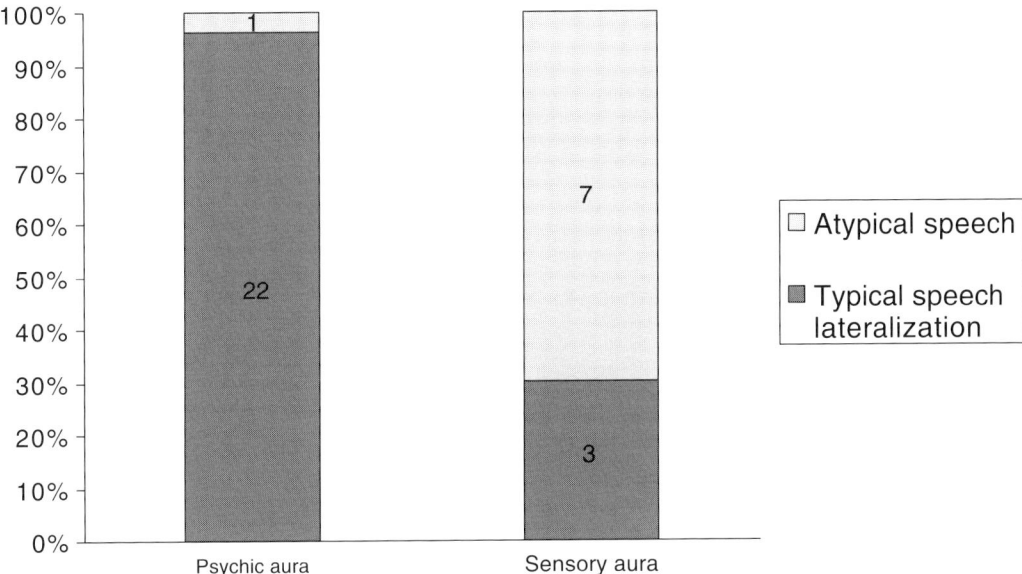

**Figure 2. Wada test study.**
Psychic auras representing a temporo-medial limbic seizure spread are associated with typical language lateralization. Sensory (auditory, vertigous, somatosensory) auras representing temporo-lateral seizure spread are associated with atypical speech confirmed by Wada test.

Conclusively, in this study, we found that in patients with focal epilepsy, not only the known factors, *i.e.* the age at which the brain injury occurred and its localization, but also the epileptic activity itself, *i.e.* interictal discharges and seizure spread – may influence speech reorganization. Our findings also suggest that not only structural elements but also the functional factors have an effect on the language organization of the brain.

The Wada test is an invasive procedure and crossflow to the opposite anterior cerebral artery may also influence the clinical effects. Thus, by using the Wada test we can investigate only a minority of selected patients. On the other hand, fMRI is a safe non-invasive procedure; we can investigate patients consecutively and we can analyze the speech lateralization as a continuous phenomenon, which may be much closer to the biological reality than the categorical division used by the Wada test. The fundamental methodological difference between the Wada test and speech-activated fMRI is that the former is a method based on inhibition, while the latter is a tool based on the activation of investigated structures. Thus, we decided to reproduce our findings in a new series of patients by using a new investigation method: the speech-activated fMRI.

In this fMRI study we also investigated whether the interictal epileptic activity could be responsible for the evolution of atypical speech and whether this effect is independent of other known factors. As in our previous study, we investigated 28 patients with left-sided MTLE-HS. We used a verbal fluency paradigm of covertly producing words starting with certain letters. A low level reference condition of resting inactivity was chosen (Woermann et al. 2003). Activation volumes were determined in each subject by counting the significantly activated voxels in the lateral three-fourths of each hemisphere.

For each subject we calculated an asymmetry index (AI) to characterize the speech lateralization:

**AI = (activated voxels on the left − activated voxels on the right)/all activated voxels.**

Thus, positive values indicate that the activation is more pronounced on the left than on the right side.

We investigated the relationship between speech lateralization (characterized by AI) and IED frequency, controlling the other factors that may also play a role in speech lateralization [age at epilepsy onset, gender, age, seizure frequency, Wechsler IQ, and age at initial precipitating injury (IPI)]. We found that only the IED frequency had a statistically significant association with the AI ($p = 0.002$, *Figure 3*), while the other factors did not show such an association.

## ■ Plasticity of language organization and the possible role of epileptic activity in inducing atypical speech representation

Surprisingly, in our studies neither the age at the presumed brain injury, i.e. IPI, nor the age at epilepsy onset was correlated with atypical speech representation in left MTLE. These findings may be a result of a bias for the age at IPI and development of HS in early childhood (Sagar and Oxbury, 1987). Indeed, in our study most IPIs occurred before age 3 and only one patient had a history of IPI after age 3, i.e. almost all known IPIs of our patients occurred at an age when brain plasticity certainly allows for a left-right shift of speech centers. Thus the age effect of brain injury is not pronounced in MTLE because all brain injuries occur at the age of maximal brain plasticity. The question is: Why didn't all patients have a left-right speech shift due to the early brain injury? In other words, is it theoretically possible that beyond the time and localization of brain injury, the epileptic activity is a third, independent factor which is capable of inducing speech reorganization after an early brain injury affecting the left side?

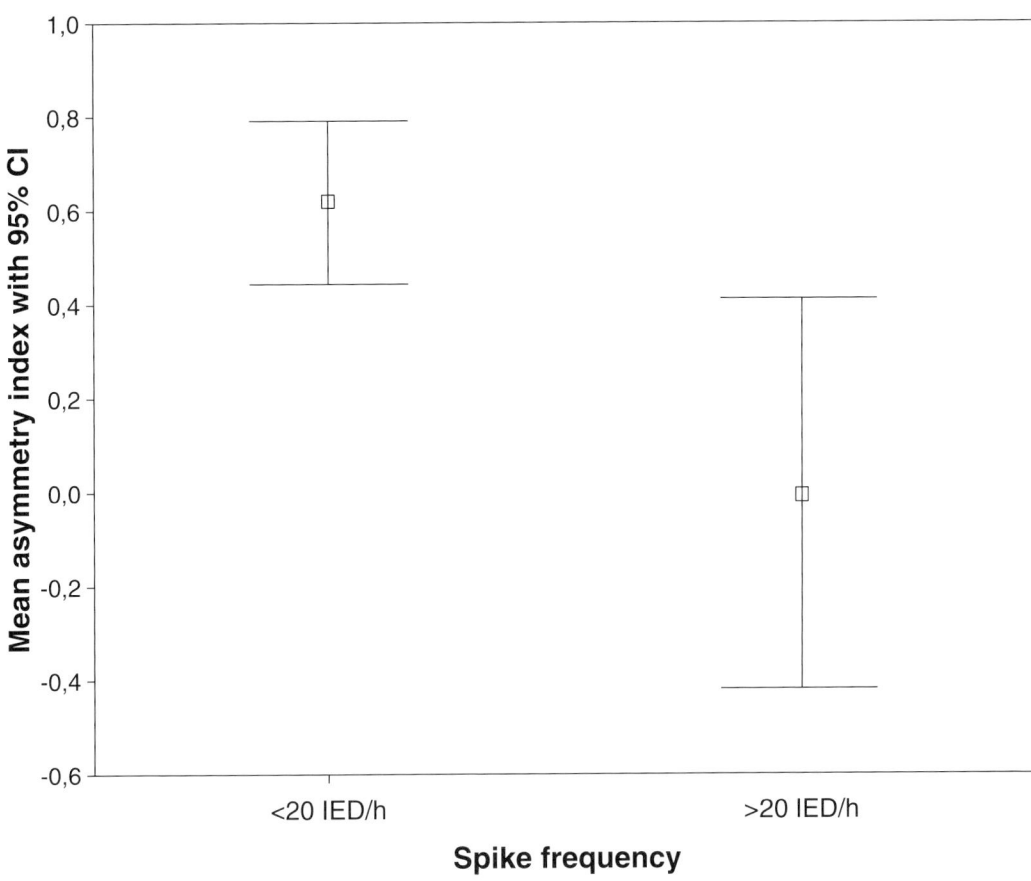

**Figure 3. fMRI study.**
Higher spike frequency is associated with more left-sided speech lateralization on fMRI. Positive values of the asymmetry index indicate that the activation is more pronounced on the left than on the right side. AI = 1 corresponds to complete left-sided lateralization, AI = –1 complete right-sided speech lateralization.

One of the arguments for the role of epileptic activity in inducing atypical speech lateralization is our finding that one-fourth of the patients with MTLE had atypical speech. Conversely, the mesiotemporal structures are rather far from the eloquent speech areas, thus, a left-sided mesiotemporal damage alone is theoretically not necessary for inducing atypical speech representation. It may be a more plausible explanation for the atypical speech seen in MTLE to say that it is caused by epileptic activity originating in the mesiotemporal structures but propagating to the speech centers.

How can the left-sided interictal or ictal epileptic activity induce a contralateral shift of language representation in a patient in whom epilepsy begins after age 6, which is thought to be the "classical" milestone for the plasticity of speech functions, as after age 6 the complete reorganization of speech functions in most cases are often incomplete? In the past few years there has been a growing amount of data to indicate that shift of language lateralization can occur to some degree in adolescence or even in adulthood. A recent fMRI study found that, although there is a negative correlation between age at brain injury and speech reorganization, there is no cut-off point after which contralateral speech reorganization does not occur in epilepsy patients (Springer et al., 1999). FMRI suggests that speech lateralization in women changes according to the menstrual cycle (Fernandez et al., 2003). Vargha-Khadem et al. (1997) reported on a 9-year-old boy suffering from left-hemispheric Sturge-Weber syndrome and severe epilepsy who failed to develop speech throughout early childhood. Following left hemsipherectomy at age 8.5, he became seizure-free and stopped receiving anti-epileptic drugs. Then he suddenly began to acquire language and speech. This case appears to challenge the widely held view that early childhood is a particularly critical period for the acquisition of speech. Thus, in this case the right hemisphere alone was capable of maintaining clearly articulated, well structured and appropriate language even after age 9.

There are other patients where a language transfer developed in adolescence age due to a left-sided epileptogenic lesion or epilepsy (Boatman et al., 1999; Hertz-Pannier et al., 2002). Improvement of aphasia in adults is paralleled by the participation of the right hemisphere in speech production, indicating some kind of contralateral speech reorganization in adulthood (Czopf, 1972; Blank et al., 2003).

Loddenkemper et al. (2002) reported on two adolescents with initial left-hemispheric language dominance proven by Wada test. In both patients Rasmussen encephalitis developed at age 8 and 11 years, respectively. Due to the effect of the chronic encephalitis or epilepsia partial continua, in both patients a right-sided language dominance developed between 9 and 15 years and between 12 and 14 years, respectively. These cases support that the role and the nature of the plasticity may be different in acute events compared to chronic disorders.

We suggest that under constant functional or slowly progressive structural disturbances such as chronic encephalitis or chronic epileptic activity, the speech representation *gradually* shifts from left to right hemisphere, without serious permanent aphasic symptoms, even in adolescence or early adulthood. Conversely, in cases of acute events, for example in left-sided stroke or hemispherectomy, the reorganization of language functions remains incomplete, and it is accompanied by speech disturbances because there may be not enough time for the right hemisphere to adapt for left-right transfer of the homologue language-related networks. This situation might be roughly similar to acute myocardial infarction. If the stenosis of a coronal artery has a slow progression due to arterosclerosis, then there may be enough time to develop a compensatory collateral circulation by bypassing the growing stenosis. In such a case a complete closing of a particular coronal artery may be accompanied by less severe myocardial damage. Conversely, if an acute coronal thromboembolia occurs without preceding a slowly progressive stenotic process, no compensatory collateral vascular system can develop and the consequence can often be a fatal myocardial infarction.

*In conclusion*, we assume that a left-right shift of speech representation in MTLE can occur in later childhood, and to some degree in adolescence, or even in adulthood under the influence of chronic and frequent epileptic activity. Our considerations and data suggest that epileptic activity may induce neuronal plasticity and functional reorganisation in an unexpected high extend that has been reglected for a long period of time.

**Acknowledgments:** This work was supported by a grant from the *Deutsche Forschungsgemeinschaft* (DFG-Eb 111/2-2, Dr. Ebner) and *Humboldt Stiftung* (dr. J. Janszky).

# References

Aarts JH, Binnie CD, Smit AM, Wilkins AJ. Selective cognitive impairment during focal and generalized epileptiform EEG activity. *Brain* 1984; 107: 293-308.

Alarcon G, Guy CN, Binnie CD, Walker SR, Elwes RD, Polkey CE. Intracerebral propagation of interictal activity in partial epilepsy: implications for source localization. *J Neurol Neurosurg Psychiatr* 1994; 57: 435-49.

Aldenkamp AP, Overwer J, Gutter T, Beun AM, Diepman L, Mulder OG. Effect of epilepsy, seizures and epileptiform discharges on cognitive function. *Acta Neurol Scand* 1996; 93: 253-9.

Balsamo LM, Xu B, Grandin CB. A functional magnetic resonance imaging study of left hemisphere language dominance in children. *Arch Neurol* 2002; 59: 1168-74.

Benbadis SR, So NK, Antar MA, Barnett GH, Morris HH. The value of PET scan (and MRI and Wada test) in patients with bitemporal epileptiform abnormalities. *Arch Neurol* 1995; 52: 1062-8.

Blank SC, Bird H, Turkheimer F, Wise RJ. Speech production after stroke: the role of the right pars opercularis. *Ann Neurol* 2003; 54: 310-20.

Boatman D, Freeman J, Vining E, Pulsifer M, Miglioretti D, Minahan R, *et al*. Language recovery after left hemispherectomy in children with late-onset seizures. *Ann Neurol* 1999; 46: 579-86.

Chassoux F, Semah F, Boilleret, *et al*. Metabolic changes and electro-clinical patterns in mesio-temporal lobe epilepsy: a correlative study. *Brain* 2004; 127: 164-74.

Chen K, Baram TZ, Soltesz I. Febrile seizures in the developing brain result in persistent modification of neuronal excitability in limbic circuits. *Nat Med* 1999; 5: 888-94.

Chiron C, Jambaque I, Nabbbout R, Lounes R, Syrota A, Dulac O. The right hemisphere is dominant in human infants. *Brain* 1997; 120: 1057-65.

Clemens Z, Janszky J, Szücs A, Bekesy M, Clemens B, Halasz P. Interictal epileptic spiking during sleep and wakefulness in mesial temporal lobe epilepsy: a comparative study of scalp and foramen ovale electrodes. *Epilepsia* 2003; 44: 186-92.

Czopf J. Über die Rolle der nicht dominanten Hemisphäre in der Restitution der Sprache der Aphasischen. *Arch Psychiatr Nervenkr* 1972; 216: 162-71.

Dehaene-Lambertz G, Dehaene S, Hertz-Pannier L. Functional neuroimaging of speech perception in infants. *Science* 2002; 298: 2013-5.

Ebner A. Lateral (neocortical) temporal lobe epilepsy. In: Wolf P, ed. *Epileptic seizures and syndromes*. Paris: John Libbey, 1994: 375-82.

Engel J, Ackermann RF. Interictal spikes correlate with decreased, rather than increased epileptogenicity in amygdaloid kindled rats. *Brain Res* 1980; 190: 543-8.

Fernandez G, Weis S, Stoffel-Wagner B, *et al*. Menstrual-cycle dependent neural plasticity in the adult human brain is hormone, task, and region specific. *J Neurosci* 23: 3790-5.

Foundas AL, Leonard CM, Gilmore RL, Fennel EB, Heilman KM. Pars triangularis asymmetry and language dominance. *Proc Natl Acad Sci USA* 1996; 93: 719-22.

Frost JA, Binder JR, Springer JA, Hammeke TA, Bellgowan PS, Rao SM, et al. Language processing is strongly left lateralized in both sex. *Brain* 1999; 122: 199-208.

Gabr M, Lüders H, Dinner D, Morris H, Wyllie E. Speech manifestations in lateralization of temporal lobe seizures. *Ann Neurol* 1989; 25: 82-7.

Gaillard WD, Hertz-Pannier L, Mott SH, Barnett AS, LeBihan D, Theodore W. Functional anatomy of cognitive development – fMRI of verbal fluency in children and adults. *Neurology* 2000; 54: 180-5.

Geschwind N, Levitsky W. Human brain: left-right asymmetries in temporal speech region. *Science* 1968; 161: 186-9.

Gotman J, Marciani MG. Electroencephalographic spiking activity, drug levels and seizure occurrence in epileptic patients. *Ann Neurol* 1985; 17: 597-603.

Hecaen H. Acquired aphasia in children and the ontogenesis of hemispheric functional specialization. *Brain Lang* 1976; 3: 114-34.

Helmstaedter C, Kurthen M, Linke DB, Elger CE. Patterns of language dominance in focal left and right hemisphere epilepsies: relation to MRI findings, EEG, sex, and age at onset of epilepsy. *Brain Cogn* 1997; 33: 135-50.

Helmstaedter C, Kurthen M. Memory and epilepsy: characteristics, course, and influence of drugs and surgery. *Curr Opin Neurol* 2001; 14: 211-6.

Hertz-Pannier L, Chiron C, Jambaqué I, Renaux-Kieffer V, Van de Moortele PF, Delalande O, et al. Late plasticity for language in a child's non-dominant hemisphere – A pre- and post-surgery fMRI study. *Brain* 2002; 125: 361-72.

Holowka S, Petitto LA. Left hemisphere cerebral specialization for babies while babbling. *Science* 2002; 297 (5586): 1515.

Hong SB, Han HJ, Roh SY, Seo DW, Kim SE, Kim MH. Hypometabolism and interictal spikes during positron emission tomography scanning in temporal lobe epilepsy. *Eur Neurol* 2002; 48: 65-70.

Janszky J, Ebner A. Interictal spikes: Signs of a negative feed-back mechanism of epilepsy? *Epilepsia* 2002; 43: 664-7.

Janszky J, Fogarasi A, Jokeit H, Ebner A. Are ictal vocalisations related to the lateralisation in frontal lobe epilepsy? *J Neurol Neurosurg Psychiatry* 2000; 69: 244-7.

Janszky J, Fogarasi A, Jokeit H, Schulz R, Hoppe M, Ebner A. Spatiotemporal relationship between seizure activity and interictal spikes in temporal lobe epilepsy. *Epilesy Res* 2001; 47: 179-88.

Janszky J, Jokeit H, Heinemann D, Schulz R, Woermann FG, Ebner A. Epileptic activity influences the speech organisation in medial temporal lobe epilepsy. *Brain* 2003; 126: 2043-51.

Janszky J, Olech I, Jokeit H, Kontopoulou K, Mertens M, Ebner A, Pohlmann-Eden B, Woermann FG. Epileptic activity influences lateralization of memory fMRI activity. *Neurology* 2004; 63: 1813-7.

Jayakar P, Bernal B, Medina S, Altman N. False lateralization of language cortex on functional MRI after cluster of focal seizures. *Neurology* 2002; 58: 490-2.

Jokeit H, Daamen M, Zang H, Janszky J, Ebner A. Seizures accelerate forgetting in patients with left-sided temporal lobe epilepsy. *Neurology* 2001b; 57: 125-6.

Jokeit H, Okujava M, Woermann G. Memory fMRI lateralizes temporal lobe epilepsy. *Neurology* 2001a; 57: 1786-93.

Kapur N, Young A, Bateman D, Kennedy P. Focal retrograde amnesia: a long term clinical and neuropsychological follow up. *Cortex* 1989; 25: 387-402.

Katz A, Marks DA, McCarthy G, Spencer SS. Does interictal spiking change prior to seizures? *Electroenceph Clin Neurophysiol* 1991; 79: 153-6.

Kertész A, Sheppard A. The epidemiology of aphasic and cognitive impairment in stroke: age, sex, aphasia type and laterality differences. *Brain* 1981; 104: 117-28.

Kotloski R, Lynch M, Lauersdorf S, Sutula T. Repeated brief seizures induce progressive hippocampal neuronal loss and memory deficits. *Prog Brain Res* 2002; 135: 95-110.

Landau WM, Kleffner FR. Syndrome of acquired aphasia with convulsive disorder in children. *Neurology* 1957; 7: 523-30.

Landau WM, Kleffner FR. Syndrome of acquired aphasia with convulsive disorder in children. *Neurology* 1957; 7: 523-30.

Librizzi L, de Curtis M. Epileptiform ictal discharges are prevented by periodic interictal spiking in the olfactory cortex. *Ann Neurol* 2003; 53: 382-9.

Loddenkemper T, Wyllie E, Lardizabal D, Stanford LD, Bingaman W. Late language transfer in patients with Rasmussen encephalitis. *Epilepsia* 2003; 44: 870-1.

Lynch M, Sayin Ü, Bownds J, Janumpalli S, Sutula T. Long-term consequences of early postnatal seizures on hippocampal learning and plasticity. *Eur J Neurosc* 2000; 12: 2252-64.

Maher J, McLachlan RS. Febrile convulsions – is seizure duration the most important predictor of temporal lobe epilepsy? *Brain* 1995; 118: 1521-8.

Marcotte AC, Morere DA. Speech lateralization in deaf populations: evidence for a developmental critical period. *Brain Lang* 1990; 39: 134-52.

Mathern GW, Babb TL, Vickrey BG, Melendez M, Pretorius JK. The clinical-pathogenic mechanism of hippocampal neuron loss and surgical outcomes in temporal lobe epilepsy. *Brain* 1995; 118: 105-18.

McGlone J. Sex differences in the cerebral organization of verbal functions in patients with unilateral brain lesions. *Brain* 1977; 100: 775-93.

Niedermeyer E, Rocca U. The diagnostic significance of sleep electroencephalograms in temporal lobe epilepsy – a comparison of scalp and depth tracings. *Eur Neurol* 1972; 7: 119-29.

Popper KR, Eccles JC. *The self and its brain*. Berlin: Springer International, 1977: 304-5, 450-6.

Ralston BL The mechanism of transition of interictal spiking into ictal seizure discharges. *Electroenceph Clin Neurophysiol* 1958; 10: 217-32.

Rasmussen T, Milner B. The role of early left-brain injury in determining lateralization of cerebral speech functions. *Ann Neurol NY Acad Sci* 1977; 299: 355-69.

Rausch R, Walsh GO. Right-hemisphere language dominance in right-handed epileptic patients. *Arch Neurol* 1984; 41: 1077-80.

Rey M, Dellatolas GJ, Bancaud J, Talairach J. Hemispheric lateralization of motor and speech functions after early brain lesion: study of 73 epileptic patients with intracarotid amytal test. *Neuropsychologia* 1988; 26: 167-72.

Sagar HJ, Oxbury JM. Hippocampal neuronal loss in temporal lobe epilepsy: correlation with early childhood convulsions. *Ann Neurol* 1987; 22: 334-40.

Savic I, Altshuler L, Baxter L, Engel J. Pattern of interictal hypometabolism in PET scans with fludeoxyglucose F 18 reflects prior seizure types in patients with mesial temporal lobe seizures. *Arch Neurol* 1997; 54: 129-36.

Schlaug G, Antke C, Holthausen H, Arnold S, Ebner A, Tuxhorn I, et al. Ictal motor signs and interictal regional cerebral hypometabolims. *Neurology* 1997; 49: 341-50.

Schulz R, Lüders HO, Hoppe M, Jokeit H, Moch A, Tuxhorn I, et al. Lack of aura experience correlates with bitemporal dysfunction in mesial temporal lobe epilepsy. *Epilepsy Res* 2001; 43: 201-10.

Shinnar S, Hauser WA. Do occasional brief seizures cause detectable clinical consequences? *Prog Brain Res* 2002; 135: 221-31.

Toth Z, Yan X, Haftoglou S, Ribak CE, Baram TZ. Seizure-induced neuronal injury: vulnerability to febrile seizures in an immature rat model. *J Neurosci* 1998; 18: 4285-94.

Vargha-Khadem F, Carr LJ, Isaacs E, Brett E, Adams C, Mishkin M. Onset of speech after left hemispherectomy in a nine-year-old boy. *Brain* 1997; 120: 159-82.

Wada JA, Clarke RJ, Hamm AE. Cerebral hemispheric asymmetry in humans. *Arch Neurol* 1975; 32: 239-46.

Walker SF. Lateralization of functions in the vertebrate brain: a review. *Br J Psychol* 1980; 71: 329-67.

Wieser HG; ILAE Commission on Neurosurgery of Epilepsy. ILAE Commission Report. Mesial temporal lobe epilepsy with hippocampal sclerosis. *Epilepsia* 2004; 45: 695-714.

Witelson SF. Neurobiological aspects of language in children. *Child Develepment* 1987; 58: 653-88.

Woermann FG, Jokcit H, Luerding R,, Freitag H, Schulz R, Guertler S, *et al*. Language lateralization by Wada test and fMRI in 100 patients with epilepsy. *Neurology* 2003; 61: 699-701.

Woods RP, Dodrill CB, Ojemann GA. Brain injury, handedness, and speech lateralization in a series of amobarbital studies. *Ann Neurol* 1988; 23: 510-8.

Wunderlich G, Schuller MF, Ebner A, Holthausen H, Tuxhorn I, Witte OW, Seitz RJ. Temporal lobe epilepsy with sensory aura: interictal glucose hypometabolism. *Epilepsy Res* 2000; 38: 139-49.

# Cognitive side-effects of antiepileptic drugs

### A.P. Aldenkamp[1,2], H.-P. Bootsma[1]

[1] Epilepsy Centre Kempenhaeghe, Heeze, The Netherlands;
[2] Department of Neurology, Maastricht University Hospital, The Netherlands

Cognitive impairment is the most common comorbid disorder in epilepsy (Aldenkamp & Dodson, 1990; Dodson & Pellock, 1993). Memory impairments, mental slowing, and attentional deficits are the most frequently reported cognitive disorders (Dodson & Trimble, 1994; Aldenkamp et al., 1995). Such consequences may be more debilitating for a patient than the seizures; thus, it is worthwhile to explore the factors that lead to cognitive impairment. The exact cause of cognitive impairment in epilepsy has not been explored fully, but three factors clearly are involved: etiology, the seizures, and the "central" side effects of drug treatment (Aldenkamp, 2002). Here we concentrate on the unwanted effects of antiepileptic medication on cognitive function. When evaluating this factor separately, it is imperative to realize that in clinical practice most cognitive problems have a multifactorial origin and that, for the most part, the three aforementioned factors, combined, are responsible for the "makeup" of a cognitive problem in an individual patient. Moreover, the factors are related, which causes therapeutic dilemmas in some patients when seizure control can only be achieved with treatments that are associated with cognitive side effects.

The interest in the cognitive side effects of antiepileptic drug (AED) treatment is of recent origin. The first studies are from the early 1970s (Ideström et al., 1972; Dodrill & Troupin, 1977) and were probably stimulated by the widening range of possibilities for drug treatment during that period (i.e., the introduction of carbamazepine and valproate). Since then, a plethora of studies have been published, the majority on the commonly used AEDs: valproate (VPA), carbamazepine (CBZ), and phenytoin (PHT).

In the last decade, several new AEDs have been introduced. Although it is claimed that these drugs have different efficacy profiles and that some drugs are particularly efficacious in specific syndromes (e.g., vigabatrin [VGB]), head-to-head comparisons between the new AEDs and between the newer drugs and the commonly used drugs (such as CBZ and VPA) are rare. Nonetheless, metaanalyses such as the influential Cochrane reviews (Marson et al., 1997; Jette et al., 2002) do not show significant differences in efficacy between the newer drugs or between newer and commonly used drugs. Also, studies analyzing long-term retention do not show differences between the drugs (Wong 1997, Stefan et al., 1998).

Several studies have shown retention rate to be the best parameter of the long-term clinical usefulness of a particular drug (Lhatoo et al., 2000). Retention rate is considered to be a composite of drug efficacy and drug safety and expresses the willingness of patients to continue drug treatment. It is therefore the best standard for evaluating the clinical relevance of side effects. The 1-year retention rate is reported to be not higher than 55% for topiramate (TPM) (Kellet et al., 1999), 60% for lamotrigine (LTG), 58% for VGB, and 45% for gabapentin (GBP) (Marson et al., 2000). Long-term (mostly 3-year) retention is about 35% for all newer AEDs (Marson et al., 2001). Side effects appear to be the major factor affecting long-term retention for most drugs (Chadwick et al., 1996; Aldenkamp, 2001). In clinical practice, tolerability is a major issue and the choice of a certain AED is at least partially based on comparison of tolerability profiles of the drugs. Also, the tolerability profiles of the newer drugs have become a more important issue in drug development, stimulated by the interest of regulatory agencies (Aldenkamp, 2001). Cognitive side effects are particularly important tolerability problems in chronic AED treatment.

## ■ Method

In evaluating studies of the cognitive effects of AEDs, we will follow an evidence-based approach (Vermeulen & Aldenkamp, 1995; Aldenkamp et al., 2003). Randomized clinical trials with monotherapy in patients with newly diagnosed epilepsy represent the most accurate procedure for assessing the cognitive impact of AEDs (Aldenkamp, 2001). These studies are not clouded by the effect of concurrent or previous AED use and permit the accurate collection of non-drug baseline data that is required for determining whether a particular treatment affects cognitive processing (i.e., to isolate drug-induced impairments from those due to other sources such as the seizures). Data from such studies can be supplemented with information from studies using add-on or polytherapy designs. In these studies, the use of two AEDs makes identifying the components of the treatment that are responsible for the observed effects more complex. In many cases, however, patients with epilepsy require dual AED therapy before adequate seizure control is obtained; therefore, data from add-on studies do warrant consideration. Also, data from healthy volunteers should be treated with caution. In general, the power of such studies is limited by small sample sizes, and drug-exposure periods are typically brief. It is possible that chronic treatment results in entirely different types of cognitive impairment that cannot be observed during short-term treatment. For example, such differences in side-effect profile between acute and long-term administration have been found with PHT. Finally, the differing cerebral substrate in patients with epilepsy and healthy volunteers suggests that cognitive responses to AEDs may be different in these populations. Nonetheless, volunteer studies may provide an early insight into the cognitive effects of an AED and therefore provide a foundation for further studies in patients with epilepsy (see Vermeulen & Aldenkamp, 1995 for a discussion of methodological aspects of cognitive drug trials in epilepsy).

# Results

## Phenobarbital (PB)

The main anticonvulsant mechanism of action is the increase of the duration (not the frequency) of the GABA activated chloride ion channel opening (Twyman et al., 1989), hence potentiating GABA mediated inhibitory neurotransmission. PB can also activate the $GABA_A$ receptor in the absence of GABA, which is sometimes considered to be a mechanism leading to its sedative properties. PB is used for the treatment of epilepsy since the discovery of its antiepileptic effect by Hauptman in 1912.

For PB one study (MacLeod et al., 1978) is available allowing the evaluation of the cognitive effects of PB relative to a non-drug condition. This study shows relative serious memory impairment (short-term memory recall) in 19 patients with epilepsy.

Comparisons with other AEDs are available from four studies (Vining et al., 1987; Callandre et al., 1990; Meador et al., 1990; Gallassi et al., 1992), all with patients with epilepsy. One of these shows more impairment for PB than for PHT or CBZ on visuomotor and memory tests (Gallassi et al., 1992) and two other study show convincing and clinically highly relevant impairments of intelligence scores after long-term PB treatment in comparison with VPA studies (Vining et al., 1987; Callandre et al., 1990). Only the study by Meador et al. (1990) does not show differences between PB and PHT or CBZ.

## Phenytoin (PHT)

The main anticonvulsant mechanism of action is use-dependent (voltage- and frequency dependent) sodium channel blocking (Schwartz & Grigat, 1989). It binds to the fast inactivated state of the channel, reducing high frequency neuronal firing. PHT has a stronger effect on the sodium-channel than CBZ, delaying recovery stronger than CBZ. PHT may also have mild effects on the excitatory glutamate system and on the inhibitory GABA system. PHT has been used as an antiepileptic drug since it was introduced for the treatment of epilepsy in 1938 by Merritt and Putnam. For 20 years PHT was (together with PB) the universal treatment of epilepsy. PHT has excellent anticonvulsant properties and is used as a broad range AED.

For PHT five studies are available (Smith & Lowrey, 1975; Thompson et al., 1980, 1981; Meador et al., 1991, 1993) comparing PHT with a non-drug condition. These studies all reveal PHT-induced cognitive impairment in the areas of attention, memory and especially mental speed. The magnitude of the reported effects is moderate to large. A caveat is, however, in order as all these studies were carried out in normal-volunteers, which opens the possibility that these effects represent short-term outcomes of the drug.

The results of head-to-head comparisons with other AEDs are somewhat more confusing. Using an ingenious long-term treatment and withdrawal design Gallassi and coworkers (Gallassi et al., 1992) found more cognitive impairment with PHT compared to CBZ. On the other hand, no difference with CBZ, VPA and even with PHB are reported (Meador et al., 1990, 1991, 1993; Forsythe et al., 1991).

## Ethosuximide (ESX)

ESX modifies the properties of voltage-dependent calcium channels, reducing the T-type currents and thereby preventing synchronized firing. The reduction is most prominent at negative membrane potentials and less prominent at more positive membrane potentials. The main effect is assumed to take place in thalamocortical relay neurons. ESX is introduced in 1960 and mainly used for the treatment of generalized absence seizures.

No controlled studies are available to evaluate the cognitive effects of ESX.

## Carbamazepine (CBZ)

The main anticonvulsant mechanism of action is similar to that of PHT with a less "slowing" effect in the recovery state than obtained for PHT. The mechanism of action is also voltage- and frequency dependent. CBZ was first synthesized in the early 1950's (Parnas et al., 1979, 1980) and introduced as an antiepileptic drug by Bonduelle in 1964 in Europe. CBZ is used for patients with partial complex seizures, with or without secondary generalization. Approval by the FDA for use in the United States followed much later (1978) because of concerns about serious hematological toxicity (e.g. aplastic anemia).

For CBZ two studies, one in normal volunteers (Thompson et al., 1980) and one in patients with epilepsy (Aldenkamp et al., 1993) report "no cognitive impairment" compared to a non-drug condition. This is challenged by the group by Meador and coworkers (Meador et al., 1991, 1993) that report impairments of memory, attention and mental speed, largely the areas that may also be affected by phenytoin.

When evaluating the comparisons of CBZ with other AEDs there are the conflicting results of the Italian study by Gallassi and coworkers, showing a more favourable profile compared with PHT and PHB (Gallassi et al., 1992) and the USA-based study by Meador and coworkers (Meador et al., 1990, 1991, 1993) that showed no differences compared with PHT and PHB.

## Valproate (VPA)

VPA, a fatty acid, is believed to possess multiple mechanisms of action. A number of studies have demonstrated an effect on sodium channels, however different from PHT and CBZ. An effect on T-type calcium channels has also been demonstrated. Recent studies have, however, demonstrated that a predominant effect concerns the interaction with the GABA-ergic neurotransmitter system. More precisely, VPA elevates brain GABA levels and potentiates GABA responses, possibly by enhancing GABA synthesis and inhibiting degradation. Furthermore, VPA may augment GABA release and block the re-uptake of GABA into glia cells. VPA is one of the most effective drugs against generalized absence seizures. It was introduced in approximately the same period as CBZ.

For VPA four studies (Thompson & Trimble, 1981; Craig & Tallis, 1994; Prevey et al., 1996) allow the interpretation of absolute effects and shows mild to moderate impairment of psychomotor and mental speed. The comparison with other drugs shows lower performance of memory and visuomotor function compared to CBZ (Gallassi et al., 1992) and a favourable profile compared to PB on tests for intelligence (Vining et al., 1987; Calandre et al., 1990). One study does not show a difference compared to PHT (Forsythe et al., 1991)

## Oxcarbazepine (OXC)

OXC is essentially a prodrug, a keto homologue of CBZ, structurally very similar to CBZ, but with a different metabolic profile. In humans, the keto group is rapidly and quantitatively reduced to form a monohydroxy derivative that is the main active anticonvulsant agent during OXC therapy. Metabolism of OXC does not result in the formation of 10,11 epoxy carbamazepine that is sometimes considered to be the main metabolite causing side-effects. The mechanism of action is similar to CBZ. However, OXC is also considered to reduce presynaptic glutamate release, possibly by reduction of high-threshold calcium currents. OXC was approved in the European Union in 1999 and is indicated for use as monotherapy or adjunctive therapy for partial seizures with or without secondarily generalized tonic-clonic seizures in patients ≥ 6 years of age.

The effects of OXC on cognitive function have been evaluated in one study in healthy volunteers and in four studies in patients with epilepsy. A double-blind, placebo-controlled, crossover study was conducted in 12 healthy volunteers (Curran & Java, 1993). The effects of two doses of OXC (300 mg/day and 600 mg/day) and placebo on cognitive function and psychomotor performance were assessed. The treatment duration for each condition was 2 weeks. Cognitive function tests were administered before treatment initiation and 4 hours after the morning doses on days 1, 8, and 15. In this study, OXC improved performance on a focused attention task, increased manual writing speed, and had no effect on long-term memory processes.

In patients with epilepsy, four monotherapy comparative studies are available to evaluate the effects of OXC on cognitive functions in adult patients with newly diagnosed epilepsy. The first study (Laaksonen et al., 1985) was a double-blind, active-control study evaluating the effects of CBZ and OXC on memory and attention in 41 patients with newly diagnosed epilepsy. The treatment duration was 1 year. Cognitive function and intelligence tests were administered before treatment initiation and after 1 year of treatment. The results indicated no deterioration of memory or attention with either CBZ or OXC. The second study was an active-control study that evaluated the effects of CBZ, VPA, and OXC on intelligence, learning and memory, attention, psychomotor speed, verbal span, and visuospatial construction in 32 patients with newly diagnosed epilepsy (Sabers et al., 1995). The treatment duration was 4 months. Cognitive function and intelligence tests were administered before treatment initiation and after 4 months of treatment. The results indicated no deterioration of cognitive function in any treatment group. Significant improvements in learning and memory tests were found for the CBZ- and OXC-treated patients. Improvements were also found in attention and psychomotor speed tests for the VPA-treated patients and partly for the CBZ-treated patients. The third study was a double-blind, randomized, active-control study that evaluated the effects of PHT and OXC on memory, attention, and psychomotor speed in 29 patients with newlydiagnosed epilepsy (Äikiä et al., 1992). The treatment duration was 1 year. Cognitive function tests were administered before treatment initiation and after 6 and 12 months of treatment. The results indicated no significant differential cognitive effects between PHT and OXC during the first year of treatment in patients with newly diagnosed epilepsy who achieved adequate seizure control. In the fourth study (McKee et al., 1994), three groups of 12 patients taking either CBZ, VPA, or PHT took a single 600 mg dose of OXC followed 7 days later by 3 weeks of treatment with OXC 300 mg thrice daily and matched placebo in random order. Seven untreated patients, acting as controls, were prescribed the single OXC dose and 3 weeks of active treatment only. There were no important changes in cognitive function test results during administration of OXC compared with placebo.

In summary, the results of these studies indicate that OXC does not affect cognitive function in healthy volunteers and adult patients with newly diagnosed epilepsy. The effects of OXC on cognitive function, however, have not been systematically studied in children and adolescents. In accordance with the latest revision of the Committee for Proprietary Medicinal Products (CPMP) Note of Guidance (CPMP EWP/566/98 rev 1, dated November 16, 2000, Sections 2.5 and 5.2), a study has recently been launched (Protocol #: CTRI476E2337) to investigate the effects of OXC on cognitive function (*i.e.*, psychomotor speed and alertness, mental information processing speed and attention, memory, and learning) in children and adolescents aged 6 to < 17 years with partial seizures.

## Topiramate (TPM)

TPM is a sulfamate-substituted monosaccharide that has clearly multiple mechanisms of action (White, 1997). TPM blocks neuronal sodium channels in a voltage- and frequency-dependent manner, it inhibits CA, it promotes the action of GABA at the $GABA_A$ receptor complex, elevates GABA brain concentrations by about 60% at 3 and 6 hours after a single dose and this increase was maintained with 4 weeks of TPM administration (Petroff et al., 1996). TPM is a carbonic anhydrase inhibiting drug. TPM has proved to be effective in patients with refractory chronic partial epilepsies (Privitera et al., 1996; Faught et al., 1996).

During the initial add-on clinical trials, central nervous system-related "cognitive" subjective complaints were frequently reported, including mental slowing, attentional deficits, speech problems, and memory difficulties (Privitera et al., 1996). It should be mentioned, however, that higher target doses and faster titration schedules were used than are now used in clinical practice (see Faught et al., 1996 for a discussion of dose and titration speed). Recent studies with TPM-treated patients have confirmed high levels of adverse cognitive effects based on subjective complaints (Ketter et al., 1999; Tatum et al., 2001). A follow-up study (Bootsma et al., 2004) showed long-term retention of 30% for a 4-year follow-up. For about half of the 70% of patients who discontinued treatment, side effects were the major reason, with cognitive side effects being most frequently mentioned. Only a few studies have psychometrically measured cognitive changes using neuropsychological tests.

A study by Martin et al. in six normal volunteers (Martin et al., 1999) used an acute dose of 2.8 mg/kg (~ 200 mg/day) followed by a titration to 5.7 mg/kg (~ 400 mg/day) in 4 weeks, resulting in weekly dose escalations of about 100 mg. The rate at which TPM was escalated in this study was very similar to the dose escalation used in the initial TPM adjunctive-therapy trials (Privitera et al., 1996), in which escalating the TPM dose to 200 or 400 mg/day over 2-3 weeks was associated with somnolence, psychomotor slowing, speech disorders, and concentration and memory difficulties (Bootsma et al., 2004). Martin et al. showed neuropsychometric changes commensurate with these CNS effects. The cognitive effects of the acute starting dose of 200 mg/day were impairments of verbal function (word finding and verbal fluency) of approximately 2 standard deviations (which represents very serious impairment) and of sustained attention. Titration to 400 mg/day in 4 weeks resulted in impairments of verbal memory and mental speed of > 2 standard deviations.

Four studies involving patients with epilepsy are available. In a study by Meador (1997) with 155 patients with epilepsy, the effects of the gradual introduction of TPM as add-on (a 50-mg starting dose, followed by increments of 50 mg per week over 8 weeks) were compared with those of more rapid dose escalation (initial dose of 100 mg, followed by two consecutive weekly increments of 100 and 200 mg). In a test battery of 23 variables representing selective attention, word fluency, and visuomotor speed, the subjects who were on a slow-titration schedule and treated with one background AED displayed TPM-associated score changes of more than one third but less than one standard deviation. A study by Aldenkamp et al. (2000) was specifically designed to compare cognitive effects of TPM and VPA added to therapeutic dosages of CBZ in 59 patients with epilepsy. In this study, a slow titration speed was used with a starting dose of 25 mg/day TPM and weekly increments of 25 mg. Moreover, the average achieved dose (approximately 250 mg) was relatively low. Neuropsychometric testing was conducted 8 weeks after the last dosage increase (20 weeks after the start of TPM therapy). The study therefore used optimal conditions (*i.e.*, slow titration, relatively low dose, and a longer treatment period), allowing for patient habituation to the effects of TPM therapy. Nonetheless, cognitive impairment was found for verbal memory function both during titration and at end point. In a study by Burton and Harden (1997), attention was assessed weekly in 10 subjects receiving TPM over a 3-month period. Four of nine subjects showed significant correlations between TPM dosage and forward digit span measured weekly, such that higher dosage was associated with poorer attention. In a retrospective study by Thompson et al. (2000), the neuropsychological test scores of 18 patients obtained before and after the introduction of treatment with TPM (median dose 300 mg) were compared with changes in test performance of 18 patients who had undergone repeat neuropsychological assessments at the same time intervals. In those patients taking TPM, a significant deterioration in many domains was found. The largest changes were for verbal IQ, verbal fluency, and verbal learning.

In summary, there is clear clinical evidence for TPM-induced cognitive impairment. Not all studies are comparable because of the confusion about dose and titration speed (see Aldenkamp, 2000 for a discussion). Moreover, the complete lack of controlled studies is remarkable.

## Lamotrigine (LTG)

LTG is a phenyltriazine with weak antifolate activity. The main anticonvulsant mechanism of action is to block voltage-dependent sodium channels that result in voltage- and frequency-dependent inhibition of the channel. This suggests that the mechanism of action is similar to that of PHT and CBZ. However much attention is focused recently on the fact that this mechanism in LTG treatment results in preventing presynaptic excitatory neurotransmitter release. It is still in debate to what extent the mechanisms of action are different from CBZ (Leach et al., 1995). Clinical evidence indicates that LTG is effective against partial and secondarily generalized tonic-clonic seizures, as well as idiopathic (primary) generalized epilepsy. LTG was introduced in Europe in 1991 and in the United States in 1994.

A large number of cognitive studies are available for LTG (see Aldenkamp & Baker, 2001 for an overview). Five volunteer studies have been conducted with LTG. Doses of 120 mg and 240 mg did not produce a significant change in cognitive function compared with baseline when administered to 12 normal volunteers in an acute study of 1 day (Cohen et al., 1985). Similarly, five volunteers received LTG (acute dose 3.5 mg/kg and then titrated to a maximum of 7.1 mg/kg) in a single-blind manner and were assessed for change in cognitive function after 2 and 4 weeks (Martin et al., 1999). There was no significant change in any of the neurocognitive measures relative to baseline performance. LTG and CBZ have been compared in 12 healthy male volunteers and associations were made between the observed cognitive effects and plasma concentrations of these drugs (Hamilton et al., 1993). The effects of these drugs were examined by means of adaptive tracking, which assesses eye-hand coordination and effects of attention, and eye movement tests. LTG treatment was not significantly different from placebo, but increased CBZ saliva concentrations were significantly associated with impaired adaptive tracking and smooth and saccadic eye movements.

The long-term effects of LTG and CBZ were compared in 23 volunteers in a 10-week crossover study (Meador et al., 2000). The neuropsychological battery in this study consisted of 19 instruments yielding 40 variables, including both subjective and objective measures. LTG showed better performance or fewer side effects in 17 (42%) of the variables, while no statistically significant differences were seen in the remaining variables. Finally, a study by Aldenkamp et al. (2002) in 30 volunteers (12 days of treatment, using a daily dose of 50 mg of LTG) showed evidence for a selective positive effect of LTG on cognitive activation, relative to both placebo and VPA. Although the results of these volunteer studies provide us with preliminary insight into the impact of LTG on cognition, the generalizability of the results from these studies to patients with epilepsy receiving long-term AED treatment is limited.

The effects of LTG on cognitive function have been compared with those of CBZ in patients with newly diagnosed epilepsy. Patients completed tests of verbal learning and memory, attention, and mental flexibility at baseline and then periodically for up to 48 weeks. Significant differences favoring LTG over CBZ were observed with semantic processing, verbal learning, and attention (Gillham et al., 2000). The authors concluded that LTG may have a favorable long-term effect on cognitive function when compared with CBZ. Other studies have reported positive cognitive effects of LTG used as adjunctive therapy. Two independent double-blind, randomized, crossover studies have examined the cognitive effects of LTG used as add-on therapy (Smith et al., 1993; Banks & Beran, 1991). Both studies included patients with a history of partial seizures (at least once weekly during the preceding 3 months) who had received no more than two other AEDs or VPA monotherapy. Both studies also used two treatment periods (12 and 18 weeks), which were separated by a washout period (4 and 6 weeks). Despite the similarity in trial design and patients, there is some inconsistency between the findings of these two studies. One study showed a marginal reduction in general "cerebral efficiency" (an indirect measure of cognitive function) following LTG treatment (Banks & Beran, 1991). Conversely, significant improvements were reported in the second study (Smith et al., 1993). In an uncontrolled add-on study (Aldenkamp et al., 1997) using CBZ as baseline drug, no deterioration on any of the cognitive tests was found after introducing LTG (200 mg). LTG therapy in seven patients with epilepsy and mental retardation caused both positive and negative psychotropic effects (Ettinger et al., 1998). These findings were based on the observations of parents and supervising staff. Positive effects included reduced irritability and increased compliance with simple instructions, while negative effects included behavioral deterioration with temper tantrums, restlessness, and hyperactivity. Similarly, a second study in 67 patients with mental retardation showed that following adjunctive treatment with LTG, social functioning was stable or improved in 90% of patients (Earl et al., 2000).

In addition to clinical studies that have assessed the impact of LTG on cognitive function, further evidence can be obtained from examining the effect of LTG on electroencephalographic (EEG) parameters. Overt EEG discharges can occur without any visible clinical correlate in many patients with epilepsy. These epileptiform episodes may be associated with transient deterioration in cognitive function (Aarts et al., 1984; Aldenkamp et al., 2001). Data from several studies indicate that LTG may reduce spontaneous epileptiform discharges, which may partially explain the favorable cognitive profile of LTG. In five patients displaying spontaneous EEG discharges, a single dose of LTG (120 mg or 240 mg in addition to existing medication) resulted in a substantial reduction in spontaneous interictal discharges within a 24-hour period (Binnie et al., 1986). The long-term effects of LTG on paroxysmal abnormalities have also been monitored with a computer-based analysis system (Marciani et al., 1996). Twenty-one patients with intractable epilepsy (twenty of whom were receiving multiple AED therapy) were evaluated before and after LTG treatment for EEG ictal events and number of spikes in a 10-minute period. Before LTG treatment, patients typically showed discharges characterized by diffuse spike-wave complexes. However, following a 4-month treatment period with LTG, ictal discharges disappeared and diffuse slow wave activity was seen with no adverse effect on background activity. Nineteen of the 21 patients also showed a reduction in seizure frequency.

The effect of LTG add-on therapy in 11 patients with refractory partial seizures with or without secondary generalization has also been reported (Marciani et al., 1998). LTG was added to existing therapy consisting of CBZ with at least one additional AED. EEG recordings were made at rest with eyes closed, during an attentive task (blocking reaction induced by several episodes of eyes open lasting 8 to 9 seconds), during cognitive tasks, and while performing mental arithmetic. In addition, a battery of neuropsychological tests was carried out. Before LTG treatment, EEG data revealed a decrease in fast activity at rest and a reduction in alpha and beta bands during attentive and cognitive tasks. LTG treatment resulted in a selective increase in alpha reactivity and beta power during the attentive tasks with no other detectable changes. During cortical activation, subtle changes were observed that were taken as indicative of a slight improvement in attention. Neuropsychological evaluation revealed that following 3 months of LTG therapy, no deterioration in cognitive function had occurred.

LTG also shows a promising cognitive profile in elderly patients suffering from age-associated memory impairment (Mervaala et al., 1995). A neuropsychological test battery in combination with auditory event-related potentials (ERPs) was used to measure the impact of LTG on cognitive function. LTG treatment caused a reduction in amplitude of the $P_{300}$ component of the ERP and a corresponding improvement in immediate and delayed visual memory and delayed logical memory. LTG may therefore improve simple memory functions in a memory-impaired elderly population.

## Levetiracetam (LEV)

LEV is a new AED, structurally and mechanistically dissimilar to other AEDs. It is believed to bind to a specific, as yet undetermined, site on the synaptic plasma membrane. Moreover LEV seems to reduce the GABA turnover in the striatum by reducing GABA synthesis and increasing GABA metabolism. It is effective in reducing partial seizures in patients with epilepsy, both as adjunctive treatment and as monotherapy. LEV has many therapeutic advantages for patients with epilepsy. It has favorable pharmacokinetic characteristics (good bioavailability, linear pharmacokinetics, insignificant protein binding, lack of hepatic metabolism, and rapid achievement of steady-state concentrations) and a low potential for drug interactions. It is licensed for use as adjunctive treatment for partial seizures, with or without secondary generalization, in people aged over 16 years.

For its impact on cognitive function, we only have data from a small pilot study that does not allow definite conclusions (Neyens et al., 1995). An international (UK/The Netherlands) cognitive study is presently carried out. In this study a first-line add-on design is used, comparing the cognitive effects of LEV with CBZ and VPA.

## Tiagabine (TGB)

Tiagabine (TGB) is a γ-aminobutyric acid (GABA) uptake inhibitor that is structurally related to the prototypic GABA uptake blocker nipecotic acid, but has an improved ability to cross the blood-brain barrier. TGB temporarily prolongs the presence of GABA in the synaptic cleft by delayed clearance. Clinical trials have shown that TGB is effective as add-on therapy in the management of patients with refractory partial epilepsy.

Three cognitive studies are available. Dodrill et al. (1997) included 162 patients who received the following treatments: placebo (n = 57), 16 mg/day TGB (n = 34), 32 mg/day TGB (n = 45), or 56 mg/day TGB (n = 26) at a fixed-dose for 12 weeks after a 4-week dose titration period. Eight cognitive tests and three measures of mood and adjustment were administered during the baseline period and again during the double-blind period near the end of treatment (or at the time of dropout). The results showed no cognitive effects of monotherapy with TGB at a low or high dose, but there was some evidence for mood effects of add-on treatment with TGB at higher dosing, possibly related to titration speed. In the add-on polytherapy study by Kälviäinen et al. (1996), 37 patients with partial epilepsy were included. The study protocol consisted of a randomized, double-blind, placebo-controlled, parallel-group add-on study and an open-label extension study. During the 3-month double-blind phase at low doses (30 mg/day), TGB treatment did not cause any cognitive changes as compared with placebo. TGB treatment also did not cause deterioration in cognitive performance during longer follow-up with successful treatment on higher doses after 6 to 12 months (mean 65.7 mg/day, range 30-80 mg/day) and after 18 to 24 months (mean dose 67.6 mg/day, range 24-80 mg/day). Finally, a study by Sveinbjornsdottir et al. (1994) was an open trial of 22 adult patients with refractory partial epilepsy followed by a double-blind, placebo-controlled, crossover trial in 12 subjects. Nineteen patients completed the initial open titration and fixed-dose phase of the study and 11 patients completed the double-blind phase. The median daily TGB dose was 32 mg during the open fixed-dose and 24 mg during the double-blind period. Neuropsychological evaluation did not show any significant effect on cognitive function in the open or double-blind phase.

## Gabapentin (GBP)

GBP (1-(aminomethyl) cyclohexane-acetic acid) is a novel AED, currently used as add-on therapy in patients with partial and generalized tonic-clonic seizures. GBP is a cyclic GABA analogue, originally designed as a GABA agonist (Macdonald & Kelly, 1995). Further research has clearly shown a specific effect of GBP on GABAergic neurotransmitter systems, especially influencing GABA turnover. Investigations using nuclear magnetic resonance imaging spectroscopy have confirmed that GBP elevates GABA concentrations, specifically in the occipital cortex of patients with epilepsy (Petroff et al., 1996).

Two volunteer studies and one clinical study are available to interpret the cognitive effects.

Martin et al. (1999) used an acute dose and rapid titration in six volunteers and did not find cognitive effects of GBP. Meador et al. (1999) compared the cognitive effects of GBP and CBZ in 35 healthy subjects by using a double-blind, randomized, crossover design with two 5-week treatment periods. During each treatment condition, subjects received either GBP 2,400 mg/day or CBZ (mean 731 mg/day). Subjects were tested at the end of each AED treatment period and in four drug-free conditions (two pretreatment baselines and two post-treatment washout periods [1 month after each AED]). The neuropsychological test battery included 17 measures yielding 31 total variables. Significantly better performance on eight variables was found for GBP, but on no variables for CBZ. Comparison of CBZ and GBP with the nondrug average revealed significant statistical differences for 15 (48%) of 31 variables. Leach et al. (1997) studied GBP in 21 patients in an add-on polytherapy study after 4 weeks of adjunctive therapy and found no change in psychomotor and memory tests. Drowsiness was more often found in higher dosing (2,400 mg). Mortimore et al. (1998) did not find a difference between continued polytherapy and an add-on with GBP in measures of quality of life.

## Zonisamide (ZNS)

The anticonvulsant properties of ZNS were discovered through extensive testing of a variety of sulfonamide compounds. Like TPM it has multiple mechanisms of action: blockade of voltage-gated sodium channels, reducing sustained repetitive firing, blocking T-type calcium channels, and inhibiting ligand binding to the $GABA_A$ receptor. Like TPM ZNS is a carbonic anydrase inhibiting drug. Although there is longer experience with ZNS in Japan (were it was developed), it was recently introduced in the USA and in Europe for partial onset seizures in refractory epilepsy.

Clinical anecdotal information shows a cognitive side-effect profile very similar to TPM but no controlled studies are available. Also no information is available about ongoing studies.

# Conclusion

A general conclusion that may be derived from most of the metaanalyses (Vermeulen & Aldenkamp, 1995) is that polypharmacy shows a relatively severe impact on cognitive function when compared with monotherapy, irrespective of the type of AEDs included. Two drugs that individually have mild cognitive effects may induce serious cognitive impairment when used together, possibly because of potentiation of tolerability problems (Trimble, 1987).

Possibly the most remarkable finding is that, although the severity of cognitive side effects is generally considered to be mild to moderate for most AEDs (Vermeulen & Aldenkamp, 1995), all commonly used AEDs have some impact on cognitive function. Such mild impact may be amplified in specific conditions and may become substantial in some patients when crucial functions are involved, such as learning in children (Aldenkamp et al., 1995) or driving capacities in adults (often requiring millisecond precision), or when functions are impaired that are already vulnerable, such as memory function in the elderly (Trimble, 1987). Moreover, the cognitive side effects represent the long-term outcome of AED therapy; therefore, the effects may increase with prolonged therapy, which contributes to the impact on daily life functioning in refractory epilepsies (American Academy of Pediatrics, 1985).

Definite evidence for drug-induced cognitive impairment has been established for phenobarbitone (memory impairment), phenytoin (mental slowing) and topiramate (mental slowing and dysphasia). Treatment with these drugs should consider these side-effects and patients should be monitored on a regular basis. Mild effects (mostly psychomotor slowing) were found for carbamazepine, oxcarbazepine, valproate and lamotrigine (with mild cognitive activating effects). The effects for ethosuximide, tiagabine, gabapentin, levetiracetam and zonisamide are inconclusive.

# References

Aarts JH, Binnie CD, Smit AM, Wilkins AJ. Selective cognitive impairment during focal and generalized epileptiform EEG activity. *Brain* 1984; 107: 293-308.

Äikiä M, Kälviäinen R, Sivenius J, Halonen T, Riekkinen RJ. Cognitive effects of oxcarbazepine and phenytoin monotherapy in newly diagnosed epilepsy: one year follow-up. *Epilepsy Res* 1992; 11: 199-203.

Aldenkamp AP. Cognitive effects of topiramate, gabapentin and lamotrigine in healthy young adults. *Neurology* 2000; 54: 270-2.

Aldenkamp AP. Cognitive and behavioural assessment in clinical trials: when should they be done? *Epilepsy Res* 2001; 45: 155-9.

Aldenkamp AP. Antiepileptic drug treatment and epileptic seizures – effects on cognitive function. In: Trimble M, Schmitz B, eds. *The neuropsychiatry of epilepsy*. New York: Cambridge University Press, 2002: 256-67.

Aldenkamp AP, Dodson WE, eds. Epilepsy and education; cognitive factors in learning behavior. *Epilepsia* 1990; 31 (suppl 4): S9-S20.

Aldenkamp AP, Alpherts WCJ, Blennow G, et al. Withdrawal of antiepileptic medication-effects on cognitive function in children: The Multicentre Holmfrid Study. *Neurology* 1993; 43: 41-50.

Aldenkamp AP, Dreifuss FE, Renier WO, Suumeijer PBM. *Epilepsy in children and adolescents*. Boca Raton, Fla: CRC Press, 1995.

Aldenkamp AP, Mulder OG, Overweg J. Cognitive effects of lamotrigine as first line add-on in patients with localized related (partial) epilepsy. *J Epilepsy* 1997; 10: 117-21.

Aldenkamp AP, Baker G, Mulder OG, et al. A multicentre randomized clinical study to evaluate the effect on cognitive function of topiramate compared with valproate as add-on therapy to carbamazepine in patients with partial-onset seizures. *Epilepsia* 2000; 41: 1167-78.

Aldenkamp AP, Baker G. A systematic review of the effects of lamotrigine on cognitive function and quality of life. *Epilepsy Behav* 2001; 2: 85-91.

Aldenkamp AP, Arends J, Overweg-Plandsoen TC, et al. Acute cognitive effects of nonconvulsive difficult-to-detect epileptic seizures and epileptiform electroencephalographic discharges. *J Child Neurol* 2001; 16: 119-23.

Aldenkamp AP, Arends J, Bootsma HP, et al. Randomized, double-blind parallel-group study comparing cognitive effects of a low-dose lamotrigine with valproate and placebo in healthy volunteers. *Epilepsia* 2002; 43: 19-26.

Aldenkamp AP, De Krom M, Reijs R. Newer antiepileptic drugs and cognitive issues. *Epilepsia* 2003; 44 (suppl 4): 21-9.

American Academy of Pediatrics. Behavioral and cognitive effects of anticonvulsant therapy. Committee on Drugs. *Pediatrics* 1985; 76: 644-7.

Banks GK, Beran RG. Neuropsychological assessment in lamotrigine treated epileptic patients. *Clin Exp Neurol* 1991; 28: 230-7.

Binnie CD, van Emde BW, Kasteleijn-Nolste-Trenite DG, et al. Acute effects of lamotrigine (BW430C) in persons with epilepsy. *Epilepsia* 1986; 27: 248-54.

Bootsma HP, Coolen F, Aldenkamp AP, Arends J, Diepman L, Hulsman J, Lambrechts D, Leenen L, Majoie M, Schellekens A, de Krom M. Topiramate in clinical practice: long-term experience in patients with refractory epilepsy referred to a tertiary epilepsy center. *Epilepsy Behav* 2004; 5 (3): 380-7.

Burton LA, Harden C. Effect of topiramate on attention. *Epilepsy Res* 1997; 27: 29-32.

Calandre EP, Dominguez-Granados R, Gomez-Rubio M, et al. Cognitive effects of long-term treatment with phenobarbital and valproic acid in school children. *Acta Neur Scand* 1990; 81: 504-6.

Chadwick DW, Marson T, Kadir Z. Clinical administration of new antiepileptic drugs: an overview of safety and efficacy. *Epilepsia* 1996; 37 (suppl 6): S17-22.

Cohen AF, Ashby L, Crowley D, Land G, Peck AW, Miller AA. Lamotrigine (BW430C), a potential anticonvulsant. Effects on the central nervous system in comparison with phenytoin and diazepam. *Br J Clin Pharmacol* 1985; 20: 619-29.

Craig I, Tallis R. Impact of valproate and phenytoin on cognitive function in elderly patients: results of a single-blind randomized comparative study. *Epilepsia* 1994; 35: 381-90.

Curran HV, Java R. Memory and psychomotor effects of oxcarbazepine in healthy human volunteers. *Eur J Clin Pharmacol* 1993; 44: 529-33.

Dodrill CB, Troupin AS. Psychotropic effects of carbamazepine in epilepsy: a double-blind comparison with phenytoin. *Neurology* 1977; 27: 1023-8.

Dodrill CB, Arnett JL, Sommerville KW, Shu V. Cognitive and quality of life effects of differing dosages of tiagabine in epilepsy. *Neurology* 1997; 48: 1025-31.

Dodson WE, Pellock JM. *Pediatric epilepsy: diagnosis and treatment*. New York: Demos Publications, 1993.

Dodson WE, Trimble MR. *Epilepsy and quality of life*. New York: Raven Press, 1994.

Earl N, McKee JR, Sunder TR, et al. Lamotrigine adjunctive therapy in patients with refractory epilepsy and mental retardation [Abstract]. *Epilepsia* 2000; 41 (suppl 1): 72.

Ettinger AB, Weisbrot DM, Saracco J, Dhoon A, Kanner A, Devinsky O. Positive and negative psychotropic effects of lamotrigine in patients with epilepsy and mental retardation. *Epilepsia* 1998; 39: 874-7.

Faught E, Wilder BJ, Ramsay RE, et al. Topiramate placebo-controlled dose-ranging trial in refractory partial epilepsy using 200-, 400-, and 600-mg daily dosages. *Neurology* 1996; 46: 1684-90.

Forsythe I, Butler R, Berg I, et al. Cognitive impairment in new cases of epilepsy randomly assigned to carbamazepine, phenytoin and sodium valproate. *Developmental Medicine and Child Neurology* 1991; 33: 524-34.

Gallassi R, Morreale A, Di Sarro R, Marra M, Lugaresi E, Baruzzi A. Cognitive effects of antiepileptic drug discontinuation. *Epilepsia* 1992; 33 (suppl 6): S41-4.

Gillham R, Kane K, Bryant-Comstock L, Brodie MJ. A double-blind comparison of lamotrigine and carbamazepine in newly diagnosed epilepsy with health-related quality of life as an outcome measure. *Seizure* 2000; 9: 375-9.

Hamilton MJ, Cohen AF, Yuen AW, et al. Carbamazepine and lamotrigine in healthy volunteers: relevance to early tolerance and clinical trial dosage. *Epilepsia* 1993; 34: 166-73.

Ideström CM, Schalling D, Carlquist U, Sjoqvist F. Acute effects of diphenylhydantoin in relation to plasma levels. Behavioral and psychological studies. *Psychol Med* 1972; 2: 111-20.

Jette NJ, Marson AG, Hutton JL. Topiramate add-on for drug-resistant partial epilepsy. *Cochrane Database Syst Rev* 2002; (3): CD001417.

Kälviäinen R, Äikiä M, Mervaala E, Saukkonen AM, Pitkanen A, Riekkinen PJ Sr. Long-term cognitive and EEG effects of tiagabine in drug-resistant partial epilepsy. *Epilepsy Res* 1996; 25: 291-7.

Kellet MW, Smith DF, Stockton PA, Chadwick DW. Topiramate in clinical practice: first year's postlicensing experience in a specialist epilepsy clinic. *J Neurol Neurosurg Psychiatry* 1999; 66: 759-63.

Ketter TA, Post RM, Theodore WH. Positive and negative psychiatric effects of antiepileptic drugs in patients with seizure disorders. *Neurology* 1999; 53 (5 suppl 2): 53-67.

Laaksonen R, Kaimola K, Grahn-Terävainen E, Waltimo O. A controlled clinical trial of the effects of carbamazepine and oxcarbazepine on memory and attention. 16th International Epilepsy Congress, Hamburg, 1985 (abstract).

Leach MJ, Lees G, Riddall DR. *Lamotrigine: mechanisms of action.* In: Levy RH, Mattson RH, Meldrum BS, eds. *Antiepileptic drugs*, 4th edition. New York: Raven Press, 1995: 861-9.

Leach JP, Girvan J, Paul A, Brodie MJ. Gabapentin and cognition: a double blind, dose ranging, placebo controlled study in refractory epilepsy. *J Neurol Neurosurg Psychiatry* 1997; 62: 372-6.

Lhatoo SD, Wong ICK, Sander JW. Prognostic factors affecting long-term retention of topiramate in patients with chronic epilepsy. *Epilepsia* 2000; 41: 338-41.

Macdonald RL, Kelly, KM. Antiepileptic drug mechanisms of action. *Epilepsia* 1995; 36 (S2): 2-12.

MacLeod CM, Dekaban AS, Hunt E. Memory impairment in epileptic patients: selective effects of phenobarbital concentration. *Science* 1978; 202: 1102-4.

Marciani MG, Spanedda F, Bassetti MA, et al. Effect of lamotrigine on EEG paroxysmal abnormalities and background activity: a computerized analysis. *Br J Clin Pharmacol* 1996; 42: 621-7.

Marciani MG, Stanzione P, Mattia D, et al. Lamotrigine add-on therapy in focal epilepsy: electroencephalographic and neuropsychological evaluation. *Clin Neuropharmacol* 1998; 21: 41-7.

Marson AG, Kadir ZA, Hutton JL, Chadwick DW. The new antiepileptic drugs: a systematic review of their efficacy and tolerability. *Epilepsia* 1997; 38: 859-80.

Marson AG, Kadir ZA, Hutton JL, Chadwick DW. Gabapentin for drug-resistant partial epilepsy. *Cochrane Database Syst Rev* 2000; (2): CD001415.

Marson AG, Hutton JL, Leach JP, et al. Levetiracetam, oxcarbazepine, remacemide and zonisamide for drug resistant localization-related epilepsy: a systematic review. *Epilepsy Res* 2001; 46: 259-70.

Martin R, Kuzniecky R, Ho S, et al. Cognitive effects of topiramate, gabapentin, and lamotrigine in healthy young adults. *Neurology* 1999; 52: 321-7.

McKee PJ, Blacklaw J, Forrest G, et al. A double-blind, placebo-controlled interaction study between oxcarbazepine and carbamazepine, sodium valproate and phenytoin in epileptic patients. *Br J Clin Pharmacol* 1994; 37: 27-32.

Meador KJ. Assessing cognitive effects of a new AED without the bias of practice effects [Abstract]. *Epilepsia* 1997; 38 (suppl 3): 60.

Meador KJM, Loring DW, Huh K, Gallagher BB, King DW. Comparative cognitive effects of anticonvulsants. *Neurology* 1990; 40: 391-4.

Meador KJM, Loring DW, Allen, ME, et al. Comparative cognitive effects of carbamazepine and phenytoin in healthy adults. *Neurology* 1991; 41: 1537-40.

Meador KJM, Loring DW, Abney OL, et al. Effects of carbamazepine and phenytoin on EEG and memory in healthy adults. *Epilepsia* 1993; 34 (1): 153-7.

Meador KJ, Loring DW, Ray PG, et al. Differential cognitive effects of carbamazepine and gabapentin. *Epilepsia* 1999; 40: 1279-85.

Meador KJ, Loring DW, Ray PG, Perrine KR, Bazquez BR, Kalbosa T. Differential effects of carbamazepine and lamotrigine [Abstract]. *Neurology* 2000; 54 (suppl 3): A84.

Mervaala E, Koivista K, Hanninen T, et al. Electrophysiological and neuropsychological profiles of lamotrigine in young and age-associated memory impairment (AAMI) subjects [Abstract]. *Neurology* 1995; 45 (suppl 4): A259.

Mortimore C, Trimble M, Emmers E. Effects of gabapentin on cognition and quality of life in patients with epilepsy. *Seizure* 1998; 7: 359-6.

Neyens LGJ, Alpherts WCJ, Aldenkamp AP. Cognitive effects of a new pyrrolidine derivative (levetiracetam) in patients with epilepsy. *Prog Neuropsychopharmacol Biol Psychiatry* 1995; 19: 411-9.

Parnas J, Flachs H, Gram L. Psychotropic effect of antiepileptic drugs. *Acta Neurol Scand* 1979; 60: 329-43.

Parnas J, Gram L, Flachs H. Psychopharmacological aspects of antiepileptic treatment. *Prog Neurobiol* 1980; 15: 119-38.

Petroff OAC, Rothman DL, Behar KL, et al. The effect of gabapentin on brain gamma-aminobutyric acid in patients with epilepsy. *Ann Neurol* 1996; 39: 95-9.

Prevey ML, Delaney RC, Cramer, JA, Cattanach, L, Collins JF, Mattson RH. Effect of Valproate on cognitive function. Comparison with carbamazepine. The Department of Veterans Affairs Epilepsy Cooperative Study 264 Group. *Arch Neurol* 1996; 53 (10): 1008-16.

Privitera M, Fincham R, Penry J, et al. Topiramate placebo-controlled dose-ranging trial in refractory partial epilepsy using 600-, 800-, and 1000-mg daily dosages. Topiramate YE Study Group. *Neurology* 1996; 46: 1678-83.

Sabers A, Moller A, Dam M, et al. Cognitive function and anticonvulsant therapy: effect of monotherapy in epilepsy. *Acta Neurol Scand* 1995; 92: 19-27.

Schwarz JR, Grigat G. Phenytoin and carbamazepine: potential- and frequency-dependent black of NA currents in mammalian myelinated nerve fibers. *Epilepsia* 1989; 30: 286-94.

Smith WL, Lowrey JB. Effects of diphenylhydantoin on mental abilities in the elderly. *J Am Geriatr Soc* 1975; 23: 207-11.

Smith D, Baker G, Davies G, Dewey M, Chadwick DW. Outcomes of add-on treatment with lamotrigine in partial epilepsy. *Epilepsia* 1993; 34: 312-22.

Stefan H, Krämer G, Mamoli B, eds. *Challenge epilepsy – new antiepileptic drugs*. Berlin: Blackwell Science, 1998.

Sveinbjornsdottir S, Sander JW, Patsalos PN, Upton D, Thompson PJ, Duncan JS. Neuropsychological effects of tiagabine, a potential new antiepileptic drug. *Seizure* 1994; 3: 29-35.

Tatum WO, French JA, Faught E, et al. Postmarketing experience with topiramate and cognition. *Epilepsia* 2001; 42: 1134-40.

Thompson PJ, Trimble MR. Sodium valproate en cognitive functioning in normal volunteers. *Br Journ Clin Pharmacol* 1981; 12: 819-24.

Thompson PJ, Huppert F, Trimble MR. Anticonvulsant drugs, cognitive function and memory. *Acta Neurol Scand* 1980; (S80): 75-80.

Thompson PJ, Huppert FA, Trimble MR. Phenytoin and cognitive functions: effects on normal volunteers and implications for epilepsy. *British Journ Clin Psychol* 1981; 20: 155-62.

Thompson PJ, Baxendale SA, Duncan JS, Sander JW. Effects of topiramate on cognitive function. *J Neurol Neurosurg Psychiatry* 2000; 69: 636-41.

Trimble MR. Anticonvulsant drugs and cognitive function: a review of the literature. *Epilepsia* 1987; 28 (suppl 3): 37-45.

Twyman RE, Rogers CJ, Macdonald RL. Differential regulation of gamma-aminobutyric acid receptor channels by diazepam and Phenobarbital. *Ann Neurol* 1989; 25: 213-20.

Vermeulen J, Aldenkamp AP. Cognitive side-effects of chronic antiepileptic drug treatment: a review of 25 years of research. *Epilepsy Res* 1995; 22: 65-95.

Vining EP, Mellitis ED, Dorsen MM, Cataldo MF, Quaskey SA, Spielberg SP, Freeman JM. Psychologic and behavioral effects of antiepileptic drugs in children: a double-blind comparison between phenobarbital and valproic acid. *Pediatrics* 1987; 80 (2): 165-74.

White HS. Clinical significance of animal seizure models and mechanism of action studies of potential antiepileptic drugs. *Epilepsia* 1997; 38 (suppl 1): S9-S17.

Wong IC. New antiepileptic drugs. Study suggests that under a quarter of patients will still be taking the new drugs after six years. *BMJ* 1997; 314: 603-4.

# Mood effects of antiepileptic drugs

B. Schmitz

*Department of Neurology, Charité, Humboldt University Berlin, Germany*

---

Antiepileptic drugs (AEDs) modify the balance between neuronal excitation and inhibition via their influence on cerebral transmitter systems and/or ion channel activities. These effects do not only selectively reduce the seizure threshold, they may also modify systems which regulate mood and behaviour. Anticonvulsant and psychotropic effects of AEDs are however not independent. Effects on seizure control have indirect effects on the mental state. Patients who are seizure free have no risk of developing seizure-related psychiatric complications. On the other hand sudden cessation of seizures may lead to an imbalance in the mental state as in "forced normalisation" (FN). Some anticonvulsants have dose related paradoxical proconvulsive properties which may cause behavioural disturbances with an underlying non-convulsive status epilepticus. Therefore psychotropic effects may be negative or beneficial in individual patients. These effects depend on the antiepileptic strength and the mode of action of the anticonvulsant and the patient's biological and psychological predisposition. With the increasing choice of AEDs behavioural drug profiles have become very important for optimal treatment in epilepsy. Recent quality of life studies have shown that the tolerability of AEDs is more important to patients than seizure reduction (Gilliam et al., 2002). Furthermore, the high psychiatric comorbidity in epilepsy often requires psychopharmacological interventions, which may be avoided when anticonvulsants are used which not only have antiepileptic but also psychotropic properties. This chapter discusses the effects of AED on behaviour and mood with a special focus on depression.

In clinical practice, adverse AED effects on mood are often overlooked. One reason for this is the complex and multifactorial aetiology of psychiatric complications in epilepsy. AEDs represent only one of several biological and psychological risk factors which need to be disentangled in every individual patient. Adverse mood effects of AED are often not recognized because many neurologists are not competent in the exploration of a mental state, or they don't have the additional time needed. Often patients do not complain about depressive symptoms unless they are specifically interviewed. Many patients are not primarily troubled by obvious depressive symptoms such as sadness or feelings of guilt. Depression in epilepsy often presents with sleep disorders or somatoform complaints and memory problems, which make the diagnosis difficult unless the full psychopathological status is explored. If delayed psychiatric adverse effects occur after months or years of treatment, the causal relationship with drug treatment is often not considered and is in fact difficult to prove, unless drug withdrawal is followed by remission of psychiatric symptoms.

AED-related mood disturbances are common in patients with epilepsy, the exact prevalence is however difficult to estimate. In a consecutive series of patients with epilepsy and major depression (Schmitz et al., 1999), 28% were considered AED-related (including intoxications, withdrawal syndromes and cases of forced normalisation). The percentage of drug induced "iatrogenic" depression was also 28% in a series of 100 patients with depressive syndromes in need of treatment (Kanner et al., 2000).

## ■ Adverse psychiatric effects of conventional AEDs

There are little systematic data on the psychiatric side effects of classical AEDs. Our knowledge is largely empirical, based on small case series or anecdotal reports. Several studies suggested a link between depression and treatment with barbiturates both in adults and in children (Robertson et al., 1987, Brent 1986). 40% of school children treated with barbiturates were diagnosed with "major depression", as compared to only 4% of children treated with carbamazepine (Brent et al., 1987).

In children, a conduct disorder resembling the attention deficit hyperactivity disorder may be provoked by many AEDs, but the most frequently implicated drug is phenobarbitone. Irritability and aggressive behaviour are side effects particularly often seen when barbiturates are used in mentally retarded patients. Withdrawal problems which present with nervousness, dysphoria and insomnia may occur even when barbiturates are very slowly tapered down.

Phenytoin may provoke schizophrenia-like psychoses at high serum levels (Mcdanal and Bolman, 1975). These psychoses are dose related, thus toxic syndromes, but they are not associated with cerebellar signs which are the most common central nervous side effects of phenytoin. In a study on 45 patients with drug related psychoses, 25 (56%) were attributed to treatment with phenytoin (Kanemoto et al., 2001). A chronic encephalopathy has also been described with phenytoin and has been referred to as "dilantin dementia" (Trimble and Reynolds, 1976).

Psychoses typically following cessation of seizures and associated with a normalisation of the EEG occur in 2% of children treated with ethosuximide. The risk of "forced normalisation" is higher (8%) in adolescents and adults treated with ethosuximide for persisting absence seizures (Wolf et al., 1984).

Affective problems are rare complications of treatment with carbamazepine (Dalby, 1975). These are either depressive disorders or mania, the latter being explained as a paradoxical effect due to the antidepressant properties of carbamazepine which is chemically related to tricyclic antidepressants (Drake and Peruzzi, 1986).

Rarely, valproate is associated with acute or chronic encephalopathies (Sackellares et al., 1979; Zaret and Cohen, 1986; Schöndienst and Wolf, 1992). These encephalopathies are related to dose and perhaps polytherapy and are reversible with dose reduction.

## Adverse psychiatric effects of newer AEDs

Nine new antiepileptic drugs have been introduced over the last 15 years. Data from premarketing studies provide information on the frequency of psychiatric side effects of these new AEDs. However, drug trials are designed to test antiepileptic efficacy and psychiatric adverse events are not systematically reported. Thus severity and psychopathological nature of drug-induced behavioural problems remain obscure. Further, differences in patients included in trials do not allow comparisons of psychiatric risks of specific drugs, particularly since following the early vigabatrin experience, patients with a psychiatric history were often excluded from trials. Drug trials have a limited duration and are therefore insensitive to delayed psychotropic effects. Furthermore, fixed titrations schemes which are used in trials are often different from those which later prove optimal in clinical practice. Therefore psychotropic profiles of new drugs are often not identified through regulatory trials and become clear only with postmarketing clinical experience. *Table I* summarises data from premarketing controlled trials suggesting a relatively high frequency of depressive reactions in vigabatrin, tiagabine and topiramate, and relative low rates for lamotrigine, gabapentin and levetiracetam.

Table I. Incidence rates of psychoses and depression in controlled trials
(Besag, 2001; Janssen Cilag, 1996; Levinson and Devinsky, 1999).

|  | Psychoses (%) | Depression (%) |
|---|---|---|
| Vigabatrin | 2.5 | 12.1 |
| Lamotrigine | 0.2 | – |
| Felbamate | 0.02 | – |
| Gabapentin | 0.5 | – |
| Topiramate | 0.8 | 9-18 |
| Tiagabine | 0.8-2 | 5 |
| Levetiracetam | 0.3-0.7 | 0.5-2% |

Obviously psychiatric risks of the newer AEDs are not the same for all compounds. Some of the drugs seem to have neutral effects, some have a relevant risk for negative effects, and some may have predominately beneficial psychotropic effects. A general comment is that the overall psychiatric risks of newer AED are not lower than those of older AEDs.

## Vigabatrin

Of the newer agents the behavioural effects of vigabatrin have been studied relatively frequent, perhaps on account of its being the first to be tested and licensed. Shortly after the introduction of vigabatrin, significant psychiatric complications occuring in 7% of treated patients were reported (Sander et al., 1991). When these cases were analysed in more detail (Thomas et al., 1995), three patterns were identified with respect to psychoses: of a total of 28 psychotic patients eleven had become seizure free (a strong indication for the role of "forced normalisation"), six had a postictal psychosis following a cluster of seizures after initial seizure control, possibly related to tolerance, and two psychoses occurred after withdrawal of vigabatrin. None of the 22 patients with vigabatrin related depression had become seizure free, suggesting that the underlying mechanisms for the provocation of psychosis and depression may be different. In children, particularly in association with learning disabilities, the most common psychiatric side effects are agitation and excitation, hyperkinesia and aggression, a behaviour syndrome similar to that seen with barbiturates. In a French study, the incidence of behavioural disturbances in children was as high as 28% (Dulac et al., 1991).

The risk of psychiatric complications caused by vigabatrin has been confirmed by two meta-analyses. When looking at psychoses and severe behavioural reactions leading to drug discontinuation in seven placebo controlled European studies (Ferrie et al., 1996) the overall incidence of these complications was 3.4% in the vigabatrin group and 0.6% in the placebo group. Remarkably, the incidence rates were rather different in different studies, ranging from 1% to 12%, suggesting that either the risk is not identical for all patient groups or that the threshold to report psychiatric side effects is not the same among different investigators.

Another meta-analysis on the psychiatric risks of vigabatrin (Levinson and Devinsky, 1999) translated psychopathological symptoms described in the investigator forms into standardized psychiatric terminology, which was then summarized into a syndromatic diagnosis. This analysis of US-American and non-US double blind studies demonstrated a significantly increased risk for psychosis and particularly for depression. Psychoses occurred in 2.5% of patients treated with vigabatrin compared to an incidence of 0.3% in the placebo group ($p < 0.05$), and depression occurred in 12.1% of patients treated with vigabatrin in contrast to only 3.5% in the placebo group ($p < 0.001$).

## Lamotrigine

Lamotrigine has gained a reputation of having positive psychotropic properties, improving both mood and cognitive functions. Severe psychiatric complications seem to be uncommon with lamotrigine, and psychosis and depression occurred only in very few cases in the trials (Fitton and Goa, 1995). Insomnia, which may be associated with irritability, anxiety or even hypomania, is the only significant psychiatric side effect, occurring in 6% of patients treated in monotherapy, compared to 2% in patients treated with carbamazepine and 3% in patients treated with phenytoin (Brodie et al., 1995).

When there were first reports that carers complained that mentally handicapped patients became more alert and demanding, this was interpreted to reflect inadequate rehabilitation facilities rather than being a negative side effect (Binnie, 1997). Besag refers to this as a "release phenomenon" (Besag, 2001). There are however a number of reports that children with learning difficulties and adults with mental handicap may develop behavioural problems such as aggression (Beran et al., 1998; Ettinger et al., 1998) and there have been reports on the induction of a reversible Tourette syndrome which in some cases was accompanied by obsessive compulsive symptoms (Lombroso, 1999).

## Felbamate

Felbamate is at present only used in a minority of patients particularly with Lennox-Gastaut syndrome due to its haematologic and hepatic toxicity. According to the manufacturer, psychoses are rare, reported as serious adverse events in 0.02% of all patients treated before 1996 (Essex Pharma, 1996). Felbamate may lead to increased alertness, inducing sleep problems and behavioural problems related to agitation in some patients, again, particularly in children with learning disabilities (McConnell et al., 1996). In an English study (Li et al., 1996) 14 of 111 patients experienced adverse psychotropic side-effects being the commonest reason for withdrawal. According to a study by Ketter et al. the psychotropic effects of felbamate may be particularly negative in anxious children, while other, primarily sedated children are likely to benefit from the stimulating properties of felbamate (Ketter et al., 1996).

## Gabapentin

Beyond somnolence, negative psychotropic effects have not been demonstrated in the controlled studies with gabapentin, which is a generally well tolerated anticonvulsant. However, there are a number of studies suggesting that gabapentin may induce behavioural problems such as aggression in children with learning disabilities and adults with a mental handicap (Lee et al., 1996; Wolf et al., 1995; Tallian et al., 1995). It has been suggested, that these behavioural effects could be explained by rapid titration of gabapentin. In elderly people with reduced creatinine clearance gabapentin may cause various neurotoxic symptoms due to its renal elimination.

## Tiagabine

A specific problem with tiagabine is the paradoxical provocation of de novo non-convulsive status epilepticus due to a relatively narrow therapeutic window (Schapel and Chadwick 1996). Therefore, EEG recordings are necessary when behavioural problems arise, particularly when clinical signs such as mutism, qualitative change in consciousness, automatisms or myoclonia suggest non-convulsive status epilepticus. Unfortunately, this complication was discovered following the initial trials and it is therefore not possible to know whether psychiatric complications in the trials were related to underlying epileptic activity or not.

In the placebo-controlled add-on studies, nervousness and depressed mood were both increased in the tiagabine group (Leppik, 1995) (12% versus 3%, 5% versus 1%). The incidence of serious adverse events presenting as psychosis was 2% versus 1% in the placebo group.

## Topiramate

In the premarketing studies and possibly related to aggressive titration schemes, topiramate was associated with a relatively high rate of neurotoxic side effects. Psychotic reactions were however relatively infrequent with a prevalence of 0.8%. In a postmarketing study comparing psychiatric side effects of topiramate, lamotrigine and gabapentin, psychotic episodes occurred in 12% of patients treated with topiramate compared to 0.7% of patients treated with lamotrigine and 0.5% of patients treated with gabapentin (Crawford, 1998). A significant proportion of topiramate associated psychoses are explained as alternative syndromes in patients who become seizure free (Mula et al., 2003a). An unusual idiosyncratic side effect of topiramate is amnesic or motor aphasia and in the controlled trials 17-28% of patients developed symptoms classified as "abnormal thinking" (Janssen-Cilag, 1996).

The rate of affective symptoms is clearly dose dependent with an incidence of 9% and 19% with a daily dose of 200 mg respectively 1,000 mg in one premarketing study (Janssen-Cilag, 1996). In Mula's analysis of topiramate related psychiatric complications, depression was significantly correlated with rapid titration and high dosages (Mula et al., 2003a). But even with careful titration schemes some patients don't tolerate topiramate. In Mula's study there was an interesting correlation between depression and cognitive side effects, suggesting that neuropsychological and affective problems are closely interlinked. The neuropsychological disorders caused by topiramate resemble a frontal lobe problem and have been interpreted as regional behavioural toxicity. It would be interesting to investigate whether patients with focal epilepsies and frontal lobe dysfunction are more vulnerable to these effects, because with respect to topiramate associated aphasia, these occur more frequently in patients with a dominant seizure origin.

## Levetiracetam

Levetiracetam is not associated with a high risk for severe psychotic or depressive reactions. Significant affective episodes were reported in 2% and psychoses in 0.7% of patients treated in preclinical trials. Some of the levetiracetam associated psychoses were explained as a manifestation of forced normalisation.

A clinically relevant psychiatric side effect of levetiracetam is the provocation of aggressive behaviour and irritability which occurs both in adults and children. In an English series of 517 adult patients treated with levetiracetam 10% developed a psychiatric complication, most frequently presenting with aggressive behaviour (Mula et al., 2003b). Aggression occurs particularly often, but not exclusively, in patients with preexisting irritability and dysphoria. Mesad and Devinsky (2002) analysed cases of severe aggressive behaviour, defined by objective verbal or physical aggression leading to withdrawal of levetiracetam. The prevalence was 18 out of 460 consecutive patients (3.9%). Seven patients had previous episodes of aggressive behaviour.

Children may be at an even higher risk to develop aggression including suicidal behaviour, with prevalence rates up to 68% (Estrada et al., 2002). In children with preexisting neuropsychiatric symptomatology levetiracetam may provoke an exacerbation of behavioural problems (Gustafson et al., 2002). Kossoff et al. (2001) reported on four adolescents who developed a psychosis secondary to treatment with levetiracetam all of which were reversible following withdrawal. All patients had preexisiting behavioural problems, and two had become seizure free, supporting the role of FN.

## Zonisamide

Beyond Japan, there is still limited experience with this novel drug, which acts via a carboanhydrase inhibition mechanism similar to topiramate. There are however reports of significant psychiatric adverse events including affective problems (*Figure 1*) and psychoses.

In a Japanese series of patients with psychotic episodes half of drug related episodes were triggered by zonisamide (Matsuura, 1999).

## Pregabaline

There is no evidence for significant psychiatric adverse events from controlled trials with pregabaline. However, clinical experience with this recently introduced drug is still limited.

## ■ Risk factors

Patients with a biographic or genetic predisposition are presumably more at risk to develop AED related psychiatric complications such as depression and psychosis (*Table II*).

Patients with previous depressive episodes are more likely to develop an affective disorder while patients with previous schiozophrenia-like psychoses are more likely to present with a psychotic reaction, suggesting that the clinical presentation of psychiatric adverse reactions depends on the individual psychopathological predisposition. In patients with previous psychiatric problems rapid titration should therefore be avoided, since aggressive titration schemes further increase the risk of behavioural toxicity.

Table II. Risk factors for depression and psychosis with vigabatrin, topiramate and levetiracetam.

|  | Vigabatrin*<br>Depression/psychoses<br>n = 22/28 | Topiramate**<br>Depression/psychoses<br>n = 46/16 | Levetiracetam***<br>Depression/psychoses<br>n = 13/6 |
| --- | --- | --- | --- |
| Psychiatric history | +/+ | +/+ | +/+ |
| Febrile seizures | ?/? | +/? | +/? |
| Status epilepticus | ?/? | ?/? | +/? |
| Titration/dosage | +/- | +/- | -/- |
| Seizure freedom | -/+ (13 cases) | -/+ (10 cases) | -/+ (4 cases) |
| Severity of epilepsy | -/+ | +/? | -/? |
| Cognitive side effects | ?/? | +/- | -/- |

* Thomas *et al.*, 1996, ** Mula *et al.*, 2003a, *** Mula *et al.*, 2003b.
+ significant relationship, – no relationship, ? not studied or too small numbers.

Some studies have shown that patients with severe epilepsies are at a higher risk for psychiatric side effects. Mula et al. (2003a) demonstrated that hippocampal sclerosis is more common in patients who develop depressive episodes secondary to treatment with topiramate as compared to patients without affective side effects, another indication for the close links between limbic dysfunction and affective disorders.

Children and adults with learning disability and multiple handicaps are particularly vulnerable to behavioural adverse effects of AED. In these patients, the exact psychiatric diagnosis may be difficult, and both depression and psychosis may manifest with aggressive behaviour. Also nonpsychiatric adverse mood effects may lead to disturbed behaviour because patients may have difficulties to express their discomfort otherwise. In these patients drug changes should be monitored carefully, and it is recommended that the behavioural changes are carefully discussed with the caring team. Sometimes interpretations of behavioural changes are different within the team and particularly when patients become more alert and active due to the positive psychotropic AED effects, these changes may be regarded negative because they request adaptations in the attitude of carers and make new treatment programs necessary.

## ■ Mechanisms

There are four major mechanisms which explain behavioural effects of AEDs: 1. dosage-dependant toxicity, 2. dose-independent idiosyncratic drug effects, 3. withdrawal effects and 4. indirect effects via anticonvulsive actions. Of these, the two most important mechanisms are pharmacodynamic side effects related to the drugs mode of action and effects which arise with seizure control, so called alternative syndromes associated with the phenomenon of forced normalisation.

### Idiosyncratic effects

There are only three gross categories of antiepileptic drug mechanisms (which however do not explain the mode of action of all AEDs): membrane stabilisation via ion channel blockade, increased inhibition by GABA-ergic effects, and decreased excitation by anti-glutamatergic effects. Trimble was the first to note that psychiatric problems and in particular depressive disorders are significantly increased with those AED which have strong GABA-ergic properties: barbiturates, vigabatrin, tiagabine and topiramate (Trimble, 1997). *Figure 1* demonstrates that not only depression but also other affective side effects of newer AEDs (including emotional lability, nervousness, agitation and irritability) which were reported in controlled trials were more common with tiagabine, vigabatrin and topiramate compared to lamotrigine, levetiracetam and gabapentin.

Trimble's hypothesis of a link between psychiatric complications and GABA-ergic mechanisms of AEDs was extended by Ketter et al. (1999) who distinguished two categories of AED, the first being GABA-ergic with sedating, anxiolytic and antimanic properties *(Table III)*.

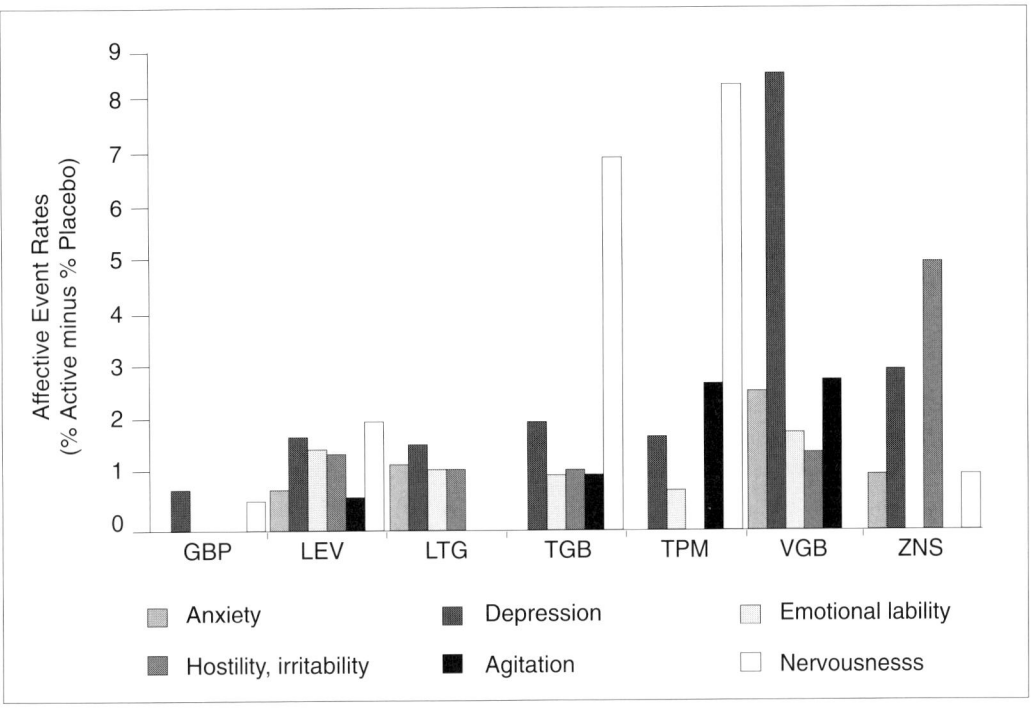

**Figure 1. Incidence of affective disorders associated with new antiepileptic drugs (Cramer et al., 2003).**
GBP Gabapentin, LEV Levetiracetam, LTG Lamotrigine, TGB Tiagabine, TPM Topiramate, VGB Vigabatrin, ZNS Zonisamide.

**Table III. Two categories of AED with different psychotropic effects depending on the preexisting mental state** (Ketter et al., Neurology, 1999).

| Mechanism | GABA-ergig drugs | Anti-glutamatergic drugs |
|---|---|---|
| Psychotropic effects | Sedating<br>Anxiolytic<br>Depressogenic<br>Antimanic | Activating<br>Anxiogenic<br>Antidepressive<br>Insomnia |
| Drugs | Barbiturates<br>Benzodiazepines<br>Valproate<br>Vigabatrin<br>Tiagabine<br>Gabapentin | Felbamate<br>Lamotrigine |
| Effect in activated patients | Positive | Negative |
| Effect in sedated patients | Negative | Positive |

This category comprises barbiturates, benzodiazepines, valproate, vigabatrin, tiagabine and gabapentin. The second category comprises anti-glutamatergic drugs which are claimed to have activating, anxiogenic and antidepressive effects: felbamate and lamotrigine. In this scheme topiramate holds an intermediate position because of its multiple mechanisms, and levetiracetam cannot be classified because of the atypical mode of action. The authors suggest that anticonvulsant drugs have different mood effects depending on the preexisting mental status of patients. They predict that patients who are primarily activated may benefit from drugs which belong to the "sedating" category and become worse with "activating" drugs. On the other hand, patients who are primarily sedated would benefit from a drug from the "activating" category, while the same patients would worsen with a "sedating" anticonvulsant. Taking the primary psychopathological status of patients into account explains the sometimes unexpected and seemingly paradoxical effects of some AED in individual patients. A scheme with only two categories of AEDs is certainly an oversimplification. Therefore, the influence of the patient's preexisting mental state on the direction of psychotropic AED effects deserves systematic research. Based on clinical experiences *table IV* suggests some "predictable" psychiatric AED risks depending on baseline psychopathology.

Table IV. Psychiatric risks of antiepileptic drugs in patients with preexisting psychiatric problems.

| Patient | Cave | Possible side effect |
| --- | --- | --- |
| Dysthymia | PHB, VGB, TPM, TGB | Major depression |
| Paranoia | DPH, VGB, TPM | Schizophrenic psychosis |
| Agitation | LTG | Insomnia, anxiety, hypomania |
| Hypermotor | LTG | Tourette-syndrome |
| Dysphoric | LEV | Aggression |
| Learning disability | All AED | Behaviour disorders |

PHB: Phenobarbitone, LEV: Levetiracetam, LTG: Lamotrigine, TGB: Tiagabine, TPM: Topiramate, VGB: Vigabatrin, DPH: Phenytoin.

## Forced normalisation

The concept of forced normalisation goes back to the publications of Landolt (1958). Cases of FN or alternative psychiatric syndromes have been reported with all conventional and novel anticonvulsants but seem to be particularly common with the more potent drugs such as vigabatrin, topiramate and levetiracetam. FN has rarely been reported with tiagabine and lamotrigine, and is extremely rare with gabapentin. The best known manifestation of FN is a psychotic state. However in a consecutive series by Wolf (1984), 50% of 36 consecutive patients presented with predominating affective symptomatology.

The phenomenon of FN is not restricted to drug induced seizure control. It is likely that in patients who develop de novo psychosis following epilepsy surgery forced normalisation plays a role, and cases of an alternative psychosis secondary to vagal nerve stimulation have also been published (Gatzonis et al., 2000).

# Positive effects of AED on mood

## Conventional AEDs

Positive psychotropic effects of carbamazepine and valproate have been confirmed in controlled trials (Muzina et al., 2002) (Table V). Carbamazepine is licensed for the prophylaxis of bipolar disorder. Other indications include impulse control disorder and alcohol withdrawal. Carbamazepine is not efficacious in anxiety disorders. Valproate is particularly useful in the management of acute mania (Walden et al., 1989). Other indications for valproate include: bipolar disorder, particularly the rapid cycling subtype, schizoaffective psychosis, and add on treatment in schizophrenia. Of the other classical AEDs only clobazam is sometimes used for psychiatric indications, as a tranquilizer.

**Table V. Positive psychotropic effects of antiepileptic drugs demonstrated in controlled trials.**

|  | Depression | Mania | Bipolar disorder | Anxiety |
|---|---|---|---|---|
| Carbamazepine | 0 | + | + | 0 |
| Oxcarbazepine | 0 | + | 0 | 0 |
| Valproate | 0 | + | + | 0 |
| Lamotrigine | 0 | 0 | + | 0 |
| Gabapentin | 0 | – | – | +/– |
| Topiramate | 0 | – | 0 | 0 |
| Tiagabine | 0 | – | 0 | 0 |
| Levetiracetam | 0 | 0 | 0 | – |
| Pregabaline | 0 | 0 | 0 | + |
| Zonisamide | 0 | 0 | 0 | 0 |

+ = positive results, – negative results, 0 = no published data.

## Newer AED

### Gabapentin

This drug was used in almost all psychiatric conditions, probably because of its good tolerability and lack of interactions with other drugs. Positive experiences were reported with respect to bipolar disorder, acute mania, anxiety diosrders, schizophrenia, obsessive compulsive disorder, episodic dyscontrol, alcohol withdrawal, somatoform pain disorder and post traumatic stress disorder (Letterman and Markowitz, 1999). The evidence for positive psychotropic effects of gabapentin is however poor. Most publications relate to small case series or open studies. Controlled studies with positive results exist only for a subtype of anxiety disorders: social phobia (Pande et al., 1999). A controlled trial in panic disorder failed to show superiority over placebo; only a post hoc analysis identified a subgroup efficacy of gabapentin in patients who were severely affected (Pande et al., 2000). A controlled study in mania was negative (Pande et al., 2000) as well as a study in uni- and bipolar affective disorder (Frye et al., 2000).

## Lamotrigine

Positive psychotropic effects of lamotrigine were described by epileptologists very early after the drug was introduced. Antidepressive effects have been confirmed in controlled trials with primary psychiatric patients and in many countries lamotrigine has been licensed for the treatment of bipolar depression. In a randomised double blinded monotherapy study with more than 1,300 patients with bipolar depression, who either received lamotrigine, lithium or placebo, lamotrigine and lithium were equally effective with respect to manic and submanic symptomatology, whereas only lamotrigine was efficacious with respect to depressive episodes (Calabrese et al., 2002). These findings were confirmed in another large controlled trial which included almost 1,000 patients who suffered from bipolar depression, and who were treated with either lamotrigine, lithium or placebo. Lamotrigine and lithium were superior to placebo with respect to the length of time until a therapeutic intervention for an affective disorder; only lamotrigine was superior to placebo with respect to the prophylaxis of depressive episodes (Yatham et al., 2002). Lamotrigine is not superior to lithium with respect to the prophylaxis of manic episodes. In the treatment of acute mania lamotrigine has no place because of its high allergenic potential with rapid titration. Lamotrigine has proven efficacy in rapid cycling bipolar disorder (Calabrese et al., 1999; Kasumakar et al., 1997). Other potentially interesting indications for lamotrigine so far include schizoaffective psychoses and borderline personality disorder (Erfurth et al., 1998; Pinto and Akiskal, 1998).

## Levetiracetam

There are no controlled data on levetiracetam in primary psychiatric disorders. The results from a large placebo controlled study in anxiety disorder have not been published so far. Positive experiences were reported with respect to acute mania and alcohol withdrawal.

## Oxcarbazepine

Small controlled studies suggest efficacy of oxcarbazepine in acute mania. For the use of oxcarbazepine in other psychiatric conditions there are only open data and case reports available (Hellewell, 2002). Oxcarbazepine has a more favourable side effect profile and less interactions than carbamazepine. Therefore, a controlled study confirming combarable efficacy in bipolar disorder would be very useful. Open studies in this indication suggest that oxcarbazepine is efficacious and well tolerated (Ghaemi et al., 2003).

## Pregabaline

This recently introduced anticonvulsant is a structural analogon of GABA, although the exact mechanism of action is not known. Pregabaline was tested in a number of anxiety disorders (generalised anxiety disorder, social phobia, panic disorder). A double blind and placebo controlled study in patients with social phobia demonstrated dose dependent efficacy in comparison with placebo (Pande et al., 2003). Another promising indication for pregabaline is insomnia.

**Table VI. Psychiatric adverse events of anticonvulsants.**

1. Two main recognised mechanisms: GABA-ergic effects (depression) and forced normalisation (psychosis).
2. Psychiatric adverse events are often overlooked (particularly affective disorders, forced normalisation and delayed effects).
3. The direction of psychotropic effects depends on the preexisting mental state.
4. Psychiatric adverse events are usually reversible with appropriate management (adjustment of anticonvulsants and/or psychopharmacological treatment).
5. The vulnerability is different in specific patient groups: *e.g.* patients with learning disability, children, elderly.
6. Psychotropic AED effects may be related to epileptic syndromes (*e.g.* depressogenic effects in "limbic" and frontal lobe epilepsies?).

*Tiagabine*

Tiagabine was tested in a small number of patients with bipolar depression and mania with negative results in an open study (Carta *et al.*, 2002). In epilepsy, tiagabine has a narrow therapeutic window with the risk for proconvulsive effects at moderate dosages and de novo seizures were observed in primary psychiatric patients (Post, personal communication, Grunze, 1999).

*Topiramate*

Initial experiences with topiramate in psychiatry seemed promising (van Kammen, 2002). The frequently observed weight loss was considered an advantage in comparison to other psychopharmacological compounds many of which induce significant weight gain. Preliminary positive results in bipolar affective disorders (Marcotte, 1998; Grunze *et al.*, 2001) could not be confirmed in a placebo-controlled study in acute mania (Boylan *et al.*, 2002).

*Vigabatrin*

Vigabatrin has no clinically useful positive psychotropic effects.

# Positive psychotropic effects of AEDs in patients with epilepsy

Unfortunately, the potentially positive psychotropic effects of AED have not been systematically studied in patients with epilepsy. This is unsatisfactory because the experience with primary psychiatric patients cannot easily be transferred to epilepsy. Many psychiatric disorders in epilepsy are different in their phenomenology and most likely also in their pathogenesis from "endogenous" disorders. Classical bipolar disorder which is the main indication for anticonvulsants in psychiatry, is extremely rare in epilepsy. The evidence for mood stabilising effects of carbamazepine and valproate when used in patients with epilepsy is based on few observations (Robertson *et al.*, 1987; Trimble and Reynolds, 1976; Schmitz *et al.*, 1999).

With respect to the newer AEDs the only convincing evidence with respect to positive psychotropic effects relates to lamotrigine. In the quality of life study by Smith et al. (1993) 81 patients were randomised according to a cross-over-design and treated with either lamotrigine or placebo. In the lamotrigine group there were improvements in two subscales ("happiness" and "mastery"). These effects were independent of effects on seizure frequency. In another study the tolerability of lamotrigine was compared to carbamazepine in patients with new onset epilepsy. Using a standardized questionnaire for side effects (Gillham et al., 2000) the lamotrigine group demonstrated better tolerability with respect to cognitive functions and psychiatric symptoms such as "dysphoria" and "worries". The study by Edwards et al. (2000) compared lamotrigine and valproate in monotherapy specifically with respect to effects on mood. All mood rating scales (Beck-Depression-Inventory, Cornell-Dysthymia-Rating Scale, Profile of Mood States) showed improved mood in the lamotrigine group after 10 weeks, and a further improvement after 32 weeks. In the valproate group there were no significant mood changes as compared to baseline. An open study investigated the effects of lamotrigine in 13 patients who suffered from comorbid depression. There were significant improvements with respect to anxiety (after five weeks) and depression (after three months) (Kalogjera-Sackellares et al., 2002).

# References

Beran RG, Gibson RJ. Aggressive behaviour in intellectually challenged patients with epilepsy treated with lamotrigine. *Epilepsia* 1998; 39: 280-2.

Besag FMC. Behavioural effects of the new anticonvulsants. *Drug Safety* 2001; 24: 513-36.

Binnie DB. Lamotrigine. In: Engel J, Pedley TA, eds. *Epilepsy. A Comprehensive Textbook*. Philadelphia, New York: Lippincott-Raven, 1997: 1531-40.

Boylan LS, Devinsky O, Barry JJ, Ketter TA. Psychiatric uses of antiepileptic treatments. *Epilepsy Behav* 2002; 3 (suppl 5): 54-9.

Brent DA, Crumrine PK, Varma RR, Allan M, Allman C. Phenobarbital treatment and major depressive disorder in children with epilepsy. *Pediatrics* 1987; 80: 909-17.

Brent DA. Overrepresentation of epileptics in a consecutive series of suicide attempters seen at a children's hospital, 1978-1983. *J Am Acad Child Psychiatry* 1986; 25: 242-6.

Brent DA, Crumrine PK, Varma RR, Allan M, Allman C. Phenobarbital treatment and major depressive disorder in children with epilepsy. *Pediatrics* 1987; 80: 909-17.

Brodie MJ, Richens A, Yuen AW. Double-blind comparison of lamotrigine and carbamazepine in newly diagnosed epilepsy. UK Lamotrigine/Carbamazepine Monotherapy Trial Group. *Lancet* 1995; 345: 476-9.

Calabrese J, Bowden C, Sachs G, Ascher J, Monaghan E, Rudd D: A double blind placebo controlled study of lamotrigine monotherapy in outpatients with bipolar I depression. *J Clin Psychiatry* 1999; 60: 79-88.

Calabrese JR, Shelton MD, Rapport DJ, Kimmel SE, Elhaj O. Long-term treatment of bipolar disorder with lamotrigine. *J Clin Psychiatry* 2002; 63 (suppl 10): 18-22.

Carta MG, Hardoy MC, Grunze H, Carpiniello B. The use of tiagabine in affective disorders. *Pharmacopsychiatry* 2002; 35: 33-4.

Cramer JA, De Rue K, Devinsky O, Edrich P, Trimble MR. A systematic review of the behavioral effects of levetiracetam in adults with epilepsy, cognitive disorders, or an anxiety disorder during clinical trials. *Epilepsy Behav* 2003; 4: 124-32.

Crawford P. An audit of topiramate use in a general neurology clinic. *Seizure* 1998; 7: 207-11.

Dalby MA. Behavioral effects of carbamazepine. In: Penry JK, Daly DD, eds. *Complex partial seizures and their treamtent*. Advances in Neurology. Vol. 11, New York: Raven Press, 1975: 331-43.

Drake ME, Peruzzi WT. Manic state with carbamazepine therapy of seizures. *J Natl Med Assoc* 1986; 78: 1105-7.

Dulac O, Chiron D, Cusmai R, Pajot N, Beaumont D, Mondragon S. Vigabatrin in childhood epilepsy. *J Child Neurol* 1991; 6 (suppl 2): 30-7.

Edwards KR, Sackellares JC, Vuong A, Hammer AE, Barrett PS. Lamotrigine monotherapy improves depressive symptoms in epilepsy: a double-blind comparison with valproate. *Epilepsy Behav* 2001; 2: 28-36.

Erfurth A, Walden J, Grunze H. Lamotrigine in the treatment of schizoaffective disorder. *Neuropsychobiology* 1998; 38: 204-5.

Essex Pharma. *Felbamate: Product Monograph*. 1996

Estrada G, Wildrick D, Prantazelli M. Neuropsychiatric complications of levetiracetam in children with epilepsy. Abstract, *American Psychiatric Association* 2002

Ettinger AB, Weisbrot DM, Saracco J, Dhoon A, Kanner A, Devinsky O. Positive and negative psychotropic effects of lamotrigine in patients with epilepsy and mental retardation. *Epilepsia* 1998; 39: 874-7.

Ferrie CD, Robinson RO, Panaziotopoulos CP. Psychotic and severe behavioural reactions with vigabatrin: a review. *Acta Neurol Scand* 1996; 93: 1-8.

Fitton A, Goa KL Lamotrigine. *Drugs* 1995; 50: 691-713.

Frye M, Ketter TA, Kimbrell TA, Dunn RT, Speer AM, Osuch EA, Luckenbaugh DA, Cora-Ocatelli G, Leverich GS, Post RM. A placebo-controlled study of lamotrigine and gabapentin monotherapy in refractory mood disorders. *J Clin Psychopharmacol* 2000; 20: 607-14.

Gatzonis SD, Stamboulis E, Siafakas A, Angelopoulos E, Georgaculias N, Sigounas E, Jekins A. Acute psychosis and EEG normalisation after vagus nerve stimulation. *J Neurol Neurosurg Psychiatry* 2000; 69: 278-9.

Ghaemi SN, Berv DA, Klugman J, Rosenquist KJ, Hsu DJ. Oxcarbazepine treatment of bipolar disorder. *J Clin Psychiatry* 2003; 64 : 943-5.

Gillham R, Kane K, Bryant-Comstock L, Brodie MJ. A double-blind comparison of lamotrigine and carbamazepine in newly diagnosed epilepsy with health-related quality of life as an outcome measure. *Seizure* 2000; 9: 375-9.

Gilliam F. Optimizing epilepsy management: seizure control, reduction, tolerability, and co-morbidities. Introduction. *Neurology* 2002; 58 (suppl 5): 1.

Grunze HC, Normann C, Langosch J, Schaefer M, Amann B, Sterr A, Schloesser S, Kleindienst N, Walden J. Antimanic efficacy of topiramate in 11 patients in an open trial with an on-off-on design. *J Clin Psychiatry* 2001; 62: 464-8.

Grunze H, Erfurth A, Marcuse A, Amann B, Walden J. Tiagabine appears not to be efficacious in the treatment of acute mania. *J Clin Psychiatry* 1999; 13: 194-9.

Gustafson MC, Ritter FJ, Frost MD, Karney V. Behavioral and emotional effects of levetiracetam in children with intractable epilepsy. Abstract, *American Psychiatric Association* 2002.

Hellewell JSE. Oxcarbazepine (Trileptal) in the treatment of bipolar disorders: a review of efficacy and tolerability. *Journal of affective disorders* 2002: 72; 23-34.

Janssen-Cilag. *Topamax. Product monograph*. 1996.

Kalogjera-Sackellares D, Sackellares JC. Improvement in depression associated with partial epilepsy in patients treated with lamotrigine. *Epilepsy Behav* 2002; 3: 510-6.

Kanemoto K, Tsuji T, Kawasaki J. Reexamination of interictal psychoses based on DSMIV psychosis classification and international epilepsy classification. *Epilepsia* 2001; 42: 98-103.

Kanner AM, Kozak AM, Frey M. The use of sertraline in patients with epilepsy: is it safe? *Epilepsy and Behaviour* 2000; 1: 100-5.

Kasumakar V, Yatham LN. An open study of lamotrigine in refractory bipolar depression. *Psychiatry Res* 1997; 19: 145-8.

Ketter TA, Malow BA, Flamini R, Ko D, White SR, Post RM, Theodore WH. Felbamate monotherapy has stimulant-like effects in patients with epilepsy. *Epilepsy Res* 1996; 23: 129-37.

Ketter TA, Post RM, Theodore WH. Positive and negative psychiatric effects of antiepileptic drugs in patients with seizure disorders. *Neurology* 1999; 53 (suppl 2): 53-67.

Kossoff EH, Bergey GK, Freeman JM, Vining PG. Levetiracetam psychosis in children with epilepsy. *Epilepsia* 2001; 42; 1611-3.

Landolt H. Serial electroencephalographic investigations during psychotic episodes in epileptic patients and during schizophrenic attacks. In: Lorentz de Haas AM, ed. *Lectures on epilepsy*. Amsterdam: Elsevier, 1958: 91-131.

Lee DO, Steingard RJ, Cesena M, Helmers SL, Riviello JJ, Mikati MA. Behavioral side effects of gabapentin in children. *Epilepsia* 1996; 37: 87-90.

Leppik E. Tiagabine: the safety landscape. *Epilepsia* 1995; 36 (suppl 6): 10-3.

Letterman L, Markowitz J S. Gabapentin: a review of published experience in the treatment of bipolar disorder and other psychiatric conditions. *Pharmacotherapy* 1999; 19: 565-72.

Levinson DF, Devinsky O: Psychiatric adverse events during vigabatrin therapy. *Neurology* 1999; 53: 1503-11.

Li LM, Nashef L, Moriarty J, Duncan JS, Sander JW. Felbamate as add-on therapy. *Eur Neurol* 1996; 36: 146-8.

Lombroso CT. Lamotrigine-induced tourettism. *Neurology* 1999; 52: 1191-4.

Matsuura M. Epileptic psychoses and anticonvulsant drug treatment. *J Neurol Neurosurg Psychiatry* 1999; 67: 231-3.

McConnell H, Snyder PJ, Duffy JD, Weilburg J, Valeriano J, Brillman J, *et al*. Neuropsychiatric side effects related to treatment with felbamate. *J Neuropsychiatry Clin Neurosci* 1996; 8: 341-6.

McDanal CE, Bolman WM. Delayed idiosyncratic psychosis with diphenylhydantoin. *JAMA* 1975; 231: 1063.

Mesad SM, Devinsky O. Levetiracetam related aggression. Abstract, *American Psychiatric Association* 2002.

Mula M, Trimble MR, Lhatoo SD, Sander JW. Topiramate and psychiatric adverse events in patients with epilepsy. *Epilepsia* 2003a; 44: 659-63.

Mula M, Trimble MR, Yuen A, Liu RS, Sander JW. Psychiatric adverse events during levetiracetam therapy. *Neurology* 2003b; 61: 704-6.

Muzina DJ, El-Sayegh S, Calabrese JR. Antiepileptic drugs in psychiatry-focus on randomized controlled trial. *Epilepsy Res* 2002; 50: 195-202.

Pande AC, Davidson JR, Jefferson JW, Janney CA, Katzelnick DJ, Weisler RH, *et al*. Treatment of social phobia with gabapentin: a placebo-controlled study. *J Clin Psychopharmacol* 1999; 19: 341-8.

Pande AC, Pollack MH, Crockatt J, Greiner M, Chouinard G, Lydiard RB, *et al*. Placebo-controlled study of gabapentin treatment of panic disorder. *J Clin Psychopharmacol* 2000; 20: 467-71.

Pande AC, Crockatt JG, Feltner DE, Janney CA, Smith WT, Weisler R, *et al*. Pregabalin in generalized anxiety disorder: a placebo-controlled trial. *Am J Psychiatry* 2003; 160: 533-40.

Pinto OC, Akiskal HS. Lamotrigine as a promising approach to borderline personality: an open case series without concurrent DSM-IV major mood disorder. *J Affect Disord* 1998; 51: 333-43.

Robertson MM, Trimble MR, Townsend HRA. Phenomenology of depression in epilepsy. *Epilepsia* 1987; 28: 364-72.

Sackellares JC, Lee SI, Dreifuss FE. Stupor following administration of valproic acid to patients receiving other convulsant drugs. *Epilepsia* 1979; 20: 697-703.

Sander JWAS, Hart ZM, Trimble MR, Shorvon SD. Vigabatrin and psychosis. *J Neurol Neurosurg Psychiatry* 1991; 54: 435-9.

Schapel G, Chadwick D. Tiagabine and non-convulsive status epilepticus. *Seizure* 1996; 5: 153-6.

Schmitz B, Robertson M, Trimble MR. Depression and schizophrenia in epilepsy: social and biological risk factors. *Epilepsy Res* 1999; 35: 59-68.

Schöndienst M, Wolf P, Zur Möglichkeit neurotoxischer Spätwirkungen von Valproinsäure. In: Krämer G, Laub M, eds. *Valproinsäure*. Berlin, Heidelberg, New York: Springer, 1992: 259-65.

Smith D, Baker G, Davies G, Dewey M, Chadwick D. Outcomes of add on treatment with lamotrigine in partial epilepsy. *Epilepsia* 1993; 34: 312-22.

Tallian KB, Nahata MC, Lo W, Tsao CZ. Gabapentin associated with aggressive behavior in pediatric patients with seizures. *Epilepsia* 1996; 37: 501-2.

Thomas L. Trimble MR, Schmitz B, Ring HA. Vigabatrin and behaviour disorders: A retrospective study. *Epilepsy Res* 1996; 25: 21-7.

Trimble MR, Reynolds EH Anticonvulsant drugs and mental symptoms: a review. *Psychol med* 1976; 6: 169-78.

Trimble MR. Neuropsychiatric consequences of pharmacotherapy. In: Engel J, Pedley TA, eds. *Epilepsy. A Comprehensive Textbook*. Philadelphia, New York: Lippincott – Raven, 1997: 2161-70.

van Kammen DP, Shank RP. New anticonvulsants in affective disorder: Topiramate. In: Trimble MR, Schmitz B, eds. *Seizures, affective disorders and anticonvulsant drugs*. Guildford: Clarius press: 143-63.

Walden J, Normann C, Langosch J, Berger M, Grunze H. Differential treatment of bipolar disorders with old and new antiepileptic drugs. *Neuropsychobiology* 1998; 38: 181-4.

Wolf P. 1984 The clinical syndromes of forced normalisation. *Fol Psychiat Neurol Jpn* 38: 187-92.

Wolf P, Inoue Z, Röder-Wanner UU, Tsai JJ. Psychiatric complications of absence therapy and their relation to alteration of sleep. *Epilepsia* 1984; 25: 56-9.

Wolf SM, Shinnar S, Kang H, Balaban gil K, Moshé SL. Gabapentin toxicity in children manifesting as behavioral changes. *Epilepsia* 1995; 36: 1203-5.

Yatham LN, Kusumakar V, Calabrese JR, Rao R, Scarrow G, Kroeker G. Third generation anticonvulsants in bipolar disorder: a review of efficacy and summary of clinical recommendations. *J Clin Psychiatry* 2002; 63: 275-83.

Zaret BS, Cohen RA. Reversible valproic acid-induced dementia: a case report. *Epilepsia* 1986; 27: 234-40.

# Can we expect a specific correlation between the type of partial epilepsy, etiology and neuropsychological deficits?

H. Jokeit, M. Schacher

*Swiss Epilepsy Center, Zurich, Switzerland*

---

The majority of children with epilepsy have normal cognitive development. Nevertheless, neuropsychological deficits are frequently observed in children and adults suffering from epileptic seizures. Deficits in both global mental functions such as consciousness, arousal and activation, as well as specific cognitive functions such as attention, memory and language may be more debilitating than the seizures themselves (Rausch, 1997). Consequently, impairments in memory, attention, and psychomotor speed are risk factors for academic underachievement in paediatric epilepsy (Fastenau, 2004).

Cognitive impairment in epilepsy results from a variety of interacting factors: aetiology, age of onset, type of epilepsy, type of seizure, seizure frequency, seizure duration, seizure severity, medication and duration of epilepsy. It is well established in children with difficult to treat epilepsies that early seizure onset, long duration of epilepsy, and high seizure frequency likely impair cognitive and behavioural development. Complex interactions between these factors and a large number of moderating variables (*e.g.* anti-epileptic drugs, coping strategies, adaptation, remediation) make it difficult to isolate the impact of a certain factor and determine its relative contribution to the complex cognitive and behavioural symptoms. Apart from animal models, it is almost impossible to differentiate between the impact of the underlying brain pathology and the impact of the epilepsy itself. In this paper we discuss the ramifications of two factors: "type of epilepsy" and "etiology" on cognitive functioning in patients with epilepsy.

The question of whether certain types of epilepsy and their underlying aetiologies are characterised by a specific profile of cognitive strengths and weaknesses is of interest for diagnostics and treatment of children and adults with epilepsy. If one postulates that certain types of epilepsy are related to specific neuropsychological profiles, it does not necessarily follow that the type of epilepsy is the casual factor leading to specific cognitive deficits. Patients suffering from a certain type of epilepsy often share a specific aetiology or location of a brain lesion, therefore, a specific neuropsychological deficit may not reflect a specific type of epilepsy but rather result from common brain pathology. However, the opposite could also be true. Epileptic seizures frequently accompany or result from acquired brain pathology. The pathology defines the seizure onset zone and impairs cognitive functions residing in the affected brain structures. It should be noted that a certain seizure onset zone and a structural lesion causing a functional deficit can, but must not, be located in the same region (Lüders, 1991). A frequent seizure spread from a functionally "silent" area into a functionally relevant remote brain region (e.g. frontal lobe) may cause neuropsychological deficits that appear to be atypical for the location of the lesion (e.g. a low grade tumour within the right lateral temporal lobe). Consequently, a circumscribed cognitive deficit does not necessarily localise the structural lesion, identify the seizure onset zone, the type of epilepsy or the etiology.

Over the course of development, aetiology and type of epilepsy interact with various developmental time lines and vulnerabilities of certain cognitive functions. Functions showing experience-dependent change throughout the lifespan can be addressed through training and remediation (e.g. knowledge acquisition). By contrast, functions that are modifiable by experience and practice during only limited developmental timeframes frequently result in life long deficits following developmental abnormalities (eg. dynamic regulation of attentional shifting, first language acquisition). On the other hand, there is longstanding evidence in children of plastic change following brain injury that results in nearly normal cognitive functioning. The same type of focal or mass brain lesions would cause permanent deficits in adults (e.g. hemispherectomy).

Knowing about such pathological and developmental complexity, can we expect to find a specific correlation between the type of epilepsy, aetiology and neuropsychological deficits? To answer this question we focus our brief review on data from adult patients with epilepsy due to two considerations: firstly, the number of studies in adult patients is higher and secondly, we avoid complexity by bypassing the major influence of brain developmental plasticity.

Epilepsy is not a unitary disease entity and refers to symptoms of paroxysmal disturbances of brain activity. Seizure onset zone, seizure frequency, seizure duration, and seizure semiology may vary considerably between and within patients. Despite this, considerable efforts have been undertaken to develop a common taxonomy of epilepsies. The fundamental dichotomy between generalised and focal or localisation-related epilepsies is well accepted and useful in diagnostics and treatment. In contrast, the sub-classification of symptomatic, cryptogenic, and idiopathic epilepsies cannot be considered as definite (Wolf, 1997). Genetic and exogenous factors also contribute to the pathogenesis of almost all types of epilepsies, but to varying degrees.

The taxonomy of epilepsies is not related to neuropsychological concepts. Other factors such as seizure severity, seizure frequency, and age of onset have a tremendous impact on cognition and are therefore more relevant than type of epilepsy. Consequently, it is not surprising that only a few studies have investigated the influence of type of epilepsy on cognition. To date, the majority of neuropsychological studies in adult patients with epilepsy have dealt with focal epilepsies. The presence of localised structural or functional lesions in focal epilepsies complements the methodological and theoretical concepts of neuropsychology. Moreover, structural lesions in a circumscribed brain structure (*i.e.* hippocampus) and its high prevalence has led mesial temporal lobe epilepsy to become the most thoroughly neuropsychologically investigated type of epilepsy. Due to these various issues, a comprehensive study comparing the specific impact of type of epilepsy on cognition has not been undertaken to date.

Finally, we will describe that the impact of aetiology on cognition in epilepsies is mediated by the location and extent of the pathology, the location of the ictal onset zone, and the spread pattern and frequency of seizures. Usually, these mediating factors are of greater importance for cognitive functioning than the specific aetiology itself.

# Type of epilepsy and neuropsychological findings

## Idiopathic generalised epilepsies

Epilepsies with generalised tonic-clonic seizures (23%), absence epilepsies (6%) and myoclonic epilepsies (3%) belong to the rather frequent idiopathic generalised epilepsies (Hauser, 1997). There is convincing evidence that generalised tonic-clonic seizures are more likely to impair cognitive functions than simple or complex partial seizures (Dikmen, 1977; Dodrill, 1986). Only the occurrence of status epilepticus increases the risk of cognitive impairments beyond that of epilepsies with generalised tonic-clonic seizures (Rausch, 1991).

There is still ongoing controversy as to whether seizures in primary generalised epilepsies originate in the cortex or in the thalamus. However, there is considerable evidence that frontal lobe structures play a major role in generating epileptic activity in generalised epilepsies (Pavone, 2000). In agreement with such electrophysiological data, neuropsychological tests demonstrate impairment of prefrontal functions such as working memory and mental flexibility (Devinsky, 1997; Swartz, 1996). These results are paralleled by functional brain imaging studies which have revealed reduced prefrontal glucose metabolism and N-acetyl aspartate concentrations (NAA) (Swartz, 1996; Savic, 2000). Additionally, MRI-morphometry has shown frontal lobe abnormalities in patients with primary generalised epilepsy (Savic, 1998). To summarise, EEG, neuropsychological tests, and functional and structural brain imaging have shown that frontal lobe structures are affected in patients with primary generalised epilepsy. However, these frontal deficits are not pathognomonic to generalised epilepsies. Focal epilepsies of temporal, parietal, and frontal origin may show similar or even more pronounced impairment of frontal functions.

## Symptomatic focal epilepsies

The "International Classification of Epilepsies" suggests four main localisation-related epilepsies: temporal lobe epilepsies, frontal lobe epilepsies, parietal lobe epilepsies, and occipital lobe epilepsies. There are no specific causes or aetiologies of these epilepsies with the exception of hippocampal sclerosis. There is widespread agreement that temporal lobe epilepsies associated with hippocampal sclerosis represent a highly prevalent discrete syndrome. Therefore, neuropsychological aspects of mesial temporal lobe epilepsies are discussed more thoroughly below.

## Mesial temporal lobe epilepsy

Temporal lobe epilepsy is the most frequent focal epilepsy. Histopathological studies have revealed that the majority of patients with temporal lobe epilepsy (70%) have hippocampal sclerosis (Babb, 1987). Mesial temporal lobe epilepsy (MTLE) is rarely sufficiently controlled by antiepileptic drugs. Therefore, patients with MTLE are likely candidates for epilepsy surgery. As neuropsychological diagnostics are included in a comprehensive presurgical workup, the neuropsychology of MTLE has been extensively investigated. The leading cognitive symptoms in patients with MTLE are impairments of episodic memory due to structural lesions of the hippocampal formation. In patients with MTLE of the speech-dominant hemisphere, word finding deficits are often prominent. It is assumed that frequent spread of epileptic activity into the temporo-lateral regions is responsible for such word-finding deficits. Moreover, MTLE is typically associated with moderate impairments in intelligence, academic achievement, language functions, and visuospatial functions (Hermann, 1997). Prefrontal lobe functions, such as attention and executive functions, are frequently spared. MTLE patients with secondarily generalised tonic-clonic seizures, however, are at considerable risk of global intellectual and prefrontal lobe function impairment (Jokeit, 1997). Patients with MTLE suffering from generalised tonic-clonic seizures may have prefrontal metabolic disturbances which are likely to be associated with intellectual and executive function impairments. *Figure 1* shows a FDG-PET scan of a patient with left-sided MTLE. Left temporo-lateral and mesial hypometabolic zones correspond with the diagnosis of MTLE. The evident prefrontal hypometabolic zones are probably related to the occurrence of secondarily generalised tonic-clonic seizures. At the time of PET imaging, the patient showed clear impairment of attention and higher order cognitive functions. More recently it has been shown that the absence of seizures may lead to a normalisation of prefrontal metabolism and performance in neuropsychological tests (Spanaki, 2000).

There is controversy as to whether chronic refractory temporal lobe epilepsies are associated with the risk of cognitive deterioration, although dementia is a very rare phenomenon in patients with MTLE. Patients with a long epilepsy duration (> 30 years), however, performed worse in intelligence tests than those with shorter epilepsy duration (Jokeit, 2002).

## Frontal lobe epilepsy

Frontal lobe epilepsy is the second most frequent localisation-related epilepsy. The initial symptomatology of frontal lobe seizures depends on the location of the epileptogenic zone. Focal clonic motor seizures result from epileptic activity within the primary motor cortex. Tonic seizures originate in the supplementary motor area (SMA), and complex partial seizures in orbital frontal, mesial frontal, frontal polar, and dorsal lateral regions. The complexity and diversity of frontal lobe functions are reflected by the variability of symptoms found in frontal lobe seizures and by the variability of related neuropsychological deficits.

Neuropsychological studies have compared patients with frontal lobe and temporal lobe epilepsy to controls to measure nonspecific effects of focal epilepsy on cognition. Frontal lobe epilepsy patients demonstrated a reduced attention span and psychomotor speed whereas patients with temporal lobe epilepsy had impaired episodic memory (Exner, 2002; Helmstaedter, 1996). The extent and quality of differences between both patient groups probably depends upon the localisation and upon age-related aspects of frontal lobe lesions. As previously mentioned, functional impairment of prefrontal structures is also frequently observed in patients with MTLE and secondarily generalised tonic-clonic seizures. In addition, age at onset of frontal lobe epilepsy may considerably influence the presence of specific frontal deficits (Upton, 1997).

## Parietal and occipital lobe epilepsy

The prevalence and incidence of occipital and parietal lobe epilepsy is rather low. Therefore, no comprehensive and systematic neuropsychological studies of such adult patients are available. Recognised parietal and occipital epilepsy syndromes include several types of benign childhood epilepsies as well as epilepsies with bilateral occipital calcification and encephalomyopathy with lactic acidosis and stroke-like episodes (MELAS) (Sveinbjornsdottir, 1993). Traumatic lesions, malformations of cortical development, and tumors are frequent causes of parietal and occipital lobe epilepsies in adults.

Paresthetic, dysesthetic, and painful symptoms, sexual sensations, apraxias, and disturbance of body image have been reported as aura or ictal phenomena in patients with parietal lobe epilepsy (Williamson, 1997). Parietal ictal activity frequently spreads into the frontal lobe which may considerably change ictal and postictal symptoms.

There is a longstanding controversy as to the exact role of the parietal lobe in spatial and verbal cognition. Lesions of the parietal lobe may cause visual associative agnosia, hemineglect, visuospatial and constructive disorders, apraxia and linguistic deficits. Mass lesion of the non-dominant parietal lobe considerably impairs performance in almost all non-verbal tasks in intelligence tests (Sands, 2000). Lesions within the temporo-parietal junction of the speech-dominant hemisphere may cause severe receptive aphasia. The cognitive symptoms of patients with parietal lobe epilepsy may vary considerably as a function of lateralisation and localisation, age of injury, and age of epilepsy onset.

In patients with occipital lobe epilepsy, auras frequently include elementary visual hallucinations. Other ictal symptoms are ictal blindness, eye deviation, blinking, sensation of eye movement and nystagmoid eye movements (Salanova, 1992). An ictal spread into frontal and temporal areas is quite frequent. The profile of neuropsychological functions in patients with idiopathic occipital lobe epilepsy does not systematically differ from that of other epilepsy patients (Gulgonen, 2000).

## ■ Etiology and neuropsychological findings

Seizures can arise from virtually any cerebral pathology that increases the excitability of brain tissue. The aetiologies can be divided into genetic and acquired brain lesions. The latter may be focal, multifocal or diffuse. As specific epilepsy syndromes with predominantly genetic basis (*e.g.* Lennox-Gastaut syndrome) develop in infancy or childhood, genetic factors will not be discussed here. The most important aetiologies in adulthood are cerebrovascular diseases, tumours, traumatic brain injuries, infections of the central nervous system, and neurodegenerative disorders. Multiple aetiologies cannot be excluded in some patients. The frequency of certain aetiologies differs with increasing age. In the age range between 20 to 40 years, head traumas, brain tumours and arterio-venous malformations are the most common aetiologies (Niedermeyer, 1990). Residual epilepsy due to early CNS damage (e.g. cerebral palsy) is more prelevant in young adults (Annegers, 1996). Over the age of sixty, cerebral arteriosclerosis and primary and metastatic brain tumours are most common (Niedermeyer, 1990), followed by neurodegenerative disorders such as Alzheimer's dementia (Forsgren, 1996).

## Cerebrovascular disease

Cerebrovascular disease is the leading cause of acquired epilepsy in western populations. In a large community-based study fifteen percent of patients with newly diagnosed epilepsy had a cerebrovascular pathology (Sander, 1990). In epilepsies developing after the age of sixty, cerebrovascular disorders are responsible for half of all cases (Annegers, 1996; Sander, 1990). Hemorrhagic strokes carry a much greater risk for epilepsy than ischemic events. The one-year risk for epilepsy after a subarachnoid hemorrhage is 20%, and increases if a middle cerebral artery aneurysm has been clipped. The incidence is even higher in patients with arterio-venous malformations (AVM), especially if they have bled or been treated surgically (Smith, 1998). Subarachnoid hemorrhage following ruptured aneurysms can be dramatic. In a prospective study, patients sustained relatively little brain damage and few cognitive deficits if the bleeding was arrested quickly (Ogden, 1993). Inspite of this, a considerable number of patients had visuospatial, memory, psychomotor speed deficits and reduced mental flexibility one-year post injury. Older subjects did not recover to the same extent as younger subjects. Cognitive deficits resulting from ruptured aneurysms differ from impairments due to ischemic cerebrovascular accidents: the damage is likely to be more widespread and does not necessarily follow anatomically well-defined or neuropsychologically common patterns (Lezak, 1995). An additional but rare source of hemorrhagic stroke is the AVM. If cognitive effects of non-hemorrhagic AVMs are prominent, they show the expected lateralised pattern of impairment in verbal or visuospatial processing, depending on which hemisphere was affected. Deficits typically associated with damage to the hemisphere contralateral to the AVM may also be present (Mahalick, 1991). Cognitive functions in patients with AVM treated with radiosurgery demonstrated preserved performance in follow-up tests up to three years post-op and improvements in memory and attention were observed (Steinvorth, 2002).

Stroke patients are characterised by enormous variability with respect to the depth, extent, and site of tissue damage. As most strokes are unilateral, cognitive deficits are frequently lateralised. In left-sided infarcts, speech and language disorders are common residuals. Their specific nature depends on the site and extent of the lesion. With lesions on the right, perceptual and visuospatial deficits tend to be among the most prominent impairments (Lezak, 1995).

## Traumatic brain injury

In three to four percent of patients with epilepsy seizures are the result of traumatic brain injury (Annegers, 1996; Smith, 1998). In adults with severe head trauma (intracranial mass lesions or loss of consciousness for more than 24 h) and no early seizures, the risk of developing posttraumatic epilepsy is about ten percent. If early seizures occur within the first week, the risk of developing an epilepsy increases up to 36%. No increased risk has been found for subjects with mild head injuries (amnesia or loss of consciousness of less than half an hour). Mild head injuries account for approximately 80% of all civilian head injuries (Annegers, 1980).

Those patients who survive severe traumatic brain injuries can show the full range of cognitive dysfunctions at varying levels of severity. The relationship between age and the two most important predictors of severity (duration of coma and posttraumatic amnesia) is complex, with advancing age associated with greater morbidity and mortality (Lezak, 1995). Memory, attention and information processing speed and efficiency are the domains most likely to be affected by head injury (Capruso, 1992). Prolonged reaction times in dual-tasks have suggested pronounced deficits in divided attention (Leclercq, 2000). The ability to store new material in long-term-memory and the ability to retrieve stored information may be affected (Bennett-Levy, 1984; Gronwall, 1981). Deficits associated with frontal lobe injury are often the most debilitating as they interfere with the patient's ability to use knowledge and skills fluently, appropriately or adaptively (Lezak, 1995). Other cognitive deficits may be present depending on the site, extent, depth and nature of the lesion. Language and perceptual skills tend to be relatively preserved (Capruso, 1992).

A large scale prospective study of patients with severe brain injury demonstrated that epilepsy can result in neurobehavioural disorders such as disinhibited behaviour, irritability, aggressivity and agitated behaviour (Mazzini, 2003). The high incidence of behavioural disorders, particularly the aggressive and agitated behaviours, may be explained by the finding of a hypoperfusion of the anterior temporal lobes in patients with epilepsy.

## CNS infection

Two to three percent of all epilepsies are attributed to CNS infections (Annegers, 1996; Sander, 1990). This aetiology is among the most common causes of epilepsies in infants, with a second peak occurring in elderly populations (Nicolosi, 1986). The highest risk for acute and chronic epileptic seizures follows viral encephalitides. The most common and most severe form of encephalitis, the Herpes Simplex encephalitis, has frequent epileptic manifestations in the acute stage and temporal lobe involvement is a common presenting feature (Smith, 1998; Fujii, 1999). Temporal lobe epilepsies are among the most common sequelae following Herpes Simplex encephalitis (Smith, 1998). The 20-year risk of epilepsy increases from 10% to 22% if symptomatic seizures occur during acute state. While patients with aseptic meningitis have no subsequent discernible increase in risk for epilepsy, bacterial meningitis increases the risk of epilepsy approximately fivefold (Annegers, 1996). If the acute illness is complicated by seizures, the 20-year risk of epilepsy is 13.4% compared to 2.4% if it is not (Smith, 1998). Among CNS infections, encephalitides are especially prone to cause severe cognitive decline in patients. Patients, who survived a Herpes Simplex encephalitis demonstrate severe memory impairments with profound anterograde amnesia and considerable retrograde amnesia which corresponds to brain tissue damage (Niedermeyer, 1990). Profound behavioural changes have been observed: hyperorality, loss of fear, diminished social responsibility, decreased social and personal inhibitions and an impaired ability to make discriminations. These behavioural changes are explained by the viral invasion of limbic structures and are probably associated with damage to the amygdala (Lezak, 1995).

## Brain tumours

Brain tumours account for four percent of all cases of epilepsy and for twelve percent of acquired epilepsies. Epilepsy from brain tumours can occur at any age but is greatest in patients aged 25 to 64 years (Annegers, 1996). The highest epileptogenicity is found in oligodendrogliomas (90%) followed by astrocytomas (69%), metastatic tumours (41%) meningioma (37%), and glioblastoma multiforme (34%). The site of the neoplasm may influence the epileptogenicity as frontal lobe tumours are most likely to cause generalised tonic-clonic seizures. Slow growing tumors in the vicinity of the rolandic fissure are most epileptogenic (Niedermeyer, 1990). Brain tumours compromise brain functioning in several ways: by increasing pressure, by inducing seizures, by destroying brain tissue through invasion or replacement and by secreting hormones or altering endocrine patterns that affect a variety of body functions (Lezak, 1995). Increased intracranial pressure may blunt the intellect and result in confusion and memory difficulties (Moore, 1988). The location of the tumour may also affect behaviour in ways similar to other discrete brain lesions. In addition to the lesion location, its size and rate of growth influences the neuropsychological profile (Lezak, 1995). Intracranial tumours frequently cause cognitive deficits, emotional disturbances, personality alterations, and diminished adaptive capabilities. Symptoms tend to be subtle at first and insidious in their development (Damasio, 1989). Most patients with brain tumours of the frontal or temporal lobes demonstrate impaired cognitive functioning at the time of diagnosis. In a recent study, 90% of patients with brain tumours of the frontal or the temporal lobes displayed impairment in at least one area of cognition such as memory, attention, language or executive functions. Impairment in executive functions was observed in 78% of patients, and impairment in memory and attention was observed in more than 60% of the patients (Tucha, 2000).

## Degenerative CNS Disease

Epilepsy associated with degenerative processes accounts for about two percent of all cases of epilepsy (Annegers, 1996). The incidence of degenerative neurologic disease increases with age. Alzheimer's affects less than one percent of the population aged 65-69 years, but increases up to eight percent in patients above 85 years (Hebert, 1995). Advanced Alzheimer's disease is an important risk factor for new-onset seizures in older adults (Romanelli, 1990); it is associated with a 10-fold increase in the risk for epilepsy (Annegers, 1996). The observed seizures were of the generalised tonic-clonic type and were not associated with clinical evidence of epileptogenic factors other than Alzheimer's disease. Among cognitive changes in Alzheimer's disease, the loss of memory functions is the most obvious early symptom. The initial symptoms include impairment of recent memory, as well as poor learning and retention of information over time. Poor learning and intrusion errors indicate an impairment in memory storage and retrieval (Pasquier, 1999). Visuoperceptual deficits are also common. While the pattern of dysfunctions can vary considerably, patients with Alzheimer's may be impaired on tests requiring visual discrimination, analysis, spatial judgements and perceptual organisation (Mendez, 1990). Attentional deficits may be an additional symptom, although not all patients display such problems, especially in the early stage of the disease (Parasuraman, 1994). Impairment in all aspects of attention have been reported: reduced span, trouble focusing and shifting and slowed choice reaction time (Lezak, 1995). As far as verbal functions are concerned, deterioration in the quality, quantity and meaningfulness of speech and impairments in verbal comprehension characterise the early stages of Alzheimer's disease (Huff, 1990). In formal testing, patients show impairments in tests of reading comprehension, verbal reasoning and verbal fluency (Pasquier, 1999). In patients with Alzheimer's and epilepsy, language functions may demonstrate an accelerated decline compared to patients without seizures (Volicer, 1995).

## ■ Conclusions

Our considerations about type of epilepsy and aetiology in adults and adolescents suggest that specific associations between neuropsychological deficits and type of epilepsy and aetiology are exceptions rather than the rule. Even the most homogenous epileptic syndrome, mesial temporal lobe epilepsy, shows a variety of neuropsychological symptoms depending on age of injury, age of epilepsy onset, side of seizure onset, and type of seizures. The case of prefrontal metabolic disturbances in patients with refractory temporal lobe epilepsy and exclusively unilateral hippocampal lesions highlights the complexity of the problem *(Figure 1)* (Lezak, 1995).

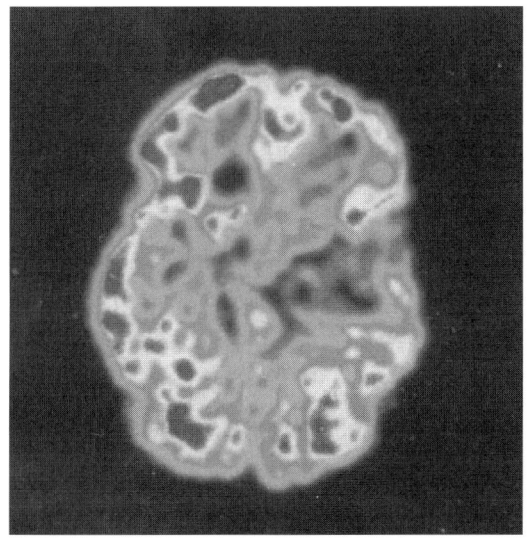

**Figure 1. An axial metabolic map (FDG-PET) of a young man with left-sided mesial temporal lobe epilepsy.**
There are corresponding left-sided temporo-lateral and –mesial hypometabolic zones. Additional remote metabolic depressions are to be seen in left prefrontal regions. Structural MRI revealed not any pathology except hippocampal sclerosis. The left brain side is to bee seen on the right hand side. Higher metabolic activity is coded by red and yellow, less metabolic activity by blue and green.

Frontal lobe functions, or more precisely executive functions, develop through adolescence. The majority of epilepsies and epileptic syndromes are associated with epileptiform brain electric activity originating within or propagating to the frontal lobes. Therefore, it is reasonable to assume that seizures and epileptiform activity likely affect the development of executive functions. Indeed, impaired regulation of cognition, attention and behaviour are frequent complaints in children with epilepsy regardless of aetiology and type of epilepsy. Moreover, these symptoms are predictors of academic underachievement. Unfortunately, impairments of executive functions are usually difficult to treat and require sensitive handling by parents and caretakers.

In summary, results of neuropsychological diagnostics rarely aid in pinpointing the specific type of epilepsy and underlying aetiology in a certain patient. Especially in newborns, infants, and children all epilepsy and aetiology related factors interact with various brain developmental time lines and vulnerabilities. Higher cognitive functions, undergoing development and maturation, are most vulnerable to the effects of seizures, most likely due to their greater neuro-developmental plasticity.

Knowledge about the type of epilepsy and the underlying pathology, however, provides vital information for neuropsychologists regarding evaluation of the nature of the deficits as either transient or chronic, in estimating probability of functional recovery, in providing therapeutic recommendations, and in guiding decisions regarding pharmacological or surgical treatment options.

# References

Annegers JF, Grabow JD, Groover RV, *et al*. Seizures after head trauma: a population study. *Neurology* 1980; 30: 683-9.

Annegers JF, Rocca WA, Hauser WA. Causes of epilepsy: contributions of the Rochester epidemiology project. *Mayo Clin Proc* 1996; 71: 570-5.

Babb TL, Brown WJ. Pathological findings in epilepsy. In: Engel J, Jr, ed. *Surgical Treatment of the Epilepsies*. New York: 1987: 511-40.

Bennett-Levy JM. Long-term effects of severe closed head injury on memory: evidence from a consecutive series of young adults. *Acta Neurol Scand* 1984; 70: 285-98.

Capruso DX, Levin HS. Cognitive impairment following closed head injury. *Neurol Clin* 1992; 10: 879-93.

Damasio H, Damasio AR. *Lesion analysis in neuropsychology*. Oxford: Oxford University Press, 1989.

Devinsky O, Gershengorn J, Brown E, *et al*. Frontal functions in juvenile myoclonic epilepsy. *Neuropsychiatry Neuropsychol Behav Neurol* 1997; 10: 243-6.

Dikmen S, Matthews CG. Effect of major motor seizure frequency upon cognitive-intellectual functions in adults. *Epilepsia* 1977; 18: 21-9.

Dodrill CB. Correlates of generalized tonic-clonic seizures with intellectual, neuropsychological, emotional, and social function in patients with epilepsy. *Epilepsia* 1986; 27: 399-411.

Exner C, Boucsein K, Lange C, *et al*. Neuropsychological performance in frontal lobe epilepsy. *Seizure* 2002; 11: 20-32.

Fastenau PS, Shen J, Dunn DW, *et al*. Neuropsychological predictors of academic underachievement in pediatric epilepsy: moderating roles of demographic, seizure, and psychosocial variables. *Epilepsia* 2004; 45: 1261-72.

Forsgren L, Bucht G, Eriksson S, et al. Incidence and clinical characterization of unprovoked seizures in adults: a prospective population-based study. *Epilepsia* 1996; 37: 224-9.

Fujii T, Yamadori A, Endo K, et al. Disproportionate retrograde amnesia in a patient with herpes simplex encephalitis. *Cortex* 1999; 35: 599-614.

Gronwall D, Wrightson P. Memory and information processing capacity after closed head injury. *J Neurol Neurosurg Psychiatry* 1981; 44: 889-95.

Gulgonen S, Demirbilek V, Korkmaz B, et al. Neuropsychological functions in idiopathic occipital lobe epilepsy. *Epilepsia* 2000; 41: 405-11.

Hauser WA. Incidence and Prevalence. In: Engel JJ, Pedley TA, eds. *Epilepsy: A comprehensive textbook*. Philadelphia: Lippincott-Raven Publishers, 1997: 47-57.

Hebert LE, Scherr PA, Beckett LA, et al. Age-specific incidence of Alzheimer's disease in a community population. *JAMA* 1995; 273: 1354-9.

Helmstaedter C, Kemper B, Elger CE. Neuropsychological aspects of frontal lobe epilepsy. *Neuropsychologia* 1996; 34: 399-406.

Hermann BP, Seidenberg M, Schoenfeld J, et al. Neuropsychological characteristics of the syndrome of mesial temporal lobe epilepsy. *Arch Neurol* 1997; 54: 369-76.

Huff FJ, Spanier C, Protetch J. Facilitation of word retrieval in Alzheimer's disease. *Adv Neurol* 1990; 51: 61-4.

Jokeit H, Ebner A. Effects of chronic epilepsy on intellectual functions. *Prog Brain Res* 2002; 135: 455-63.

Jokeit H, Seitz RJ, Markowitsch HJ, et al. Prefrontal asymmetric interictal glucose hypometabolism and cognitive impairment in patients with temporal lobe epilepsy. *Brain* 1997; 120 (Pt 12): 2283-94.

Leclercq M, Couillet J, Azouvi P, et al. Dual task performance after severe diffuse traumatic brain injury or vascular prefrontal damage. *J Clin Exp Neuropsychol* 2000; 22: 339-50.

Lezak MD. *Neuropsychological assessment* (3rd ed). New York: Oxford: Oxford University Press, 1995.

Lüders HO, Awad I. Conceptual considerations. In: Lüders HO, ed. *Epilepsy surgery*. New York: Raven Press, 1991: 51-62.

Mahalick DM, Ruff RM, U HS. Neuropsychological sequelae of arteriovenous malformations. *Neurosurgery* 1991; 29: 351-7.

Mazzini L, Cossa FM, Angelino E, et al. Posttraumatic epilepsy: neuroradiologic and neuropsychological assessment of long-term outcome. *Epilepsia* 2003; 44: 569-74.

Mendez MF, Mendez MA, Martin R, et al. Complex visual disturbances in Alzheimer's disease. *Neurology* 1990; 40: 439-43.

Moore AJ. Brain tumors. What are the general and focal effects? *Postgrad Med* 1988; 84: 163-6.

Nicolosi A, Hauser WA, Beghi E, et al. Epidemiology of central nervous system infections in Olmsted County, Minnesota, 1950-1981. *J Infect Dis* 1986; 154: 399-408.

Niedermeyer E. *The Epilepsies: Diagnosis and management*. Baltimore, Munich: Urband & Schwarzenberg, 1990.

Ogden JA, Mee EW, Henning M. A prospective study of impairment of cognition and memory and recovery after subarachnoid hemorrhage. *Neurosurgery* 1993; 33: 572-586; discussion 586-77.

Parasuraman R, Martin A. Cognition in Alzheimer's disease: disorders of attention and semantic knowledge. *Curr Opin Neurobiol* 1994; 4: 237-44.

Pasquier F. Early diagnosis of dementia: neuropsychology. *J Neurol* 1999; 246: 6-15.

Pavone A, Niedermeyer E. Absence seizures and the frontal lobe. *Clin Electroencephalogr* 2000; 31: 153-6.

Rausch R, Le MT, Langfitt JT. Neuropsychological evaluation. In: Engel JJ, Pedley TA, eds. *Epilepsy: A comprehensive textbook*. Philadelphia: Lippincott-Raven Publishers, 1997: 977-87.

Rausch R, Victoroff JI. Neuropsychological factors related to behavior disorders in epilepsy. In: Devinsky O, Theodore WH, eds. *Epilepsy and Behavior*. New York: Wiley-Liss, 1991: 213-21.

Romanelli MF, Morris JC, Ashkin K, et al. Advanced Alzheimer's disease is a risk factor for late-onset seizures. *Arch Neurol* 1990; 47: 847-50.

Salanova V, Andermann F, Olivier A, et al. Occipital lobe epilepsy: electroclinical manifestations, electrocorticography, cortical stimulation and outcome in 42 patients treated between 1930 and 1991. Surgery of occipital lobe epilepsy. *Brain* 1992; 115 (Pt 6): 1655-1680.

Sander JW, Hart YM, Johnson AL, et al. National general practice study of epilepsy: newly diagnosed epileptic seizures in a general population. *Lancet* 1990; 336: 1267-71.

Sands S, Van Gorp WG, Finlay JL. A dramatic loss of non-verbal intelligence following a right parietal ependymoma: brief case report. *Psychooncology* 2000; 9: 259-66.

Savic I, Lekvall A, Greitz D, et al. MR spectroscopy shows reduced frontal lobe concentrations of N-acetyl aspartate in patients with juvenile myoclonic epilepsy. *Epilepsia* 2000; 41: 290-6.

Savic I, Seitz RJ, Pauli S. Brain distortions in patients with primarily generalized tonic-clonic seizures. *Epilepsia* 1998; 39: 364-70.

Smith DF, Appleton RE, MacKenzie JM, et al. *An atlas of epilepsy*. New York, London: The Parthenon Publishing Group, 1998.

Spanaki MV, Kopylev L, DeCarli C, et al. Postoperative changes in cerebral metabolism in temporal lobe epilepsy. *Arch Neurol* 2000; 57: 1447-52.

Steinvorth S, Wenz F, Wildermuth S, et al. Cognitive function in patients with cerebral arteriovenous malformations after radiosurgery: prospective long-term follow-up. *Int J Radiat Oncol Biol Phys* 2002; 54: 1430-7.

Sveinbjornsdottir S, Duncan JS. Parietal and occipital lobe epilepsy: a review. *Epilepsia* 1993; 34: 493-521.

Swartz BE, Simpkins F, Halgren E, et al. Visual working memory in primary generalized epilepsy: an 18FDG-PET study. *Neurology* 1996; 47: 1203-12.

Tucha O, Smely C, Preier M, et al. Cognitive deficits before treatment among patients with brain tumors. *Neurosurgery* 2000; 47: 324-34.

Upton D, Thompson PJ. Age at onset and neuropsychological function in frontal lobe epilepsy. *Epilepsia* 1997; 38: 1103-13.

Volicer L, Smith S, Volicer BJ. Effect of seizures on progression of dementia of the Alzheimer type. *Dementia* 1995; 6: 258-63.

Williamson PD, Engel J, Jr, Munari C. Anatomic classification of lacalization-related epilepsies. In: Engel J, Jr, Pedley TA, eds. *Epilepsy: A comprehensive textbook*. Philadelphia: Lippincott-Raven Publishers, 1997: 2405-16.

Wolf P. Isolated seizures. In: Engel JJ, Pedley TA, eds. *Epilepsy: A comprehensive textbook*. Philadelphia: Lippincott-Raven, 1997: 2475-81.

# Restored cognitive functions: what can we expect following resective surgery?

I. Tuxhorn[1], H. Freitag[1], H. Holthausen[2]

[1] *Epilepsy Center Bethel, Pediatric Epilepsy Section, Bielefeld*
[2] *Behandlungszentrum Vogtareuth, Vogtareuth, Germany*

---

Surgery for epilepsy has become a realistic therapeutic option for selected children with the aim of controlling seizures and preventing secondary epilepsy-related damage (Aicardi, 1997). The spectrum of surgically treatable epilepsies in childhood has been expanded to include various forms of early onset catastrophic epilepsy, focal epilepsy associated with tuberous sclerosis and other phakomatoses, developmental tumors, malformation of cortical development and mesial temporal lobe epilepsy due to hippocampal sclerosis (Duchowny, 1998; Tuxhorn, 2001).

Besides the technological advances in imaging, neurophysiology, anesthesia and surgical techniques improving the selection process of potential surgical candidates and making surgery a safer procedure, early selection of suitable candidates for temporal lobectomy has been facilitated by studies on the age-related features of seizure semiology arising from the temporal lobe in infancy and childhood (Brockhaus & Elger, 1995; Fogarasi & Tuxhorn, 2002; Wyllie, 1996). Moreover, recent outcome studies have specified predictive prognostic variables for good seizure outcome in children with temporal and extratemporal epilepsy more clearly (Wyllie, 1998; Bourgeois, 1999; Paolicchi, 2000).

The developmental prognosis after epilepsy surgery is a central issue with regard to timing of surgical procedures for optimal long-term outcome (Caplan, 1995, 2002; Vasconcellos, 2001). In this chapter we will discuss what may be expected with regard to restoration of cognitive function after temporal lobectomy in childhood based on published data and add experiences we have gained from individual cases at our center.

## ■ Diagnosing temporal lobe epilepsy in children

Biological factors including drug resistance and the biographical prognosis including poor school performance, behavior difficulties and social adjustment to chronic disability were already focused on in the 70's and 80's by Lindsay, Ounsted & Richards (1984). Besides pointing out the poor social outcome of adolescents with intractable temporal lobe epilepsy, these authors evaluated long-term data about the low seizure remission rate of chronic temporal lobe epilepsy due to hippocampal sclerosis once adolescence was reached. They also emphasized the role of early surgery to improve the overall social prognosis in children with temporal lobe epilepsy.

The clinical, EEG and neuroimaging findings which are specific for temporal lobe epilepsy in childhood have been well delineated in a number of publications in recent years (Harvey, 1997; Duchowny, 1998; Wyllie, 1998; Bourgeois, 1998). While the clinical features in school-aged and adolescent children are quite similar to those of adult patients (see also Arzimanoglou in this volume), the features of temporal lobe epilepsy in early childhood with regard to age-related seizure semiology, EEG findings and specific pathologic substrates have become more apparent in the last decade (Brockhaus & Elger, 1995; Wyllie, 1996; Bourgeois, 1998; Fogarasi & Tuxhorn, 2002).

A recent detailed video EEG analysis of children under 7 years with well localized temporal lobe epilepsy underscores that seizure semiology is highly influenced by age-related neural mechanisms. It is characterized by a greater variability and less stereotypical ictal manifestations. This includes early motor features with tonic and myoclonic components at times resembling epileptic spasms, subtle behavioral changes and a paucity of automatisms. The transformation from this immature semiology pattern suggesting a generalized or extratemporal focus to the mature limbic or automotor pattern, which characterizes complex partial seizures of temporal lobe origin of the adult type, occurs in a linear fashion as a function of age in the preschool years as shown in *figure 1*. Before 4 years of age the motor seizure components will be the dominant seizure symptom which may mask the diagnosis of temporal lobe epilepsy, while at and after 4 years of age, the nonmotor, behavioral hallmarks will predominate and facilitate the diagnosis (Fogarasi & Tuxhorn, 2002).

## ■ Patterns of cognitive function in children with temporal lobe epilepsy. Is there evidence for a progressive disease?

A number of cross sectional and longitudinal group studies as well as case reports of single developmental trajectories give supportive evidence that epilepsy in general may be a progressive disorder in childhood (Bailet 2000, Bjorneas, 2001, 2002; Lah, 2004).

In contrast some large prospective studies provide little evidence for a change in the developmental rate after the onset of epilepsy when IQs of affected children were compared at 4 and 7 years after onset with siblings or nonaffected children (Bourgeois, 1983; Ellenberg, 1986). These epilepsies were however not classified as severe, which most likely explains these findings, at least in part.

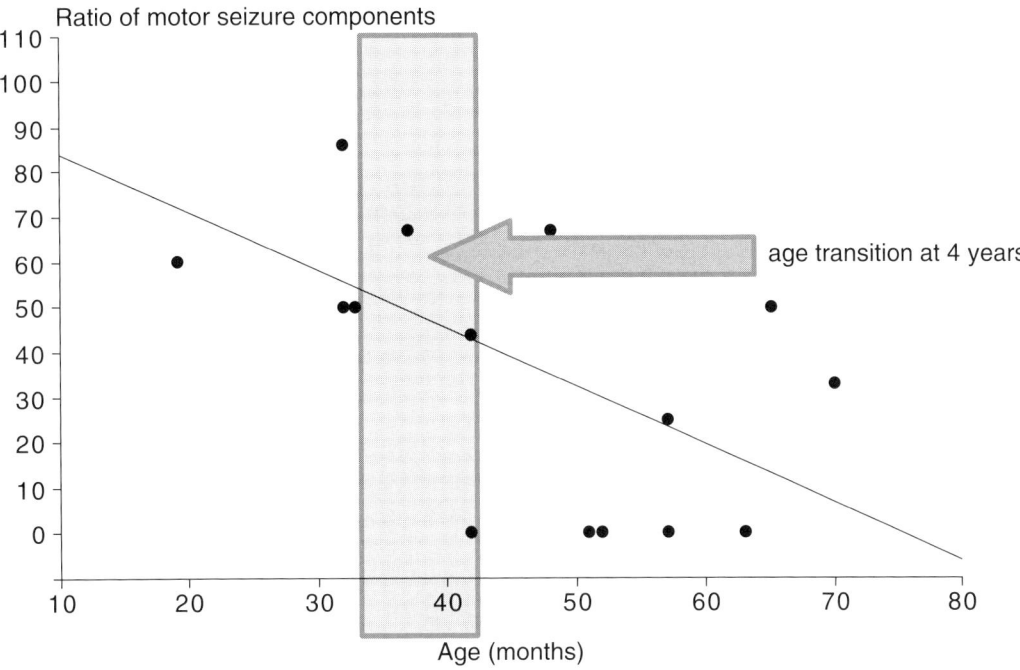

**Figure 1.** The ratio of motor to behavioral features during seizures arising from the temporal lobe in young children is highly age dependent with a transition to the adult pattern at 4 years of age.

Core risk factors for developmental delay that have been identified include an early onset, severe seizure disorder with a high seizure frequency, polytherapy and extensive pathologic substrates (Jensen, 1979; Bourgeois, 1998; Schoenfeld, 1999; Battaglia, 1999; Smith, 2002; Tromp, 2003; Lutz, 2004).

A recent comparative and prospective study of children and adults with severe focal epilepsy including temporal lobe cases awaiting surgery, has shown declines in IQ over 3.5 years in the pediatric group suggesting a more dynamic vulnerability to the negative effects of seizures on cognition in children compared to adults (Bjornaes, 2002).

In a recent study from our centre, of 50 patients treated surgically with severe epilepsy between the ages of 3 to 7 years, over 70% were retarded and only 16% displayed average intelligence prior to surgical treatment. The patients all had early onset temporal or extratemporal epilepsy. In fact, age at seizure onset and extent of the etiologic lesions were predictive variables for preoperative cognitive development (Freitag & Tuxhorn, 2005). We interpret our findings as evidence for static "etiology based" as well as dynamic "epilepsy-related" factors contributing to the presence of cognitive delay in these patients while the overriding factor may vary in the various subgroups of patients. The issues of age-related changes affecting intellectual abilities and learning efficiency as well as memory dysfunction in TLE need to be addressed in future research as has been pointed out by other authors (Mabbott & Smith, 2003).

Single case studies have reported catastrophic forms of temporal lobe epilepsy with evidence of severe autistic regression in association with seizure onset and may represent a subtype of patients who would benefit from very early surgical treatment (Deonna, 1993; Neville, 1997). In this context, we have documented the developmental profile of a preschool child who showed a gradual loss of general cognitive ability, language function and communication abilities after onset of TLE caused by a well circumscribed right-sided limbic tumor. After surgically-induced seizure remission the patient again started acquiring milestones but at a retarded level *(Figure 2)*. This manifestation is reminiscent of the acquired autism seen in patients with Landau Kleffner syndrome (Neville, 1997).

Based on a number of reports intellectual functioning in children with temporal lobe epilepsy appears quite heterogeneous, ranging from normal to severely handicapped. The potential impact of a number of clinical variables such as age of onset, etiology, seizure type, duration and severity of epilepsy as well as neuropathology obviously plays a role in this regard (Adams, 1990; Pascual-Castroviejo, 1996; Bigel, 2001; Alpherts, 2004; Lutz, 2004). For instance, early onset of and longer exposure to seizures was associated with poorer cognition in the children with complex partial seizures examined by Schoenfield (1999). Other authors have failed to find specific patterns of impairment in their series of children with temporal lobe epilepsy, although school problems were often reported, constituting a major source of concern to parents (Camfield, 1986).

Evaluating our patients with temporal lobe epilepsy of early onset who were treated surgically before the age of 16 years we have found a high incidence of mental retardation. The latter correlated positively with age of onset and severity of epilepsy (with daily seizures), but negatively with age at surgery and was essentially independent of the pathologic etiology. In our series, even children with well localized mesial lesions but catastrophic infantile forms of temporal lobe epilepsy were often mentally retarded. Of 96 school-age children with TLE, 42 had IQs below 70 (unpublished data). Disorders of learning and memory are also seen in children with TLE but the laterality effect appears not to be as prominent as it is in adults although it has been clearly reported in pediatric patients: children with left TLE have relatively greater deficits in verbal memory, children with RTLE greater impairment of visual spatial memory or memory for faces (Fedio & Mirski, 1969; Beardsworth & Zaidel, 1994; Elger, 1997; Jambaque, 2001).

Language impairment in the form of naming disorders and limitations in vocabulary and phonological processing, which is important for reading development, appears to be quite common in children with TLE suggesting more extensive dysfunction due to neocortical involvement of the temporal lobe (Williams, 1998a; Jambaque, 2001; Lah, 2004; Vanasse et al., 2003).

Taking these findings as a whole, children of any age with early onset and severe epilepsy arising from the temporal lobe may be considered at substantial risk for handicap due to the cumulative negative impact of a number of seizure-related variables on cognitive development. After intractability becomes clear despite aggressive drug treatment, presurgical assessment for evaluation of surgical treatment should not be delayed in cases with a potentially good prognosis *(Figure 2)*.

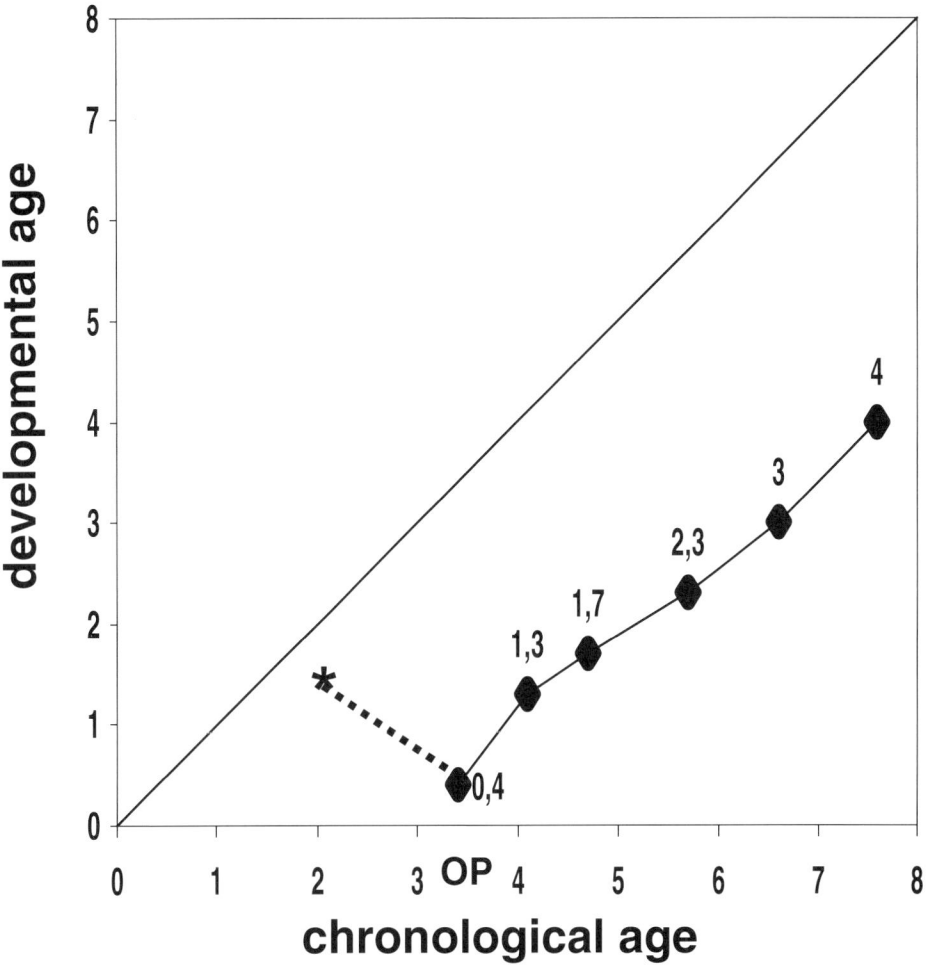

Figure 2. After dramatic developmental regression seizure remission led to restart of cognitive development, albeit in the retarded range.

## Cognitive outcome after temporal lobectomy. What can we expect?

This question is not a simple one to answer, as we are only now beginning to collect long-term data on children that have undergone temporal lobectomy at various ages. It is becoming more evident that although temporal lobe epilepsy is a fairly homogenous condition *in terms of localization*, there may be subtypes of clinical pathologic syndromes with a variable natural history regarding seizure and developmental outcome after epilepsy surgery (Jambaque, 2001; Bigel, 2001; Lah, 2004).

The collective results are encouraging however as they suggest that temporal lobectomy will not have adverse effects on intelligence in the majority of surgically treated patients (Hermann, 1990, 1997; Lassonde, 2000; Bigel, 2001; Kuehn, 2002; Alpherts, 2004).

Enhanced overall *intellectual function* however appears not to be one of the benefits to be expected in the majority of children after temporal lobectomy (Miranda & Smith, 2001). In the latter study the group results of 50 patients showed small positive changes in performance IQ, but not in verbal IQ. Analysis of individual cases however did show positive gains in verbal IQ, which were usually noted in children that were older at surgery, had lower preoperative VIQ and had a positive seizure outcome. Decline of IQ scores in a few children was not felt to necessarily reflect a true loss of function after surgery but rather the slow rate of progress seen in children with neurological dysfunction. The benefits of surgery on cognition were studied prospectively with a comparison non-surgical group by the same authors, confirming the results of previous studies that little discernible change in cognitive function can be attributed specifically to surgery in the short term (Meyer, 1986; Dluglos, 1990; Lewis, 1996; Gilliam, 1997; Williams, 1998b; Westerveld, 2000; Mabbott & Smith, 2003; Smith, 2004).

Despite the paucity of long-term post operative studies, indirect evidence is emerging that successful surgery may stabilize cognitive decline and that gains may only appear over longer follow up periods (Westerveld, 2000; Lah, 2004; Freitag & Tuxhorn, 2005). In one such study, memory losses were initially found at 3 months but some recovery was seen at 12 months after surgery, suggesting that recovery is driven by a number of factors manifesting functional reorganization (Gleissner, 2002). Results from our study of preschool children, which included 16 temporal lobectomies, showed that significant postoperative increases in DQs were seen only after 2 to 3 years and that the only significant predictor for this gain was a shorter interval between onset of epilepsy and time of surgery (Freitag & Tuxhorn, 2005). This critical issue needs to be explored further by comparing appropriate nonsurgical and surgical groups longitudinally and by collecting serial data of more individual cases as shown in *figures 2-5*.

Postoperative *effects on memory and learning* have been quite mixed with evidence of stable function, decline and improvements (Meyer, 1986; Adams, 1990; Szabo, 1998; Williams, 1998b; Mabbot, 1998; Lendt, 1999; Westerveld, 2000; Gleissner, 2002, 2005). Some studies have used global memory indices, which may not be sensitive enough to document changes so that methodology may be an issue as well as patient heterogeneity.

There is some evidence that children may be less vulnerable to memory decline after surgery compared to adults and that surgery type and timing of the postsurgical assessment plays a role in memory outcome (Gleissner, 2002). Drops in verbal memory were invariably seen after left temporal lobectomy (Szabo, 1998; Williams, 1998b) and a similar laterality impact has been noted for delayed recall (Meyer, 1986; Gleissner, 2002). Paradoxically, a significant increase in verbal memory was noted in one study after right temporal lobectomy, a finding which may secondarily derive from improved functioning of the "released" (from seizure effects) left temporal structures

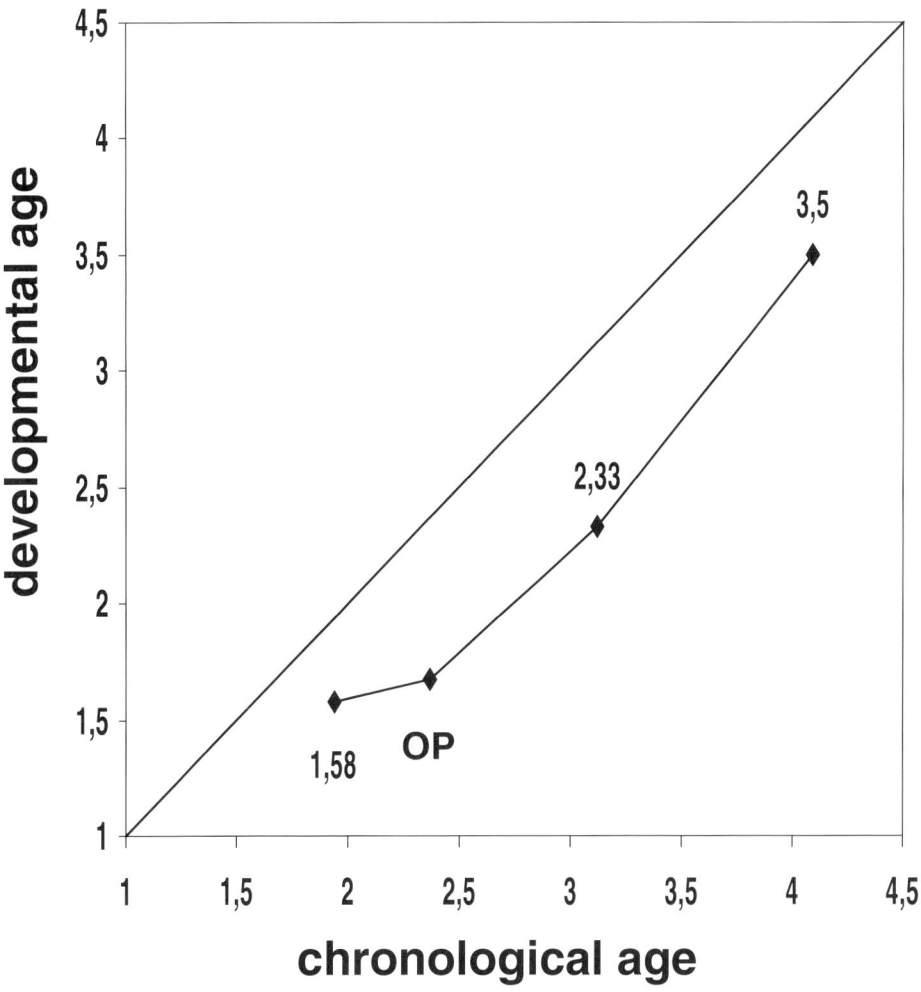

**Figure 3. Repeated developmental assessments prior to surgery revealed a slowing of cognitive development.**
After seizure remission developmental velocity increased, leading to an almost age-appropriate level of cognitive functioning about 20 months after surgery.

(Robinson, 2002). Age at seizure onset, duration of seizure disorder, seizure frequency, antiepileptic medication, sparing lateral structures with selective surgical techniques, surgical seizure outcome and time of postoperative evaluation may influence the reported memory outcome (Lendt, 1999; Westerveld, 2000; Robinson, 2002; Mabbott & Smith, 2003; Gleissner, 2002).

Little work has been published on other aspects of cognition such as attention, problem solving and academic skills after temporal lobectomy in children (Smith, 2004). Language outcome and regain of language skills after left temporal lobectomy associated with different types of early focal or more diffuse injuries needs to be further investigated (Dlugos, 1999).

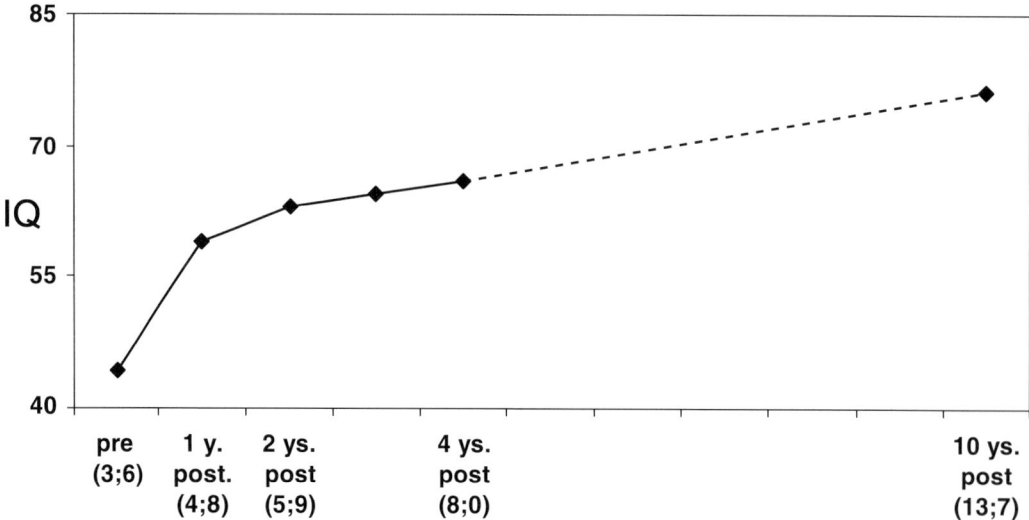

**Figure 4. Developmental gains after early surgery were maintained in the long-term.** (Age in years and months).

*In conclusion*, overall cognitive function including memory and language function may remain stable, improve or decline after temporal lobectomy. Although normalization of significant pre-operative deficits appears unlikely, developmental decline may be halted in early onset catastrophic epilepsy and normal developmental velocity may be restored after a process of regression. Early surgery may be protective and facilitate restoration of function in some cases, where functional reserve due to lack of bilaterality and less extensive damage exists. The case trajectories in *figures 2, 3* and *4* are highly suggestive that early surgery may be protective and facilitate some restoration of function. Here it will be imperative to diagnose these cases early so that patients may benefit maximally from seizure control through surgery.

However, the question that also needs to be answered is whether there may be a critical timeframe when early surgery may be detrimental to development as some preliminary data may suggest. This could imply that surgery may disrupt dynamic developmental processes in an analogous fashion to the epileptic process. This subgroup of patients needs to be more clearly defined and carefully selected with a view to optimizing timing of surgery depending on the natural history of the epilepsy and sequential cognitive profiles.

## ■ Issues of timing of surgery

The disruptive effects of frequent seizures on the developing brain, which result in clinical evidence of brain damage and significant mental handicap, present a pressing clinical problem for all child neurologists taking care of children with early onset

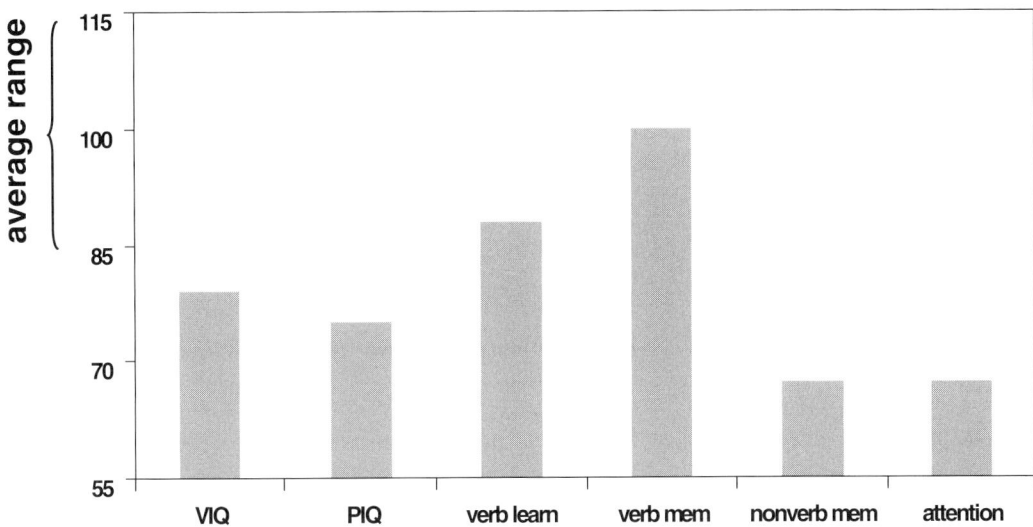

**Figure 5.** Ten years after seizure remission through early right temporal lobectomy a lateralized neuropsychological profile with spared verbal and impaired nonverbal memory was found.
(Same patient from *figure 4*).

medically resistant temporal lobe epilepsy. Therefore early syndrome diagnosis and referral to a tertiary epilepsy center will be paramount if we wish to improve the long-term overall prognosis of these patients.

However, is early surgery always beneficial in all cases?

As a general principle, we have to consider protective (positive prognostic) factors *versus* non-protective (risk) factors for overall development and weigh these into the scale which may tip the window of opportunity towards good outcome. On the one hand we have early surgery, functional reserves generated by release phenomena, lack of bilaterality, plasticity and re-organization, more localized deficits and early seizure control, while on the other hand we have the noxious effects of early seizure onset, polytherapy, high seizure burden in a dynamically developing brain, extensive etiologies and disruption of biological processes underlying critical developmental time frames.

To be able to answer the question as to what we can expect in the individual patient, a better understanding of the longitudinal impact of each of these factors will be paramount to reduce the secondary sequelae on cognitive development associated with uncontrolled temporal lobe epilepsy.

# References

Adams CBT, Beardsworth ED, Oxbury SM, et al. Temporal lobectomy in 44 children: outcome and neuropsychological follow-up. *J Epilepsy* 1990; 3 (suppl): 157-68.

Aicardi J. Paediatric epilepsy surgery: how the view has changed. In: Tuxhorn I, Holthausen H, Boenigk H, eds. *Paediatric Epilepsy Syndromes and their Surgical Treatment*. London: John Libbey, 1997: 3-7.

Alpherts WCJ, Vermeulen J, Hendriks MP, et al. Long-term effects of temporal lobectomy on intelligence. *Neurology* 2004; 62 (4): 607-11.

Bailet LL, Turk WR. The impact of childhood epilepsy on neurocognitive and behavioral performance: a prospective longitudinal study. *Epilepsia* 2000; 41 (4): 426-31.

Battaglia D, Rando T, Deodato F, et al. Epileptic disorders with onset in the first year of life: neurological and cognitive outcome. *Eur J Paediatr Neurol* 1999; 3 (3): 95-103.

Beardsworth ED, Zaidel DW. Memory for faces in epileptic children before and after brain surgery. *J Clin Exp Neuropsychol* 1994; 16 (4): 589-96.

Bigel MG, Smith ML. The impact of different neuropathologies on pre- and postsurgical neuropsychological functioning in children with temporal lobe epilepsy. *Brain Cogn* 2001; 46 (1-2): 46-9.

Bjornaes H, Stabell K, Henriksen O, et al. The effects of refractory epilepsy on intellectual functioning in children and adults. A longitudinal study. *Seizure* 2001; 10 (4): 250-9.

Bjornaes H, Stabell K, Henriksen O, et al. Surgical versus medical treatment for severe epilepsy: consequences for intellectual functioning in children and adults. A follow-up study. *Seizure* 2002; 11 (8): 473-82.

Brockhaus A, Elger CE. Complex partial seizures of temporal lobe origin in children of different age groups. *Epilepsia* 1995; 36 (12): 1173-81.

Bourgeois BF, Prensky AL, Palkes HS, Talent BK, Busch SG. Intelligence in epilepsy: a prospective study in children. *Ann Neurol* 1983; 14 (4): 438-44.

Bourgeois BF. Temporal lobe epilepsy in infants and children. *Brain Dev* 1998; 20 (3): 135-41.

Bourgeois M, Sainte-Rose C, Lellouch-Tubiana A, et al. Surgery of epilepsy associated with focal lesions in childhood. *J Neurosurg* 1999; 90 (5): 833-42.

Camfield PR, Gates R, Ronen G, et al. Comparison of cognitive ability, personality profile, and school success in epileptic children with pure right versus left temporal lobe EEG foci. *Ann Neurol* 1984; 15 (2): 122-6.

Caplan R. Epilepsy in early development: the lesson from surgery for early intractable seizures. *Sem Pediatr Neurol* 1995; 2 (4): 238-45.

Caplan R, Siddarth P, Mathern G, et al. Developmental outcome with and without successful intervention. *Int Rev Neurobiol* 2002; 9: 269-84.

Deonna T, Ziegler AL, Despland PA, et al. Autistic regression in relation to limbic pathology and epilepsy: report of two cases. *Dev Med Child Neurol* 1993; 35: 166-76.

Dlugos DJ, Moss E, Duhaime AC, et al. Language-related cognitive declines after left temporal lobectomy in children. *Pediatr Neurol* 1999; 21 (1): 444-9.

Duchowny M, Jayakar P, Resnick T, Harvey AS, et al. Epilepsy surgery in the first three years of life. *Epilepsia* 1998; 39 (7) 737-43.

Elger CE, Brockhaus A, Lendt M, et al. Behavior and cognition in children with temporal lobe epilepsy. In: Tuxhorn I, Holthausen H, Boenigk H, eds. *Paediatric Epilepsy Syndromes and their Surgical Treatment*. London: John Libbey, 1997: 311-25.

Ellenberg JH, Hirz DG, Nelson KB. Do seizures in children cause intellectual deterioration? *N Engl J Med* 1986; 314: 984-1085.

Fedio P, Mirsky A. Selective intellectual deficits in children with temporal lobe or centrencephalic epilepsy. *Neuropsychologia* 1969; 7: 287-300.

Fogarasi A, Jokeit H, Faveret E, Jansky J, TuxhornI. The effect of age on seizure semiology in childhood temporal lobe epilepsy. *Epilepsia* 2002; 43 (6): 638-43.

Freitag H, Tuxhorn I. Cognitive function in preschool children after epilepsy surgery: rationale for early intervention. *Epilepsia* 2005; 46 (4): 561-7.

Gleissner U, Sassen R., Lendt M, et al. Pre- and postoperative verbal memory in pediatric patients with temporal lobe epilepsy. *Epilepsy Research* 2002; 51: 287-96.

Gleissner U, Sassen R, Schramm J, et al. Greater functional recovery after temporal lobe epilepsy surgery in children. Submitted to *Brain* 2005.

Harvey AS, Berkovic SF, Wrennall JA, et al. Temporal lobe epilepsy in childhood: clinical, EEG, and neuroimaging findings and syndrome classification in a cohort with new-onset seizures. *Neurology* 1997; 49: 960-8.

Hermann B, Seidenberg M, Bell B, et al. The neurodevelopmental impact of childhood-onset temporal lobe epilepsy on brain structure and function. *Epilepsia* 2002; 43 (9): 1062-71.

Hermann BP. Psychosocial outcome following focal resections in childhood. *J Epilepsy* 1990; 3 (suppl): 243-52.

Jambaqué I. Neuropsychology of temporal lobe epilepsy in children. In: Jambaqué I, Lassonde M, Dulac O, eds. *Neuropsychology of childhood epilepsy*. New York: Kluver Academic/Plenum Publishers, 2001: 97-102.

Jensen I, Larsen K. Mental aspects of temporal lobe epilepsy. *J Neurol Neurosurg and Psychiatry* 1979; 42: 256-65.

Kuehn SM, Keene DL, Richards PMP, Ventureya ECG. Are there changes in intelligence and memory functioning following surgery for the treatment of refractory epilepsy in childhood? *Childs Nerv Syst* 2002; 18: 306-10.

Lah S. Neuropsychological outcome following focal cortical removal for intractable epilepsy in children. *Epilepsy Behav* 2004; 5: 804-17.

Lassonde M, Sauerwein HC, Jambaque I, et al. Neuropsychology of childhood epilepsy: pre- and postsurgical assessment. *Epileptic Disord* 2000; 2: 3-13.

Lewis DV, Thompson RJ, Santos CC, et al. Outcome of temporal lobectomy in adolescents. *J Epilepsy* 1996; 9: 198-205.

Lindsay J, Ounstead C, Richards P. Long-term outcome in children with temporal lobe seizures. *Dev Med Child Neurol* 1984; 26: 25-32.

Lutz MT, Elger CE, Helmstaedter C. Effects of age at onset and duration of epilepsy on cognition in the framework of Cattell's theory of fluid and crystallized abilities. *Epilepsia* 2004; 45 (suppl 7): 7-346.

Mabbott DJ, Smith ML. Memory in children with temporal or extra-temporal excisions. *Neuropsychologia* 2003; 41: 995-1007.

Meyer FB, Marsh W, Laws ER, Sharbrough F. Temporal lobectomy in children with epilepsy. *J Neurosurg* 1986; 64: 371-6.

Neville BG, Harkness WF, Cross JH, et al. Surgical treatment of severe autistic regression in childhood epilepsy. *Pediat Neurol* 1997; 16: 137-40.

Miranda C, Smith ML. Predictors of intelligence after temporal lobectomy in children with epilepsy. *Epilepsy Behav* 2001; 2: 13-9.

Pascual-Castroviejo I, Garcia Blazquez M, Gutierre Molina MB, et al. 24-year preoperative evolution of a temporal astrocytoma. *Childs Nerv Syst* 1996; 12: 417-20.

Paolicchi JM, Jayakar P, Dean P, et al. Preditors of outcome in pediatric epilepsy surgery. *Neurology* 2000; 54: 642-7.

Robinson S, Park TS, Blackburn LB, Bourgeois BF, Dodson WE. Transhippocampal selective hippocampal amygdalo-hippocampectomy in children and adolescents: efficacy of the procedure and cognitive morbidity in patients. *J Neurosurg* 2000; 93: 402-9.

Schoenfeld J, Seidenberg M, Austin W, et al. Neuropsychological and behavioral status of children with complex partial seizures. *Dev Med Child Neurol* 1999; 41: 724-31.

Smith ML, Elliott IM, Lach L. Cognitive skills in children with intractable epilepsy: comparison of surgical and nonsurgical candidates. *Epilepsia* 2002; 3 (6): 631-7.

Smith ML, Elliott IM, Lach L. Cognitive, psychosocial and family function one year after pediatric epilepsy surgery. *Epilepsia* 2004; 45 (6): 650-60.

Szabó CA, Wyllie E, Stanford L, et al. Neuropsychological effect of temporal lobe resection in preadolescent children with epilepsy. *Epilepsia* 1998; 39 (8): 814-9.

Tromp SC, Weber JW, Aldenkamp AP, et al. Relative influence of epileptic seizures and of epilepsy syndrome on cognitive function. *J Child Neurol* 2003; 18 (6): 407-12.

Tuxhorn I, Moch A, Holthausen H. Pediatric epilepsy surgery: state of the art, recent developments and future perspective. *Epileptic Disord* 2000; 2: 53-5.

Vanasse, CM, Beland R, Jambaque I, Lassonde M. Impact of temporal lobe epilepsy on phonological processing and reading: A case study of identical twins. *NeuroCase* 2003 9 (6): 515-22.

Vasconcellos E, Wyllie E, Sullivan S, et al. Mental retardation in pediatric candidates for epilepsy surgery: the role of early seizure onset. *Epilepsia* 2001; 42 (2): 268-74.

Westerveld M, Sass KJ, Chelune GJ, et al. Temporal lobectomy in children: cognitive outcome. *J Neurosurg* 2000; 92: 24-30.

Williams J, Griebel ML, Dykman RA. Neuropsychological patterns in pediatric epilepsy. *Seizure* 1998a; 7: 223-8.

Williams J, Griebel ML, Sharp GB, Boop FA. Cognition and behavior after temporal lobectomy in pediatric patients with intractable epilepsy. *Pediatr Neurol* 1998b; 19 (3): 189-94.

Wyllie E. Surgical treatment of epilepsy in children. *Pediatr Neurol* 1998; 19 (3): 179-88.

Wyllie E, Comair YS, Kotagal P, et al. Epilepsy surgery in infants. *Epilepsia* 1996; 37 (7): 625-37.

# Temporal lobe epilepsy in children and cognitive dysfunction: comprehensive methodologies for a comprehensive research and care

## A. Arzimanoglou

*Epilepsy Unit, Child Neurology and Metabolic Diseases Department, University Hospital Robert Debré (AP-HP), Paris, France*

In recent years, the identification and classification of epilepsy syndromes and epilepsies allowed a better definition of the types of investigation for a precise diagnosis and a better knowledge of the most appropriate therapeutic strategies. Furthermore, the work furnished for the definition of epilepsies and epilepsy syndromes also facilitated a better characterization of some of the cognitive and behavioural deficits encountered. This is particularly true for generalized symptomatic epilepsies and epileptic encephalopathies. The devastating character of entities like West, Dravet, Lennox-Gastaut syndromes and clinical entities associated to continuous spike waves during slow sleep, stimulated the scientific investment of highly specialized child neurology centres. Consequently, a number of contributions focused specifically on the cognitive outcome of epileptic encephalopathies (Jambaqué et al., 2001, Dulac et al., 1994, Delgado-Escueta et al., 2005, Beaumanoir et al., 1995). Recent studies (Metz-Lutz et al., 1999; Massa et al., 2001) also assessed the neuropsychological profile of patients with idiopathic partial epilepsies, a category considered as benign in terms of global evolution. Given the fully justified importance the child neurology community attributes to socio-cognitive development in children, one could expect that advances would be at least similar in the vast domain of cognitive and behavioural evolution of children with non-idiopathic focal epilepsies, the most prevalent category of epilepsy in both children and adults.

However, although the incidence of focal seizure disorders is around 20/100000 per year, with a prevalence around 4/1000 (Crawford, 2000), the studies discussing cognition and behaviour in patients with non-idiopathic partial epilepsies remain relatively limited (Schoenfeld et al., 1999; Lassonde et al., 2000; Bulteau et al., 2000; Nolan et al., 2003; Hernandez et al., 2003; Freitag and Tuxhorn, 2005). Those available are usually devoted to the neuropsychological status of adults with intractable temporal lobe epilepsy (Hermann *et al.*, 1997; Hennessy *et al.*, 2001; Helmstaedter *et al.*, 2003; Rausch *et al.*, 2003), mainly because the condition may be amenable to surgical treatment. These patients usually have a long history of epilepsy and, the important difference between those with an epilepsy onset in childhood, adolescence or adulthood is rarely taken into account. These studies are certainly of value in identifying functional deficits in surgical candidates and in forecasting cognitive outcome following surgery. But what these, pre- and post-surgical, assessments are not designed to provide is a solid answer to a number of other crucial questions:

- To what extent early identification of a degenerative process, in terms of cognitive development, allows rehabilitation or at least prevention of further deterioration? What orientation should rehabilitative measures take, what functions should be reinforced, when and how?
- How will functional plasticity integrate modifications of a given developmental process (physiological, pathological or a combination of both) as a result of rehabilitative measures?
- To what extent mental competences can develop based on other neural cortical associative networks than those involved in normal development, the activity of the later being supposed to be altered by the epilepsy process?
- To what extent the neuropsychological profile of a candidate to surgery reflects the result (or is independent) of his/her seizures, or of a causative disorder or of both?
- Is early surgery fully justified from a neuropsychological point of view?

A "comprehensive" neuropsychological evaluation of non-idiopathic focal epilepsies is one that includes and considers everything that is essential or necessary for identifying specific cortical regions or networks that are dysfunctional in patients with a given type of epilepsy.

*In everyday clinical practice* the aim would be, whenever possible, to suggest adequate measures for rehabilitation (total or partial).

*In terms of clinical research*, the aim would be to further identify the installation process and the underlying mechanisms of such dysfunctions, a prerequisite for a preventive attitude towards future patients.

The recent "Villa Grazioli" workshop at the origin of the present volume, discussed in detail issues related to cognitive function and dysfunction in children with temporal lobe epilepsy. Every effort was made to integrate available current knowledge from studies in adults or from basic science. The conclusion was that despite the complexity of the issues involved and the numerous parameters to be considered, studies in children, performed from the very onset of their epilepsy, can provide valuable clues for treatment and global care.

In this chapter, and in order to better define practice and research parameters for neuropsychological assessment in patients with non idiopathic focal epilepsy, we briefly review some of the reasons explaining current paucity of robust answers to the above mentioned crucial questions. Some are directly related to the heterogeneity and complexity of the focal epilepsies. Others are related to the limits of current knowledge on the developmental processes. On the basis of available data we discuss rational attitudes for everyday care and suggest methodologies for future research.

# Issues related to the diagnostic difficulties of focal non-idiopathic epilepsies

Focal non-idiopathic epilepsies represent one of the major problems among childhood epilepsies because of their frequency and the difficult therapeutic problems they raise. This group is highly heterogeneous with respect to aetiology, pathology and clinical presentations. As a result it is more difficult to establish precise semeiological and prognostic criteria (Arzimanoglou et al., 2004), than for the idiopathic focal epilepsies. Most non-idiopathic focal syndromes are defined mainly by the electro-clinical characteristics of the seizures rather than, as is the case for other syndromes, by the association of several symptoms not randomly associated. This is the case for the topographic syndromes reflecting the involvement - although not necessarily the origin - of various regions of the brain, that have been proposed by the ILAE classification. They are based essentially on description of the *seizures*. As a result, the causes and the prognosis often have to be determined on the basis of an *individual* combination of signs and symptoms, and on the results of multiple investigations.

Particularly in children, precise topographic diagnosis of non-idiopathic partial epilepsies may prove to be difficult for a number of age-related particularities (Kahane et al., 2005):

- Collection of concrete information on clinical manifestations and their analysis may prove to be difficult. Particularly regarding alteration, or not, of consciousness and description of possible subjective symptoms. Description of the signal-symptom, when found in children, is usually much less detailed than in adults, especially for hallucinations. This may only reflect the more limited expressive abilities of children, especially young ones, and the different interpretation they make of a given subjective symptom, often in relation to their inability in early development to dissociate external from internal sources of stimulation.

- A partial seizure in a child, especially if very young, can manifest itself with a rather unusual clinical presentation, compared to what we observe in adult patients. In a number of cases the semeiology can pass practically unnoticed, while in others it may be rather "explosive", probably due to the rapidity of propagation of the ictal discharges. It is thus that, focal seizures in very young children are often reported to present a global motor semeiology which masks the partial character of the seizure, or which precedes the more clearly partial semeiology. Symptoms concerning a whole hemi-body are also frequent. It remains no less true that partial seizures resembling very closely those in adults can be observed even in very young children.

- The clinical expression of seizures at a given age evolves with time. Several factors, such as progression of the maturational process, increasing capacity of children to describe subjective feelings (Marchini et al., 1988; Minotti et al., 1998) and eventually drugs administered, may influence changes in expression of seizures.

- Interictal EEG abnormalities tend to be more diffuse; it implies that EEG recordings should be repeated over time in the search of focal, particularly slow abnormalities that may appear or become more evident during evolution.

- Whether or not an epileptogenic lesion (particularly a small dysplastic lesion) will be detected with MR imaging depends on the quality of the images, and the expertise of the reader. Particularly in very young children, changes of appearance due to the dynamics of brain myelination may make early (or late) identification of abnormalities of cortical development difficult.

## Issues related to the diagnostic difficulties of temporal lobe epilepsies

Little data is available on the characteristic semeiology of different lobar epilepsies in children (Lawson et al, 2002; Fogarasi et al., 2002; 2003; Villanueva and Serratosa 2005). Consequently, one often tends to extrapolate semeiology described in adolescent or adult patients, usually surgical candidates. Such extrapolations, although sufficient to roughly orient the topographic diagnosis, are undoubtedly insufficient for defining topographic syndromes and for drawing up an evolution profile.

Temporal lobe epilepsies in children can start at any age but sometimes can only be diagnosed at the time of a secondarily-generalized seizure. The semeiological expression of seizures can be misleading, particularly when the fits resume in isolated visceral autonomic manifestations or psychological and sensory manifestations, leading to confusion with gastro-intestinal complaints or with behavioural problems of a non-epileptic nature.

The seizures are often grouped over several days, rarely manifest during sleep and secondary generalization is rather infrequent. Episodes of status are rare but they may inaugurate the disease or punctuate its course in the first years of evolution. Particularly in very young children, clinical expression of the seizures may be rather discrete, limited to changes in facial expression, motionless staring with minor or no automatisms (also defined as 'hypomotor seizures' - Lüders et al., 1998), thus leading to the erroneous diagnosis of "absences". In other cases the manifestations may be rather "noisy" with motor signs in the foreground due to the rapidity of discharge propagation (Brockhaus and Elger, 1995; Wyllie 1993; Wyllie et al., 1995). However, in the majority of school-age children, the symptomatology of the seizures is relatively close to what is observed in adults.

The seizures are usually prolonged (1-2 min), initiated by a "signal symptom" which typically takes the form of autonomic ("I have a pain in my stomach") or psychic ("I'm afraid") manifestations or olfactory hallucinations. The presence of auditory hallucinations ("I hear music") may suggest an early implication of the neocortical structures. Alteration of consciousness is more or less marked, usually appearing late in the course of the seizure, although sometimes it may initiate the seizure in the form of motor arrest or staring. The automatisms are more distinct the more the child is older, typically oro-alimentary (chewing) or simple gestures, and more rarely verbal. The post-ictal phase is often long-lasting. Postictal sleep is common, particularly in young children. Total amnesia of the incident is possible (Arzimanoglou et al., 2004; Kahane et al., 2005).

Propagation of seizures with *mesio-basal* onset is rapid and mainly to the contra lateral hippocampus, but some attacks spread to the cingulate gyrus or to the orbital and lateral frontal cortex (Lieb *et al.*, 1976, 1981). *Lateral (or neocortical) temporal origin* is often characterized by auditory or complex perceptual visual hallucinations, illusions, a dreamy state or vertiginous symptoms. Impairment of consciousness may begin with motor arrest, or staring, followed by oro-alimentary automatisms. However, automatisms may appear while the patient is still responsive or consciousness is fluctuating. Amnesia for the ictal event is the rule after alteration of consciousness but may be present even when the patient had apparently remained conscious. Post-ictal confusion and, in small children, post-ictal sleep are frequent.

Temporal lobe seizures of neocortical origin are less frequent than limbic attacks. Such seizures often spread to the ipsilateral mesiobasal-limbic regions, which can act as secondary "pacemaker areas," permitting maintenance and further propagation of the ictal events thus relayed (Wieser and Kausel, 1987). The generation of a dreamy state requires simultaneous involvement of both the temporal neocortex and the mesial limbic structures (Munari and Bancaud, 1985; Munari *et al.*, 1979). Dual pathology, with dysplastic or tumoral lesions of the neocortex and associated hippocampal sclerosis, is not rare (Levesque *et al.*, 1991; Raymond *et al.*, 1994). Language impairment indicates involvement of the dominant hemisphere.

Aetiologies are extremely variable, dominated - unlike in the adult - by the migration and tumoural pathologies (Arzimanoglou *et al.*, 2004). A hippocampal sclerosis is moreover not rare and in this case, antecedents of prolonged febrile convulsions are frequently reported, especially in epilepsies described as mesio-temporal (for a review see Cendes *et al.*, 2005).

*In summary*, seizures implicating the temporal structures have a rich and complex semeiology. Early recognition of a definitely "temporal lobe epilepsy" might prove to be difficult. Propagation of ictal and interictal abnormalities is the rule rather than the exception. All the above, represent additional difficulties when designing prospective studies aiming to evaluate cognitive development.

## ■ Issues related to the variable evolution of TLE in children

Natural evolution and prognosis of non-idiopathic temporal lobe epilepsies in children is extremely variable. Factors such as age at onset, frequency of seizures, history of episodes of status and the presence, and type, of an underlying lesion may influence both the control of seizures and cognitive outcome. As a result, attempting to draw up a development profile of all childhood temporal lobe epilepsies would be futile, there being so many localizations of seizures and multiplicity of aetiologies. Available data almost exclusively concerns either mesial temporal lobe epilepsy (MTLE) with hippocampal sclerosis (HS) or evolution of some lesional epilepsies (due to dysplastic, vascular or tumoural lesions).

*Concerning evolution and treatment of mesial TLE*, a recent report of the ILAE subcommission on MTLE with HS (Wieser, 2004) concluded *"it is clear that some patients who have MTLE with HS have seizures that are easily controlled with medication, but only those with severe forms are well characterized, because they are commonly first seen at tertiary epilepsy centers. Prospective studies are necessary to characterize benign MTLE with HS, define its incidence and prevalence relevant to the severe form, and determine whether the benign and severe forms represent two different pathophysiologic conditions, or a spectrum of a single pathophysiologic condition."* Such a differentiation is of extreme importance particularly when discussing evolution not only in terms of seizures but also in terms of socio-cognitive development.

In the same report the commission also underscored the following remarks, which are certainly of interest for the present discussion:

- Retrospective studies from surgical series have demonstrated a high incidence of "initial precipitating incidents", including febrile seizures, trauma, hypoxia, and intracranial infection, usually, but not always, before age 5 years.

- Although patients classically have a *latent* period between the "initial precipitating incident" and onset of habitual seizures, some patients have no identifiable initial incident, and some have habitual seizures that begin immediately after what is considered the initial precipitating incident. It would be important to understand the difference between the patients who demonstrate a latent period and those who do not, and whether this is influenced by brain maturation or other factors such as laterality and gender.

- A *silent* period occurring between the first habitual seizure and the onset of intractability also has been well described and exists in a high percentage of patients (Berg et al., 2003). The silent period indicates that seizures are initially easily controlled for some time before they become medically refractory, strongly suggesting that the pathologic substrate is progressive. It would be important to know whether the existence of a silent period might differentiate MTLE with HS from MTLE due to other lesions.

- Evidence strongly suggests that progressive behavioural changes occur, particularly increasing memory deficit and an increased appearance of contralateral EEG spikes, over time with MTLE with HS, but it is not clear whether this differentiates this condition from MTLE due to other lesions. The same is true of the silent period, which suggests progression, and some data indicate that surgical outcome is worse with longer duration.

- Several studies have concluded that patients who have MTLE with MRI-identified HS are more likely to have intractable seizures than are patients with other MRI-identified lesions. A large study, from a tertiary center in Paris (Semah et al., 1998), found that only 11% of patients with HS and only 3% with dual pathology had been seizure free in the past year, whereas another study, from a primary center in Glasgow (Stephen et al., 2001), which also found HS to be associated with the most intractable seizures, reported that 46% of these patients had been seizure free in the past year. The difference between these observations in the tertiary and primary centers confirms a view that a relatively high incidence of benign MTLE with HS is found, although it is unclear how many of these patients appearing at the primary center were in their "silent" period, and in whom refractory epileptic seizures would eventually develop.

The ILAE subcommission also extensively reviewed available data on surgical outcome in MTLE with HS (see also Engel *et al.*, 2003 and McIntosh *et al.*, 2001) and provided a state-of-the-art report for the various conditions encountered and the most appropriate surgical approaches.

Recently, Schmidt, Baumgartner and Loscher (2004) reviewed 13 retrospective and five prospective clinical observations published since 1980 that provided data on long-term seizure control off AEDs in a total of 1,658 patients. No randomized studies were found. According to this analysis, following temporal lobe surgery, approximately one in four adult patients and approximately one in three children or adolescents were shown to be seizure-free for 5 years without AEDs (25%, mean of eight studies in adults, 95% CI: 21-30%, and 31%, mean of three studies in children, 95% CI: 20-41%). The rate of seizure control off AEDs seemed to be stable after 2 years of follow-up. However, the authors noted that as 55% of patients free of disabling seizures preferred not to discontinue their medication completely as late as 5 years after surgery, it is impossible to know if they are cured or not. No features predictive of surgical cure were detected except for better cure outcome in children versus adults with hippocampal sclerosis and in patients with typical versus atypical Ammons horn's sclerosis or tumour in one small study each.

*Concerning other than HS lesions*, any type of tumour can give rise to seizures. Recent studies have emphasized the role of neuronal glial tumours especially *gangliogliomas and developmental neuroepithelial tumors (DNT)* in the causation of chronic epilepsy that may remain monosymptomatic in the form of recurrent partial seizures for many years. Taylor type cortical dysplasias are another frequent cause. All these lesions are highly epileptogenic and related epilepsy is resistant to drugs in most of the cases. Prognostic factors and outcome following surgery are currently under evaluation and reports from various epilepsy groups recently started to emerge (Chassoux *et al.*, 2000; Clussman *et al.*, 2004; Hennessy *et al.*, 2001; Kral *et al.*, 2003; Cohen-Gadol *et al.*, 2004; Kloss *et al.*, 2002; Hader *et al.*, 2004; Francione *et al.*, 2003; Fauser *et al.*, 2004; Tassi *et al.*, 2002; Hamiwka *et al.*, 2005; Nolan *et al.*, 2004; Sakuta *et al.*, 2005).

*In summary*, the natural evolution of focal epilepsies implicating the temporal lobe is extremely variable. Available data suggests that the majority of patients with hippocampal sclerosis or highly epileptogenic lesions will have an intractable course or will remain drug dependent. Although results from epilepsy surgery studies are promising, with regard to seizure control, prospective controlled studies are still needed. Coupled to a comprehensive neuropsychological assessment, such studies could provide some answers to crucial questions.

## ■ Neuropsychological evaluation in children with TLE: general principles and particular problems

Evaluation of cognitive capacities and "treatment" of possible incapacities call for understanding of the mechanisms and neural networks involved. Complexity of the processes involved in brain and cognition relationships is addressed by developmental cognitive neurosciences and can certainly not be reviewed in the present, much less ambitious, chapter.

To summarize, the following 3 issues must be taken under consideration:

1. When studying cognitive function one studies how the brain transforms environmental signals, process and "build" information, programs behaviour (including mental state).

2. "Maturation" refers to *a dynamic process*, of unknown duration, involving interactions between genetics and environment at every level of observation, from molecules to the behaviour of the organisms. Apparently, the sensitive periods of the cerebral cortex, during which the functional connections laid out according to the genetic blueprint can be sculpted, spans the first 3 years of human life and more (see for instance for speech and for face processing Pallier et al., 2003; Sangrigoli et al., 2005). This plasticity can last into puberty for some of the higher cognitive and linguistic functions, which imply learning in a more formal sense; aspects of other sensori-motor and cognitive functions might also be concerned. Plastic changes are only possible within the framework of the genetically determined design of connectivity, which in turns limits and solicits interaction with the respective environment.

3. *Neuropsychological research*, through studies of normal and abnormal processing, reveals the mechanisms of information processing and building. *Neuropsychological assessment* seeks to evaluate adaptive behavioural insufficiencies and abnormal developmental trajectories by considering key variables including the type, number, combination, and degree of any cognitive deficits, the presence or absence of associated or contributory impairments, the known or suspected aetiology, and the significance of any ability-related strengths. Neuropsychological assessment depends closely on knowledge on normal mechanisms of information processing and building by the brain. As this domain of knowledge is presently progressing very quickly, new issues and new tools are appearing for neuropsychological assessment.

In its turn, *epilepsy*, of any type, *is also a dynamic process* evolving with brain maturation and development of cognitive capacities. It can then be expected that epilepsy can adversely influence learning and developmental processes, as a result of episodic, but repetitive, disruption of neural activity, usually against a background of chronic neurophysiological dysfunction. The question of whether certain types of epilepsy and their underlying aetiologies are characterized by a specific profile of cognitive strengths and weaknesses is of interest for diagnostics and treatment of children and adults with epilepsy.

Current knowledge on neuropsychological deficits in children with TLE is thoroughly reviewed in this volume by Sauerwein *et al.* Their review demonstrates that TLE in children affects the same structures and functions as in adults. Among the typical temporal lobe functions, verbal memory and language-related functions appear to be most affected in children. Attention and language problems may be, at least in part, responsible of the memory deficits. As discussed in Chapter 3 by Dunn and Kronenberger, we dispose of no evidence that children with TLE are more likely to have symptoms of ADHD than children with other epilepsies, but the studies that addressed symptoms of ADHD in children with epilepsy have consistently found a higher prevalence of problems in children with epilepsy as compared to controls or population based norms. Speech organization and when and how it can be influenced by interictal and ictal TLE activities is further discussed by Janszky and collaborators.

Another important point, underscored by Sauerwein *et al.*, is the fact that the impact of prolonged exposure to potentially damaging epileptic activity extends beyond the functions mediated by the temporal lobes, with frontal lobes apparently being the preferred target. Cristoph Helmstaedter, when extensively reviewing the effects of chronic temporal lobe epilepsy on memory functions, reaches a similar conclusion. *Taking into account the extreme variety of temporal lobe seizure patterns in terms of, ictal propagation, interictal activity and type of lesion (see previous paragraphs), these well documented conclusions are probably not a surprise.* The chapter by Zilbovicius and Meresse on temporal lobe and social abilities and the discussion by Cross *et al.*, on autism spectrum disorders in children with TLE shed new light on the interactions that influence overall cognitive development. Furthermore, data reviewed by Laurent *et al.*, together with recent preliminary data, suggest that unilateral temporal lobe epilepsy can generate deficit in early-developing social competences, such as face processing, while sparing other kinds of visual competences.

The impact of antiepileptic drugs is another issue to be considered when discussing how a given epilepsy influences socio-cognitive development (Hirsch *et al.*, 2003). Schmitz reviewed in detail the effects of AED on behaviour and mood with a special focus on depression. As argued, effects on mood are often overlooked and although the exact prevalence is difficult to estimate, it looks as high as 30 per cent. As for the "central" side effects of antiepileptic drug treatment, Aldenkamp and Bootsma rightly insist that, when evaluating their effect we must realize that in clinical practice most cognitive problems have a multifactorial origin. Their review of recently existing data concludes that, although the severity of cognitive side effects is generally considered to be mild to moderate for most AEDs, all commonly used AEDs have some impact on cognitive function. *Issues related to drug effects should be taken into account when evaluating socio-cognitive development.* Absolute effects of drugs (effects of a given treatment as against no treatment) can only be evaluated at onset of an epilepsy, ideally before administration of any treatment. As for relative effects (comparison of the cognitive side-effects of one drug with the effects of another), studies can be conclusive only if a number of rules are rigorously respected (Aldenkamp and Van Bronswijk, 1999).

The review by Jokeit and Schacher, suggested that specific associations between neuropsychological deficits and type of epilepsy and aetiology are exceptions rather than the rule. One of the reasons that related studies provide arguments for a similar conclusion stems from *the ambiguous role attributed to those neuropsychological studies.* Neuropsychology has two aims:

- one is to increase our knowledge on normal and abnormal neuro-cognitive functioning;
- the other is to evaluate a given person at a given period of time.

Children and adults with epilepsy are involved in a society and have to be emotionally and cognitively evaluated, to be appropriately supported in their process of social integration. Standardized tests are used for this evaluation which provides good and reliable information on each individual's coarse competences. But the standard tests used for such an evaluation are presently unable to help us finding out what kind of cognitive deficit results *systematically* from each given type of epilepsy. Only scientific research, addressing new questions on the relationships between epilepsy and cognitive deficit, can uncover reliable relationships.

For decades, cognitive assessment has categorized deficits in terms of gross cognitive functions and their relationships with cortical areas. Such a coarse correspondence inescapably showed no clear relationships between types of epilepsy and kinds of deficits. But, during the last decade, our knowledge in cognitive neurosciences is changing. These changes are based on data coming from studies on healthy infants, children and adults as well as from brain injured young and adult individuals. Cognitive competences are being splitted and dissociated into several components that involve different neural networks and develop along different timetables. The new landscape is departing from a simple straightforward correspondence where language competences as a whole were associated uniquely with left hemisphere; visuo-spatial competences with the right hemisphere; attention with the prefrontal cortex; Papez's circuit with emotions and plasticity systematically associated with a unique window during the two first years of age, just to mention a few. As our knowledge is departing from this simple view, cognitive deficits associated with non-idiopathic focal epilepsies might become more and more interesting and informative. For instance, the kind of questions addressed and the situations used to assess deficits in frontal epilepsy has changed with increasing knowledge on mechanisms of cognitive functions of the pre-frontal cortex. This also applies to temporal lobe epilepsies.

Consequently, what is of interest to the physician in estimating probability of functional recovery and in providing therapeutic recommendations, is *knowledge on when and how* the various epilepsy-related factors interact with brain developmental timelines and vulnerabilities. Given the complexity of the developmental processing this can only be answered, most probably still only partially, by neuropsychological assessments performed as early as possible in the course of the disease and repeated in sufficiently reasonable intervals to allow a better understanding of the overall evolution and of the means to modify it. The first step in assessing a cognitive/behavioural profile lies in deciding *what* to measure, and in evaluating as rigorously as possible the type of the underlying epilepsy.

## ■ Concluding remarks: Towards a comprehensive methodology

As discussed above and in other chapters of this volume, studies mainly conducted in adults with focal epilepsy showed that a variety of factors, *i.e.*, underlying pathology, age of onset, psychosocial problems, origin of seizures, treatment side effects, genetic factors, sleep disturbances- contribute to the development of cognitive and behavioural deficits. Although this conclusion is most probably correct, it must be taken into account that the above mentioned parameters are probably the only measurable ones when patients are tested after a long (or short) history of ongoing epilepsy.

What is more difficult to measure is *at what moment of the developmental process a child's brain is more vulnerable to the epileptic process, what are the competences that are altered without any possibility to be developed elsewhere* and *at what stages of development, and whether and how, the specific changes of some of the cognitive functions influence the rest of the process.*

As discussed by Nehlig, Ben-Ari and Hasson *et al.*, the question of whether seizures can cause neuronal damage, the sequences that are relevant to seizure generation and their effects on the construction of networks according to their time of occurrence, have been more directly addressed in experimental animal models. Equivalent studies must be carried in humans and animal models of epilepsy, a true translational undertaking.

The choice of epilepsy global treatment attitudes - which drug and for how long; on-time implementation of which educational interventions; surgery, yes or no; and, above all, an answer to the crucial question *"do we dispose of sufficient data to praise early surgery"* in children with focal non-idiopathic epilepsies - requires a much more profound understanding of the impact of seizures and/or interictal abnormalities on the developing brain and of the methods to precociously identify specific cognitive deficits. Assuming that the overall effects on developmental processes will be identical whatever the origin and propagation of a seizure, is an unproven short-cut.

## What attitude in everyday clinical practice

In everyday clinical practice systematic neuropsychological testing of patients with non-idiopathic focal epilepsy can certainly yield invaluable information on their cognitive profile and on the specific domains necessitating rehabilitative measures. But, neuropsychologists having time for research and with a special interest in epilepsy are not that many, costs for testing are relatively high and it would be difficult to suggest for each patient a systematic testing of all possibly affected domains. What can be concluded here is that in everyday practice the need for neuropsychological testing must be raised in the initial evaluation of every child with epilepsy and it should be left to the clinician and parents to decide which children will actually be referred (Buelow and McNelis, 2002). In pre- and post-surgical evaluation testing must remain systematic as it certainly provides valuable information on specific risks and care strategies for the surgical candidate, as well as important elements for a better understanding of the various cognitive processes.

## Future research

In order to answer, at least partly, some of the clinical questions asked above, **comprehensive, multi-centric, research programs are required, including prospective evaluation of various aspects and levels of** *somesthesic, olfactive, visual, auditory, spatial and temporal regulation and cognition; speech and language including arithmetics; social and emotional cognition; attention and memory; decision taking; reasoning.*

*Selection of patients to be included in prospective studies should not be based on a, sometimes arbitrary, categorization between temporal, frontal, parietal, central or occipital epilepsies. As shown, this is not always easily identifiable at onset. If one waits for a clear-cut topographic diagnosis to assess these patients he/she unavoidably introduces a bias. It should* also be taken into account that a clinically recognizable semeiology may only reflect implication of a given brain region and not obligatorily designate the origin of the seizures. Furthermore, we still do not dispose of sufficient data allowing to identify to what extent cognitive dysfunction is more influenced by the site of origin of a seizure than by its propagation pathways or by both. We know even less about the possible indirect influence of the epileptic process on brain regions, and networks, at a distance from the epileptogenic area.

*Parallel to the initial neuropsychological assessment and follow-up, efforts should continue for a better individual topographic diagnosis, to allow homogeneous groups for final analysis.* Clinical assessment should systematically include a detailed description of seizure semeiology and its evolution with time; sufficient data on interictal activity during daytime and sleep and its possible modifications during follow-up; data on seizure onset and ictal propagation. Frequency and duration of seizures must be evaluated at regular intervals.

*Electro-clinical assessment must be coupled to modern, high quality, anatomical and functional neuroimaging* tagging the impairment of specific functional circuitries, as clearly demonstrated in the chapters by Cendes, Weber et al., Asano and Chugani and Ryvlin. Such a multi-technical approach will not only help in a better localization of given epilepsies but will also allow us to follow the possible progression of structural and functional deficits in patients with epilepsy. Appropriate and consensual design may reduce the variable impact of antiepileptic drugs used. Last but not least, as discussed by Tuxhorn et al., data from research projects of the kind will enrich the debate on the well-founded or not of early epilepsy surgery.

All the above mentioned protocol requirements are realistic for the majority of large epilepsy centres. What looks more difficult to realize is a full battery of all possible tests to evaluate all domains of cognitive development. This would be time consuming for both the patient and the neuropsychologists and would inconsiderably increase the cost of such research programs. Another option would be to perform for each patient to be included only some of the evaluation tests, on the basis of our hypothesis on the brain structures primarily involved in his epilepsy. It is easily understood that such an approach would introduce a number of biases. To avoid the above mentioned difficulties and biases, *centres participating in such multi-centric studies should agree upon a number of neuropsychological batteries* including tests measuring "overall intelligence", such as IQ measures, various aspects of language functions, visual-spatial and auditory processing, memory, attention and, executive functions. Information from families and school teachers should be systematically collected. Questionnaires on everyday life competencies, similar to those used for personality studies, could be built. Such a global approach would provide a common basis for analysis of results and it would still leave place for innovative ideas in centres wishing to explore other, more specific, domains.

# References

Aldenkamp A, Van Bronswijk K. Cognitive side-effects as an outcome measure in antiepileptic drug treatment: the current debate. In: M. Sillanpää, L. Gram, S. Johannessen, T. Tomson, eds. *Epilepsy and Mental retardation*. Wrightson Biomedical Publishing, 1999: 135-46.

Arzimanoglou A, Guerrini R, Aicardi J. *Aicardi's Epilepsy in children*. 2004. Philadelphia: Lippincott Williams & Wilkins.

Beaumanoir A, Bureau M, Deonna T, et al. *Continuous spikes and waves during slow sleep. Electrical status epilepticus during slow sleep*. Mariani Foundation Pediatric Neurology Series. Paris: John Libbey Eurotext 1995.

Berg AT, Langfitt J, Shinnar S, et al. How long does it take for partial epilepsy to become intractable? *Neurology* 2003; 60: 18690.

Brockhaus A, Elger CE. Complex seizures of temporal lobe origin in children of different age groups. *Epilepsia* 1995; 36: 1173-81.

Buelow JM, McNelis A. Should every child with epilepsy undergo a neuropsychological evaluation? *Epilepsy Behav* 2002; 3: 210-3.

Bulteau C, Jambaque I, Viguier D, Kieffer V, Dellatolas G, Dulac O. Epileptic syndromes, cognitive assessment and school placement: a study of 251 children. *Dev Med Child Neurol* 2000; 42: 319-27.

Cendes F, Kahane P, Brodie M, Andermann F. The mesio-temporal lobe epilepsy syndrome. In: Roger J, Bureau M, Dravet Ch, Genton P, Tassinari CA, Wolf P (eds). *Epileptic syndromes in infancy, childhood and adolescence*. Paris: John Libbey Eurotext, 3rd edition, 2002: 513-30.

Chassoux F, Devaux B, Landre E, Turak B, Nataf F, Varlet P, Chodkiewicz JP, Daumas-Duport C. Stereoelectroencephalography in focal cortical dysplasia: a 3D approach to delineating the dysplastic cortex. *Brain* 2000; 123: 1733-51.

Clusmann H, Kral T, Fackeldey E, Blumcke I, Helmstaedter C, von Oertzen J, Urbach H, Schramm J. Lesional mesial temporal lobe epilepsy and limited resections: prognostic factors and outcome. *J Neurol Neurosurg Psychiatry* 2004; 75: 1589-96.

Cohen-Gadol AA, Ozduman K, Bronen RA, Kim JH, Spencer DD. Long-term outcome after epilepsy surgery for focal cortical dysplasia. *J Neurosurg* 2004; 101: 55-65.

Crawford PM. Epidemiology of intractable focal epilepsy. In: Oxbury J, Polkey C, Duchowny M, eds. *Intractable focal epilepsy*. London: W.B. Saunders, 2000: 25-40.

Delgado-Escueta A, Guerrini R, Medina MT, Genton P, Bureau M, Dravet C. (Eds). *Myoclonic Epilepsies*. Advances in Neurology, Vol. 95, Philadelphia: LWW 2005.

Dulac O, Chugani HT, Dalla Bernardina B. *Infantile spasms and West syndrome*, Saunders London, 1994.

Engel J Jr, Wiebe S, French J, et al. Practice parameter: temporal lobe and localized neocortical resections for epilepsy: report of the Quality Standards Subcommittee of the American Academy of Neurology, in association with the American Epilepsy Society and the American Association of Neurological Surgeons. *Neurology* 2003; 60: 53847.

Fauser S, Schulze-Bonhage A, Honegger J, Carmona H, Huppertz HJ, Pantazis G, Rona S, Bast T, Strobl K, Steinhoff BJ, Korinthenberg R, Rating D, Volk B, Zentner J. Focal cortical dysplasias: surgical outcome in 67 patients in relation to histological subtypes and dual pathology. *Brain* 2004; 127: 2406-18.

Fogarasi A, Boesebeck F, Tuxhorn I. A detailed analysis of symptomatic posterior cortex seizure semiology in children younger than seven years. *Epilepsia* 2003; 44: 89-96.

Fogarasi A, Jokeit H, Faveret E, Janszky J, Tuxhorn I. The effect of age on seizure semiology in childhood temporal lobe epilepsy. *Epilepsia* 2002; 43: 638-43.

Francione S, Nobili L, Cardinale F, Citterio A, Galli C, Tassi L. Intra-lesional stereo-EEG activity in Taylor's focal cortical dysplasia. *Epileptic Disord* 2003; 5 (suppl 2): S105-14.

Francione S, Vigliano P, Tassi L, Cardinale F, Mai R, Lo Russo G, Munari C. Surgery for drug resistant partial epilepsy in children with focal cortical dysplasia: anatomical-clinical correlations and neurophysiological data in 10 patients. *J Neurol Neurosurg Psychiatry* 2003; 74: 1493-501.

Freitag H, Tuxhorn I. Cognitive function in preschool children after epilepsy surgery: rationale for early intervention. *Epilepsia* 2005; 46: 561-7.

Hader WJ, Mackay M, Otsubo H, Chitoku S, Weiss S, Becker L, Snead OC 3rd, Rutka JT. Cortical dysplastic lesions in children with intractable epilepsy: role of complete resection. *J Neurosurg* 2004; 100 (2 suppl Pediatrics): 110-7.

Hamiwka L, Jayakar P, Resnick T, Morrison G, Ragheb J, Dean P, Dunoyer C, Duchowny M. Surgery for epilepsy due to cortical malformations: ten-year follow-up. *Epilepsia* 2005; 46: 556-60.

Helmstaedter C, Kurthen M, Lux S, Reuber M, Elger CE. Chronic epilepsy and cognition: a longitudinal study in temporal lobe epilepsy. *Ann Neurol* 2003; 54: 425-32.

Hennessy MJ, Elwes RD, Honavar M, Rabe-Hesketh S, Binnie CD, Polkey CE. Predictors of outcome and pathological considerations in the surgical treatment of intractable epilepsy associated with temporal lobe lesions. *J Neurol Neurosurg Psychiatry* 2001; 70: 450-8.

Hermann BP, Seidenberg M, Schoenfeld J, Davies K. Neuropsychological characteristics of the syndrome of mesial temporal lobe epilepsy. *Arch Neurol* 1997; 54: 369-76.

Hernandez MT, Sauerwein HC, Jambaque I, de Guise E, Lussier F, Lortie A, Dulac O, Lassonde M; Attention, memory and behavioral adjustment in children with frontal lobe epilepsy. *Epilepsy Behav* 2003; 4: 522-36.

Hirsch E, Schmitz B, Carreno M. Epilepsy, antiepileptic drugs (AEDs) and cognition. *Acta Neurol Scand Suppl* 2003; 180: 23-32.

Jambaqué I, Lassonde M, Dulac O (eds.). Neuropsychology of childhood epilepsy. New York: Kluver Academic/Plenum Publishers, 2001.

Jokeit H, Schacher M. Neuropsychological aspects of type of epilepsy and etiological factors in adults. *Epilepsy Behav* 2004; 5: S14-20.

Kahane P, Arzimanoglou A, Bureau M, Roger J. Non-idiopathic focal epilepsies in children. In: Roger J, Bureau M, Dravet Ch et al., eds. *Epileptic Syndromes in childhood and adolescence*. Paris: John Libbey Eurotext, 4th edition 2005.

Kloss S, Pieper T, Pannek H, Holthausen H, Tuxhorn I. Epilepsy surgery in children with focal cortical dysplasia (FCD): results of long-term seizure outcome. *Neuropediatrics* 2002; 33: 21-6.

Kral T, Clusmann H, Blumcke I, Fimmers R, Ostertun B, Kurthen M, Schramm J. Outcome of epilepsy surgery in focal cortical dysplasia. *J Neurol Neurosurg Psychiatry* 2003; 74: 183-8.

Lassonde M, Sauerwein HC, Jambaque I, Smith ML, Helmstaedter C. Neuropsychology of childhood epilepsy: pre- and postsurgical assessment. *Epileptic Disord* 2000; 2: 3-13.

Lawson JA, Cook MJ, Vogrin S, Litewka L, Strong D, Bleasel AF, Bye AM. Clinical, EEG, and quantitative MRI differences in pediatric frontal and temporal lobe epilepsy. *Neurology* 2002; 58 (5): 723-9.

Levesque MF, Nakasato N, Vinters HV, Babb TL. Surgical treatment of limbic epilepsy associated with extrahippocampal lesions: The problem of dual pathology. *J. Neurosurg* 1991; 75: 364-70.

Lieb JP, Dasheiff RM, Engel J. Role of the frontal lobes in the propagation of mesial temporal lobe seizures. *Epilepsia* 1991; 32: 822-37.

Lieb JP, Walsh GO, Babb TL. A comparison of EEG seizure patterns recorded with surface and depth electrodes in patients with temporal lobe epilepsy. *Epilepsia* 1976; 12: 137-60.

Luders H, Acharya J, Baumgartner C, Benbadis S, Bleasel A, Burgess R, et al. Semiological seizure classification. *Epilepsia* 1998; 39: 1006-13.

Marchini M, Munari C, Bancaud J. Epilessie temporali gravi ad insorgenza infantile: valore localizzatorio della semeiologia critica iniziale (studio retrospettivo). *Boll Lega It Epil* 1988; 64: 197-8.

Massa R, de Saint-Martin A, Carcangiu R, Rudolf G, Seegmuller C, Kleitz C, Metz-Lutz MN, Hirsch E, Marescaux C. EEG criteria predictive of complicated evolution in idiopathic rolandic epilepsy. *Neurology* 2001; 57: 1071-9.

McIntosh AM, Wilson SJ, Berkovic SF. Seizure outcome after temporal lobectomy: current research practice and findings. *Epilepsia* 2001; 42: 1288307.

Metz-Lutz MN, Kleitz C, de Saint Martin A, Massa R, Hirsch E, Marescaux C. Cognitive development in benign focal epilepsies of childhood. *Dev Neurosci* 1999; 21: 182-90.

Minotti L, Kahane P, Tassi L, Lo Russo G, Sivelle G, Joannard A, Benabid AL (1998): Peut-on simplifier les investigations préchirurgicales chez l'enfant? In: Bureau M, Kahane P, Munari C (eds). *Epilepsies partielles graves pharmaco-résistantes de l'enfant: stratégies diagnostiques et traitements chirurgicaux*, pp. 181-94. Montrouge: John Libbey Eurotext.

Munari C, Bancaud J, Bonis A, Buser P, Talairach J, Szikla G, Philippe A. Rôle du noyau amygdalien dans la survenue de manifestations oro-alimentaires au cours des crises épileptiques chez l'homme. *Rev. EEG. Neurophysiol* 1979; 9: 226-40.

Munari, C, and Bancaud, J. The role of stereoelectroencephalography (SEEG) in the evaluation of partial epileptic seizures. In: R.J. Porter, P.L. Morselli, eds. *The Epilepsies*, Butterworths, London 1985; pp. 267-306.

Nolan MA, Redoblado MA, Lah S, Sabaz M, Lawson JA, Cunningham AM, Bleasel AF, Bye AM. Intelligence in childhood epilepsy syndromes. *Epilepsy Res* 2003; 53: 139-50.

Nolan MA, Sakuta R, Chuang N, Otsubo H, Rutka JT, Snead OC 3rd, Hawkins CE, Weiss SK. Dysembryoplastic neuroepithelial tumors in childhood: long-term outcome and prognostic features. *Neurology* 2004; 62: 2270-6.

Pallier C, Dehaene S, Poline JB, LeBihan D, Argenti AM, Dupoux E, Mehler J. Brain imaging of language plasticity in adopted adults: can a second language replace the first? *Cereb Cortex* 2003; 13: 155-61.

Rausch R, Kraemer S, Pietras CJ, Le M, Vickrey BG, Passaro EA. Early and late cognitive changes following temporal lobe surgery for epilepsy. *Neurology* 2003; 25; 60 (6): 951-9.

Raymond AA, Fish DR, Stevens JM, Cook MJ, Sisodiya SM, Shorvon SD. Association of hippocampal sclerosis with cortical dysgenesis in patients with epilepsy. *Neurology* 1994; 44: 1841-5.

Sakuta R, Otsubo H, Nolan MA, Weiss SK, Hawkins C, Rutka JT, Chuang NA, Chuang SH, Snead OC 3rd. Recurrent intractable seizures in children with cortical dysplasia adjacent to dysembryoplastic neuroepithelial tumor. *J Child Neurol* 2005; 20 (4): 377-84.

Sangrigoli S, Pallier C, Argenti AM, Ventureyra VA, de Schonen S. Reversibility of the other-race effect in face recognition during childhood. *Psychol Sci* 2005; 16: 440-4.

Schmidt D, Baumgartner C, Loscher W. The chance of cure following surgery for drug-resistant temporal lobe epilepsy. What do we know and do we need to revise our expectations? *Epilepsy Res* 2004; 60: 187-201.

Schoenfeld J, Seidenberg M, Woodard A, Hecox K, Inglese C, Mack K, Hermann B. Neuropsychological and behavioral status of children with complex partial seizures. *Dev Med Child Neurol* 1999; 41: 724-31.

Semah F, Picot M-C, Adam C, et al. Is the underlying cause of epilepsy a major prognostic factor for recurrence? *Neurology* 1998; 51: 125662.

Stephen LJ, Kwan P, Brodie MJ. Does the cause of localisation-related epilepsy influence the response to antiepileptic drug treatment? *Epilepsia* 2001; 42: 35762.

Tassi L, Colombo N, Garbelli R, Francione S, Lo Russo G, Mai R, Cardinale F, Cossu M, Ferrario A, Galli C, Bramerio M, Citterio A, Spreafico R. Focal cortical dysplasia: neuropathological subtypes, EEG, neuroimaging and surgical outcome. *Brain* 2002; 125: 1719-32.

Villanueva V, Serratosa JM. Temporal lobe epilepsy: clinical semiology and age at onset. *Epileptic Disord* 2005; 7: 83-90.

Wieser HG, Kausel W. Limbic seizures. In: HG Wieser, CE Elger (Eds). *Presurgical Evaluation of Epilepsies*. Springer Berlin 1987; pp. 227-48.

Wieser HG; ILAE Commission on Neurosurgery of Epilepsy. ILAE Commission Report. Mesial temporal lobe epilepsy with hippocampal sclerosis. *Epilepsia* 2004; 45: 695-714.

Wyllie E, Chee M, Granstrom ML, DelGiudice E, Estes M, Comair Y, Pizzi M, Kotagal P, Bourgeois B, Luders H. Temporal lobe epilepsy in early childhood. *Epilepsia* 1993; 34: 859-68.

Wyllie E. Developmental aspects of seizure semiology: problems in identifying localized-onset seizures in infants and children. *Epilepsia* 1995; 36: 1170-2.

Achevé d'imprimer par Corlet, Imprimeur, S.A.
14110 Condé-sur-Noireau
N° d'Imprimeur : 85841 - Dépôt légal : août 2005

*Imprimé en France*